Explain Pain *Supercharged*

The clinician's manual | Moseley & Butler

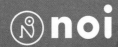 **noi**

Noigroup Publications | 19 North Street, Adelaide City West, South Australia 5000

Knowledge driving health | noigroup.com

Published by Noigroup Publications
for NOI Australasia Pty Ltd

Printed and bound in South Australia

Produced by van Gastel Total Print Management

Copyright © 2017 Noigroup Publications

A catalogue record for this book is available from the National Library of Australia.

A catalogue record for this book is available from the State Library of South Australia.

Moseley, G. Lorimer and Butler, David S.
Explain Pain Supercharged
First edition February 2017
Reprinted May 2017, August 2018
Includes index

ISBN 978-0-6480227-0-1

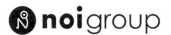

Noigroup Publications
NOI Australasia Pty Ltd
19 North Street, Adelaide City West
South Australia 5000, AUSTRALIA

www.noigroup.com
Telephone +61 (0)8 8211 6388
Facsimile +61 (0)8 8211 8909
noi@noigroup.com

Acknowledgements

Lorimer wishes to acknowledge...

Of course I thank my beautiful family and heartbeat – Anz, Browns and Gubs. Thank you to the many students, colleagues, clinicians and people in pain (special mention here to Brett) who keep me honest and stop me from climbing some ivory tower of decreasingly relevant ponderings. You have also kept me energised for the long journey towards truly reducing the burden of persistent pain, something about which I am even more hopeful now than I was a decade ago – your phone calls, visits, emails, questions at conferences, even your confused or dazed looks in courses, are the real reasons Explain Pain Supercharged has made it.

This is the third book I have coauthored with my inspirational and unswerving comrade Dave. His integrity, unexampled passion AND compassion is truly awesome. Finally, thanks from me to Jules, Hayles, Az, Tim and the Noigroup team – just sooooo good to work with.

Dave wishes to acknowledge...

The NOI team for bringing this project to fruition – Tim (contributions, reading, rereading and intellectual input), Ariane (design and typesetting with the ultimate care and skill), Hayley (reading, rereading, research and intellectual support), Ali (artwork, design and maintaining zen equilibrium), Karin (handling the dough and stuffing her back), and Fran (keeping the show on the road and the buyers calm).

Thanks to the extended NOI team of Zahra (art), Paula (infographics), James (cover art), Jeannie (reading), Wayne (printing), Neville (cleaning) and Malcolm (DHL).

Supercharged has been five years in the making, the culmination of a long and enjoyable journey with Lorimer. Much gratitude to Lozzie – a giant of the research world AND translator to the clinical battlefront with his inexhaustible desire to listen to everyone's pain story with compassion and understanding to give those narratives a place in the hearts and minds of researchers and clinicians around the globe.

A super big thanks to Juliet Gore – editor, manager, wife and all-round hot sheila! This book would not be alive without her.

Acronyms, abbreviations and jargon

It might seem daft, but there are actually good reasons to use acronyms in life – perhaps this is best demonstrated by the fact that LOL, OMG and IMHO have rocketed to the top of the most used 'words' list. We too have adopted acronyms here in EP Supercharged – in part because if we didn't then this book would be three times as heavy and twice as expensive. If you come across an acronym that doesn't mean anything to you, here is what you do: put your finger on it, keep one finger on it and with your other hand turn back to this list of acronyms, find the acronym concerned, remind yourself what it is, go back to where your finger is and write the acronym's meaning in the margin.

AMP   associated molecular pattern

The 'AMP gang'

- **BAMP** behavioural associated molecular pattern
- **CAMP** cognitive associated molecular pattern
- **DAMP** damage associated molecular pattern
- **PAMP** pathogen associated molecular pattern
- **XAMP** xenobiotic associated molecular pattern

ASIC   acid sensing ion channel

Ca²⁺   calcium

CATS   catastrophic thoughts about pain scale

CBT   cognitive behavioural therapy

CGRP   calcitonin gene related peptide

CI   confidence interval

CRPS   complex regional pain syndrome

CV   cardiovascular

DIM   danger in me

DNIC   descending noxious inhibitory control

DRG   dorsal root ganglion

EP   Explain Pain *(the book)*

EPH   Explain Pain Handbook: Protectometer *(the book)*

EPS   Explain Pain Supercharged *(the book)*

FABQ   fear-avoidance beliefs questionnaire

GMI   Graded Motor Imagery

GPPT   Grand Poobah Pain Theory

HADS   hospital anxiety and depression scale

IASP   International Association for the Study of Pain

IES-R   impact of event scale: revised

IFN   interferon

IL   interleukin

K⁺   potassium

LAFT   living adaptable force transducer

LTP   long term potentiation

M1   primary motor cortex

MME   morphine milligram equivalents

Na⁺   sodium

NGF   nerve growth factor

NMT   neuromatrix theory

NNE   number needed to educate

NNH   number needed to harm

NNK   number needed to kill

NNT   number needed to treat

NPQ   neurophysiology of pain questionnaire

NRS   numerical rating scale

PCS   pain catastrophizing scale

PMC   pre motor cortex

PY   Painful Yarns *(the book)*

QST   quantitative sensory testing

RCT   randomised controlled trial

S1   primary sensory cortex

S2   secondary sensory cortex

SIM   safety in me

TLR   toll-like receptors

TNF   tumour necrosis factor

TPD   two point discrimination

TRP   transient receptor potential

VAS   visual analogue scale

Contents

1

Why supercharge Explain Pain?

Fifteen years of Explain Pain

Explain Pain (EP) was first published in English well over a decade ago. It has now been translated into five other languages and converted to an ebook and an audio book. A second edition arrived in 2013 and although it looked pretty much the same as the first and the key messages remained intact, the 'implications' section underwent a significant revamp. Additions came mainly on the back of another 100 new scientific articles and evidence that its clinical effects had been endorsed by a number of independent research groups in several different countries and languages.

EP was and still is, in many ways a revolutionary addition to the pain library – with striking artwork from Sunyata, it provides an entertaining and somewhat irreverent introduction to modern pain science. We aimed to make it a conversation piece, in some ways lighthearted, yet entirely respectful of the complexity and magnificence of our in-built protective systems.

Since EP was first published, we have had countless conversations with clinicians, patients, health departments, sports people, politicians and artists about what works and what remains a challenge, about their favourite (and least favourite!) pictures and their most useful chapters; about patient responses (good and not so good) and about their own attempts to more effectively integrate the material with their clinical practice.

One theme that has emerged time and time again is the need for another resource. Something that fills the void that sits between EP and the scientific literature. This is, remarkably, a substantial void – many have pleaded in frustration for something that takes them beyond EP but doesn't put them to sleep or intimidate the whoopsies out of them – something that is written in a way that does not bamboozle but does not condescend. It became very clear from:

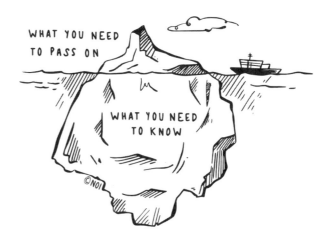

Figure 1.1 The clinician's iceberg of knowledge

- **students** – who are increasingly expected to have an understanding of pain science that exceeds what is presented in EP, to
- **clinicians** – who appreciate that what they need to know greatly outweighs what they need to pass on (Figure 1.1) and that they require educational skills and language to transfer an effective EP story, to
- **scientists** – who need a language with which they can bring their science alive in the hands of those at the coalface, and finally to
- **curious, clever and highly committed people in pain** – who just want to know more.

We needed a kind of EP Plus, or EP In More Detail. So here it is... *Explain Pain Supercharged.*

We want *Explain Pain Supercharged (EP Supercharged)* to be the go-to resource for people who seek more knowledge about pain, and who want to learn more about how to Explain Pain. As you may realise, we have taken on a very ambitious and serious challenge. It is a challenge made all the more important by a worrying trend we see emerging across the world, of people seeing the commercial value of the Explain Pain Revolution without seeing the critical importance of *actually understanding* what is going on. 'Brands' have emerged and products are being aggressively marketed, with what seems to be little care for quality control and for really equipping clinicians with the resources to Explain Pain well. We have seen clinicians fork out precious dough, only to be given scripts and low quality imitations. They arrive at our email door with comments such as *'I did the* [insert branded name of explaining pain here] *and it didn't work'*. Of course it didn't! You need to 'get it'[1] and getting it can be hard.

We all know that 'Entrepreneurs sans Scruples' emerge whenever something seems truly good, but here the stakes are really high because we are messing with the lives of real people in real need. We want you to deeply understand Explain Pain, or therapeutic neuroscience education, or pain neuroscience education[2] or whatever you want to call it. We want you to be able to think and to adapt as new knowledge emerges. We want you to be able to use *EP Supercharged* every time you stumble, to work out why you stumbled and how to get back up.

Figure 1.2 gives you an idea of where we see this book fitting. It builds on *Explain Pain* [1] and refers to it. It utilises *The Explain Pain Handbook: Protectometer* [2] – an interactive guidebook for taking on the EP journey. It also draws on the metaphors and stories in *Painful Yarns* [3]. *EP Supercharged* provides the reader (or we prefer to think of you as an adventurer) with the more complete scientific story that underpins these other resources, their content and their application.

A note on referencing

Throughout this book we will be referring to the other Explain Pain tools. Look out for these symbols, for example [EP11] refers to page 11 of Explain Pain, and [PY55] refers to page 55 of Painful Yarns.

---

1   To 'get it' means you really understand it so well you can feel it in your bones.

2   Although let's face it Dorothy – you are not just in neuroscience anymore.

The Explain Pain resources

Scientific Jargon Meter

— *More*
— *A bit*
— *Almost none*

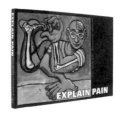

EXPLAIN PAIN
For pain sufferers, their clinicians and anyone interested in pain.

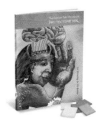

EXPLAIN PAIN HANDBOOK: PROTECTOMETER
For pain sufferers to use on their own or with clinicians.

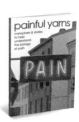

PAINFUL YARNS
Metaphors and stories for pain sufferers and anybody interested in pain.

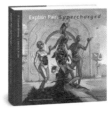

EXPLAIN PAIN SUPERCHARGED
For clinicians and interested pain sufferers.

Figure 1.2 The Explain Pain resources

Explain Pain in a nutshell

To put *EP Supercharged* into context as you embark on this adventure, it is worth iterating six of the key themes in EP.

1. Pain is very normal and very amazing

The systems that serve to protect our body are very sophisticated. The most sophisticated of these systems is the *feeling* system – the system that produces our feelings. Pain,[3] one of these feelings, is perhaps the most potent experience as far as making us behave in a certain way. It depends on a glorious system that is predictive, intuitive, evaluative, infinitomodal,[4] dynamic and modifiable. It is also however, a brutally effective system for the very reason that pain is usually so unpleasant. Pain hurts!

If you have pain right now you are not alone – about 20% of humans have pain that has persisted for more than 3 months. For everyone in pain we can say one thing for sure – it hurts because your brain is convinced that *your body needs protecting.* This is the simple bit – it really is simple.

If your brain thinks a part of your body is in danger and needs protecting, then the brain will make that part of your body hurt. You have no say in this. It is happening outside of your awareness or control. It is your brain's conviction.[5]

Simple? This is also the *huge* challenge of pain – there are many situations in which pain does not seem to match the amount of danger your body tissues are truly in. The massive amount of scientific research on this is clear – pain depends on your brain's evaluation of danger and the likely benefit of protective behaviour, not on the true danger level and the true benefit of protective behaviour. EP walks us through some of these amazing pain stories.

---

3 Anger and lust might also be considered for the gold medals here.

4 Infinitomodal is a word we just made up. We had written 'multimodal' but that seems to downplay the reality that pain can be influenced by anything really, so long as it has some danger or safety relevance (keep reading), so infinitomodal seemed more fitting.

5 We are not really as brain-centric as this sounds and we clarify our language throughout the book. That we can attribute this to your brain is a simplification, but it is a passable simplification at this stage. Hang in there...

2. Nerves are loaded with mechanical, thermal and chemical sensors

Most sensors are in the brain. However, all over the body there are sensors that are opened by a potentially dangerous change in their environment. The nerves on which these sensors ('danger receptors') are placed are called nociceptors. If enough sensors are opened a signal is triggered in the nociceptor and an alarm signal saying 'danger' is sent to the spinal cord.

At the spinal cord the danger message causes chemicals ('neurotransmitters') to be released at a synapse. These chemicals join a gaggle of other chemicals which together might have an effect on the second neurone – the spinal nociceptor ('danger messenger') which travels to the brain. A word of warning – we will dig deeper into this stuff and you will realise that Explain Pain presents a rather substantial simplification of what really happens. This synapse is the first place at which the danger signal from the tissues is processed (see box below). If it does send a danger message to the brain, the brain then draws on a huge array of inputs and may or may not decide '*yes, this body part is in danger and this organism* (that's you) *needs to do something to protect itself'*. If it decides this, the orchestra in the brain (using EP speak) produces protective responses, including pain in that body part.

[handwritten annotation: allows a neuron to transmit an electrical or chemical signal to another neuron]

[handwritten annotation: A cluster of neurons in the dorsal root of a spinal nerve.]

Here is the first obvious example of *EP Supercharged* taking you beyond EP. The notion that the synapse in the spinal cord is the first processing site as we clearly articulated in EP needs expanding. Incoming messages are actually processed to some extent in the dorsal root ganglion (DRG). Here they interact with immune-mediated processing such that quite profound computational capacity is possible at this level. The principles driving that processing are complicated and beyond our capacity to fully understand. Moreover, they are not as clearly predictable and intuitive as events occurring at the spinal nociceptor, which is why we told that little fib in EP. That is not all – the interaction between the primary nociceptor and the spinal nociceptor, and between descending projection neurones and the spinal nociceptor is also not that simple. Recent research has uncovered an extensive system of interneurones within the dorsal horn that seem to be very important in generating that initial stage of central sensitisation that occurs in a couple of hours. *EP Supercharged* will give you the 'behind the news' version rather than the more superficial 'breaking news' sound bite. We aim to give you a more complete understanding of the biology of pain.

3. The danger detection sensors have adjustable sensitivity

If body tissue is inflamed or damaged the danger sensors become more sensitive. The pattern of sensitivity varies according to the type of tissue involved. EP describes these variabilities and some of the characteristic patterns that emerge depending on where the danger sensors are located (muscle, skin, nerve, etc).

4. The danger transmission system has adjustable sensitivity

The sensitivity of spinal neurones that carry danger messages to the brain can also increase. EP covers the basics of this sensitivity change, which results in allodynia and hyperalgesia, hallmarks of central sensitisation. If pain persists, then we see changes in the brain too – the networks of brain cells that produce pain – or an immune response or a movement response – become more sensitive. It is, as we say in EP, as though the orchestra in the brain is stuck on the pain tune [EP78-79].

Remember that *any credible evidence of danger* to body tissue triggers protection. If the brain networks that actually produce pain become more sensitive, then *all* of the cues have a larger effect on pain – the thoughts, beliefs, movements, behaviours, sights, sounds, smells etc. etc. They have a larger effect on other protective outputs as well. Think of this as an internal protection meter, the level of which determines protective outputs.

5. Pain is just one of our protective systems

There are many protective systems – others include the sympathetic, motor, immune and cognitive systems. They all work together, influencing each other, changing the way our body works, the way we feel, all in an orchestrated attempt to move us out of a dangerous situation and help us learn and heal as quickly as possible.

6. Complex problems sometimes need complex solutions!

There is a range of methods of engaging with the process of recovery. EP talks about the orchestra model and we expand on that model in this book. It also discusses the 'onion skin model', in which nociception is integrated with attitudes, beliefs, behaviour – and all of these influence pain.

In our experience, there are usually no quick fixes for chronic pain,[6] but there are slow fixes that require patience, persistence, courage and coaching. The tried and tested route to recovery is centred around threat identification and graded exposure. Threats can hide in very difficult to spot places. Graded exposure is not rocket science, but it is also not unimodal. Graded exposure has historically been confined to physical upgrading only, but we think that this must change and our view on this is supported by the vast body of scientific data. Now that we know pain is infinitomodal, to presume a solely physical graded exposure is daft. It requires merging with the complexity of context, and for us the most powerful and liberating context of all is knowledge.

In EP the Twin Peaks Model (Figure 1.3) captures the idea of graded exposure and it is the figure that most often has tongues wagging (in a good way). Before injury, the buffer between the 'protect by pain' line and 'tissue tolerance' line is far smaller than the buffer after injury. Here, our bioplastic bodies have lifted protection and pain is just one of our enhanced protective systems.

These six themes are elaborated and expanded in *EP Supercharged* where you will recognise them as Target Concepts – integral parts of an Explain Pain intervention.

---

6   Although the idea of radical/rapid conceptual change is becoming more viable (Chapter 5).

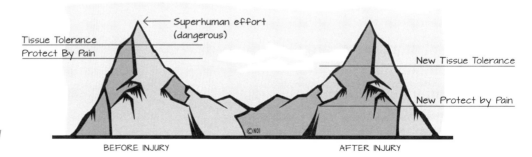

Figure 1.3 The Twin Peaks Model from Explain Pain [1]

The bio-revolution revs up!

Finally, we heartily welcome you to *EP Supercharged*. We really hope that as you read you feel part of something bigger, you feel part of a kind of revolution – something we called a 'neuro-revolution' in 2003, but what we now realise is more like a '*bio*-revolution'. This revolution is resulting in fundamental and wide-reaching changes in the way that pain is managed and treated around the world. The revolution is injecting significant and true hope into the lives of millions of people suffering from pain. What is more, it is transforming their lives – slowly but surely.

As you read, remember that the power behind the revolution lies in the hands of the large number of people slowly uncovering the mysteries of human experience and behaviour – the scientists. It lies in the hands of the rapidly growing group of clinicians who have moved beyond their comfort zone and embraced the complexity of human experience and behaviour. Most of all though, the power of the revolution lies in the hands of the vast number of people who can now say, after weeks, months, years or decades of pain, that they get it and that they have switched paths from a downward spiral of pain and suffering to a slow and steady road to recovery. We receive dozens of emails every week from people telling this kind of story. They are all different – occasionally miraculous overnight recoveries, to weeks, months or even years of gradual improvement, but every single story reminds us how lucky we are to be researchers, clinicians and educators in the pain field at this moment in history.

So, read on fearless adventurer and Supercharge yourself...

¡Viva la (bio) Revolución!

References

1. Butler DS & Moseley GL (2013) Explain Pain. 2nd Edn. Noigroup Publications: Adelaide.

2. Moseley GL & Butler DS (2015) The Explain Pain Handbook: Protectometer. Noigroup Publications: Adelaide.

3. Moseley GL (2008) Painful Yarns: Metaphors and stories to help understand the biology of pain. Dancing Giraffe Press: Canberra.

Notes...

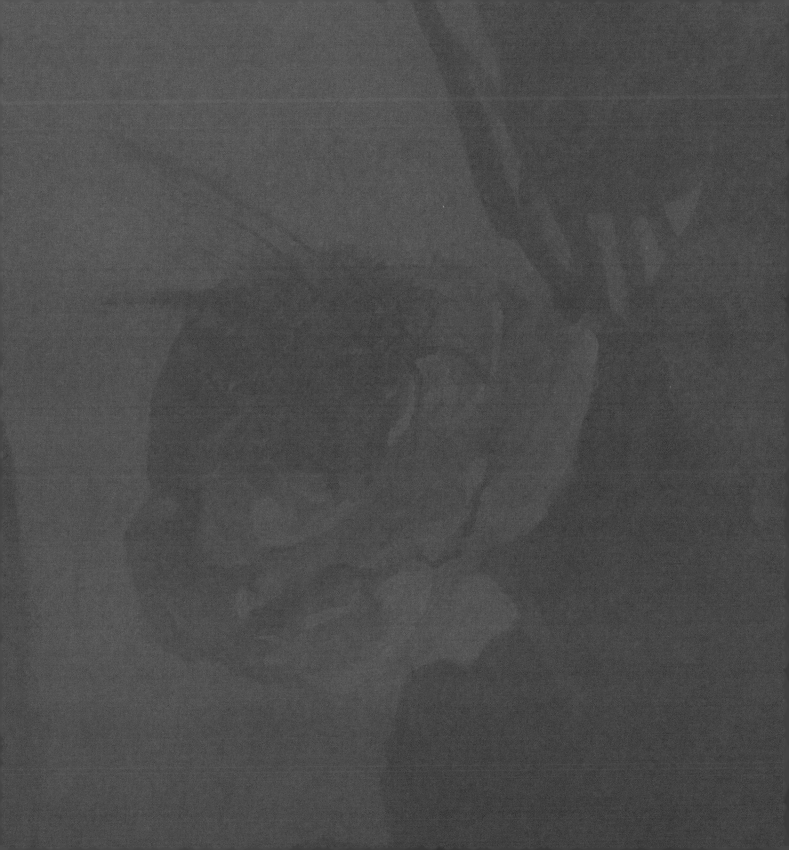

2

You and your sneaky theories

Theory: a system of ideas intended to explain something

Why on earth might we start the guts of this book by talking about theories? Well, like it or not, theories govern much of our clinical behaviour. We want you to get up close and personal with your own theories. We want you to embark upon this journey of *EP Supercharged* with a clear picture of the theories that support it and inform it. So don't be tempted to skip this little section – we have made it as light as we can to keep you on board and provide the critical base for the rest of the book. It will set you up with a *way of thinking* as you proceed.

How are theories like farts?

a) We have far more theories than we think we do.

b) We have a very low tolerance of other people's theories, particularly if they stink.

c) We sometimes think our theories don't stink even when everyone else tells us they do.

d) When we do realise our theory stinks, we tend to attribute it to someone else.

Why worry about theories?

We all have theories and those theories influence how we interpret events, how we look for things and what things we look for; what we do when we find what we were looking for, or indeed when we don't. As clinicians, we have theories about all sorts of things – risk factors, treatment moderators, treatment mediators, prognostic indicators. In clinical practice we seldom stop to identify our theories and articulate them and we seldom set out to prove them wrong. We do however, construct our thoughts and behaviours around names such as McKenzie, Mulligan, Maitland, McConnell[1], Jung, Kabat-Zinn, Zumba; or around geography – the Norwegian approach, or Eastern approaches; or perhaps around a particular tissue – the psoas major approach, the core stability approach; or around a process

– the narrative approach, the solution-focused approach; or a biological property – the neuroplasticity approach. In each case, we test something in a patient according to what our favoured theory would predict. We might see a particular outcome occur as we predicted and make a mental note (often unconsciously) that the theory has been supported.

Theories are also tested in scientific practice. In fact, theories play such a critical role in science that without them, the scientific process would be rendered pretty much useless (see [1] and [2] for interesting accounts of this). So if your eyes are glazing over at the mere thought of a theory, hang in there. Theories, paradigms, or frameworks are at the heart of clinical practice and each patient you see is, in a way, the sole participant in an *N* of 1 experiment. If you are to understand the bulk of the rest of this book then first understanding the basics of the most relevant theories will prepare you well.

Throughout this book we will refer to the relevant theories that underpin the topic of our reflection. We hope that you can quickly turn back to this section as and when you need, to remind yourself of the theoretical underpinnings of what we are discussing in each section.

Theories as thinking frameworks

Some theories are very well supported by evidence. Many would say that a theory *must* be based on a fairly solid block of evidence, but there is much conjecture about how much evidence constitutes a 'solid block'. Examples that are based on very solid blocks of evidence include the theory of gravity, the muscle length-tension relationship theory, the drink-water-upside-down-alleviates-hiccups theory.[2] Other theories are based on less solid blocks of evidence. For example, take the famous[3] 'specific cortical stupidity theory' devised and described here by Lorimer.

This 'specific cortical stupidity theory' was based on the data available to me at the time it was conjured. Like most theories it was probably not really very original, but the name I gave

---

1   One of us became quite nervous when he realised he was (a) from Australia/NZ, (b) had a name starting with M, and (c) trained as a physiotherapist, and set out from that time on to avoid the risk of ever becoming 'a guru'.

2   Okay, the upside down drink of water theory may not have been fully interrogated yet.

3   Not actually that famous, but read on.

it made it sound quite novel. The primary data on which the specific cortical stupidity theory was based was mostly observations and N of 1 experiments, interpreted in light of the available 'knowledge' (well, again, available to me). Those of you who have worked in a manual therapy field will relate to this: I could increase someone's hip range of motion by 30 degrees in 2 minutes (the N of 1 experiment). Biological evidence (knowledge) that muscles can't grow longer in two minutes meant that the theory to which I previously subscribed had to be wrong. That theory, given to me by learned teachers as it so happens, was that these techniques were increasing muscle length. So here I was with a disconnect between the theory underpinning my practice and the evidence. Even on the basis of N of 1 studies, one can prove a theory categorically wrong. Take for example the theory that pigs never fly. It would only take one flying pig to prove that theory wrong.

Back to the specific cortical stupidity theory: *In people who would substantially increase their joint range in response to my therapeutic techniques, the major contribution to their limited range of motion was their brain being too stupid to work out how to let the joint move into more range.* My interpretation of the rapid effect of my therapeutic techniques was that I was tricking the brain by perturbing the information it received about the relationship between joint angle and proprioceptive feedback.

Now, the specific cortical stupidity theory has, to my knowledge, never been published nor tested in rigorous experiments. However, the theory did provide a framework for testing because it presents clear and testable predictions or *hypotheses*. One of those hypotheses would be that *it is possible to increase one's range of motion by intensively and continually imagining a movement.* This hypothesis can be tested, and if it is true then there is a small tick in favour of the specific cortical stupidity theory. It does not prove the theory correct. But importantly, it fails to prove it wrong.

> One of the fundamental tenets of scientific process is that hypotheses are only useful if they are *testable*. That is why a hypothesis such as **penguins never get back pain** is not a very good one – you can't prove it wrong. Another fundamental tenet, for studies in biology at least, is that the hypothesis must be *biologically plausible*. That **woodpeckers suffer from headaches** is biologically plausible but not very testable;[4] that **one can treat another's aura** is neither biologically plausible nor very testable.

---

4   I was intrigued to learn recently that the assumption that woodpecker's *don't* get headaches is well endorsed [3, 4] but surely it is a very difficult assumption to verify or refute.

Hypotheses are made to be broken

The whole point of constructing a hypothesis on the basis of a theoretical framework is to try to prove it wrong. That is in many ways the essence of scientific progress – that theories and hypotheses are proposed and then attempts are made to disprove them [5]. How often is that done clinically? Have you ever had a theory about a patient and tried to work out a way of proving your theory wrong? Pragmatically, it might be difficult to justify taking this classical approach to your clinical practice. The alternative is to work at proving the theory right. There is a problem here though – the 'prove it right' approach is highly prone to making false conclusions, which is why science doesn't like it. The priority for science is to discover the truth – to explore the bounds of the knowledge universe. The priority for clinical practice is to give patients what they most want without compromising your own integrity or theirs in the process.

Our clinical interactions are really a dynamic dance between our theories, values, needs, intuitions, expectations and biases, and those of the client, those of the social environment in which we both operate and our need to feed the kids and make a dollar. However, being aware that a complex reality exists is one thing, but to engage with each and every facet in the most complete and honest way we can is another thing altogether. As Dr Mick Thacker, Research Fellow at King's College London, neuroimmunological aficionado and physiotherapist extraordinaire would say, '*How hard is your job?*' [5]

Theory as metaphor

Metaphorical theories are great – but it's important to recognise their metaphorical nature. Chapter 7 focuses on identifying metaphors and their sometimes ridiculous assumptions. Pain rehabilitation, at least the type with which we are both most familiar, is built on several theories. Some are purely conceptual and rely on metaphors, like the gate control theory and the muscle imbalance theory. In fact, most of our theories are metaphorical, and so are their descriptive labels – take concepts such as attention, hypervigilance and homunculus for example. These theories are no less valuable for their metaphorical nature, but their value to us as clinicians or scientists is different from those of non-metaphorical theories. Metaphorical theories often have built in subtle and not so subtle assumptions; they often summarise and connect several non-metaphorical theories; they are often broader and conceptually slippery; they can be more

---

5   This is one of our favourite quotes from Mick because it captures what some clinicians feel when their eyes are opened to the true complexity of the human and the challenge that this complexity presents to us when we try to work out why someone is in pain.

easily applied to similar but distinct contexts and extrapolated beyond their initial application. Metaphorical theories can still provide a framework into which complex biological events can fit and from which the scientist, the clinician and the person in pain can make and test predictions. You will gain the most out of *EP Supercharged* if you first get a grip on the theories that lie beneath and within it. However, the true power of the Explain Pain Revolution lies within the connection between science and clinical practice, between the thinker and the doer, between the rational and the intuitive. Our own professional journeys and the interaction between the two of us has been built on our unyielding conviction that both solid theory and risky exploration, both reasoned and imaginative interpretation, both accountability and speculation, are essential for knowledge growth and the pursuit of better outcomes for people in pain. With that in mind we are compelled to balance our apparent love affair of theories with discussion of why they are, on their own, somewhat impotent.

The trouble with theories

Some people find theories to be very powerful and indeed quite beautiful. To tackle the massive challenge of pain and perhaps also stress, fatigue and anxiety (the so-called 'survival perceptions' [6]), we need excellent theories, but we require real world change. And therein lies some of the trouble with theories. We can become bound up in theories to such an extent that our creativity is compromised and the opportunities for true innovation become elusive. This is where the switched on clinician has a real advantage over the pure scientist. The latter is relatively removed from the lived experience of pain and therefore misses the triggers for truly great scientific innovation. Clinicians beware though; don't breathe easy just yet – the Jurassic clinicians, naive to the theories that guide their treatments yet buried deeply within them, will also miss opportunities for truly great clinical innovation.

Relevant here are reflections on how important the theories that disrupt the status quo really are, for example the classic books *The Structure of Scientific Revolutions* [5] and *The Logic of Scientific Discovery* [1] and newer more provocative accounts, such as *Antifragile* [7] and *Surfing Uncertainty* [8]. In *Antifragile*, Nassim Taleb argues that science has lost its way by adhering too closely to theories such that 'risky science' has been stamped out and therefore so has the chance of critical shifts in thinking. As a card-carrying clinical scientist, Lorimer hopes it is not quite that depressing a situation. David, as a card-carrying scientific clinician shares Lorimer's hope, but is less confident. Both of

us think that Taleb has a point: the importance of a discovery may well be negatively related to how confidently it was predicted according to prevailing theory. But there needs to be a balance here and both scientists and clinicians can safeguard themselves from being buried or bamboozled by theory by being intentionally self-reflective and committing themselves to carefully observe what is going on in the laboratory or clinic.

Careful observation

'First and foremost observe. Clinically, observation refers to careful appraisal of the patient and their situation; to ask questions and to listen carefully to the responses. To really listen is to conjure your focus on the patient, on what they say (and indeed on what they do not) and how they say it – not just the words they use, but the entire behavioural package; their manner, their posture, their ease of articulation, their expression and the attributions they provide for their pain.' [9]

Observation and indeed 'focusing' on someone or something is no easy task. It requires practice and energy. Alain de Botton captured some of this in his reflections on listening: *'good listeners are no less rare or important than good communicators… an unusual degree of confidence is the key – a capacity to not be thrown off course by, or buckle under the weight of, information that may challenge certain settled assumptions'* [10]. These descriptions provide an excellent way to benefit from the wisdom of theories while keeping free of their potential shackles. We'll return to this later in this book – our editors have correctly pointed out that *this is the theories bit, not the clinical skills bit* – but we have sneakily changed our angle so as to keep it here at least in some form. The *theory* is that if we are to truly embrace a biopsychosocial model of pain, then carefully observing the person in pain in all of their biopsychosocial complexity will lead to better outcomes for you, for them and for the world. Everyone is a winner!

Careful observation has been captured by mindfulness – the *new black* in popular health. Neither of us are highly trained in mindfulness, but we can certainly vouch for how easily one can practice careful observation. Next time you have a kiwi fruit don't peel it, cut it cross ways down the middle, then carefully observe the spectacular arrangement of the seeds and flesh, taking particular note of where the seeds give way to flesh and the flesh abuts the skin. Once you have taken all that in, take a bite of it and carefully observe the feeling of the skin in your mouth – the little villi as they give way to your chew, as the skin mixes with the flesh and gives way to the soft moist pulp. This has nothing to do with pain?

The biopsychosocial model of pain

Now for something completely different – but incredibly sensible! If you only take one theory deep into your guts and let it penetrate everything else, then we reckon it ought to be this one. That is why we start with it. This is the first pain book we know of, including our own *Explain Pain*, that has taken this completely different but incredibly sensible approach. We think it should come before nociception. Before C fibres or TRPV1 receptors. Before peripheral or central sensitisation (Version 1 or Version 2.0 – see Chapter 3). Before glial cells and cortical reorganisation too.

The biopsychosocial model categorises the potential influences on pain into those that occur in the biological domain, the psychological domain and the social domain. In short, biological contributors are bodily events that activate nociceptors or drive tissue states outside of the safe homeostatic zone; psychological contributors are everything else – the things we think, say, believe, predict, feel and do (don't mistakenly think that 'do' is only in the 'bio' domain – what we do might have biological impact but the act of doing it we consider a psychological event because it is driven by the brain); social contributors relate to any interactions one has with others and the roles a person plays in his or her social world. The true state of a person's health can be captured by the intersect of these three categories (Figure 2.1).

There is no doubt in our minds that the transition from a structural-pathology, or pathoanatomical model of pain, to the biopsychosocial model of pain was a truly revolutionary one. Although it sometimes feels like the biopsychosocial model is new, it is not. In fact, in a remarkable twist of circumstance, Engel's landmark paper on it [11] was published on the same day as Lorimer's seventh birthday party, at which his dad made a serious pitch for 'Coolest Dad in the World' by standing motionless while Lorimer and fifteen friends shot at a lump of toothpaste on the tip of his ample nose, using water pistols that *we all got to keep!*

A new Engel: half a century later, George's concept of the biopsychosocial human is still fresh and refreshing

Engel was actually writing about the imperative to take a new angle on human health and disease [12] almost two decades before the landmark 1977 paper [11]. In our view, his 1960 paper should be required reading for every health professional – in fact, it should be required reading for every high school student. We will of course later revisit the aspects of the biopsychosocial model that need modification[6] on the basis of developments in the biological sciences of pain. For now, check out a few of George's gems – they hold as much clout now as they must have held back then. They offer sensible explanations for many of the challenges that those of us embracing the biopsychosocial model face every week. They are worth sticking on your fridge.

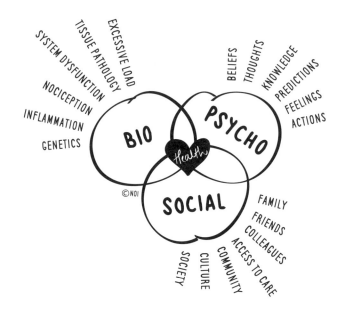

Figure 2.1 The biopsychosocial model

6   For example, that there are problems calling chronic pain a disease or that pain itself is modulated by all manner of things. Engel, like his contemporaries, mistook nociception for pain and the initial application of the biopsychosocial model to pain took that view. It was a marriage of convenience rather than wisdom – that nociception and pain are different was clearly demonstrated well before the biopsychosocial model made it into the pain world.

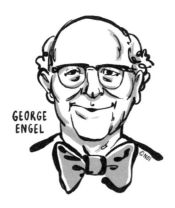

GEORGE ENGEL

George's Gem Number 1

'To be able to think of disease as an entity, separate from man and caused by an identifiable substance, apparently has great appeal to the human mind. Perhaps the persistence of such views in medicine reflects the operation of psychological processes to protect the physician from the emotional implications of the material with which he deals.' [12]

Clearly, 'physician' could be replaced with 'health professional' – physicians are no more to blame here than the rest of us. And patients are not spared the wrath:

George's Gem Number 2

'Patients, certainly, regardless of their level of education and sophistication, prefer to blame their illness on something... that happened to them and to think of disease as something apart.' [12]

Remembering that we are talking about pain here and, even though pain is entirely a symptom, it is felt in the body, which seems to leave pain well suited to this idea of being 'apart' from oneself. Critically, George observes that this perspective is not taken because people are undereducated or overeducated – it seems to be a human trait. Clinically, such perspectives can be important conceptual barriers to rehabilitation, what we call 'Target Concepts' later in this book. Many of you will also recognise George's observation of the fallacies that are sometimes offered when a treatment relieves pain even though it is based on outdated pain concepts:

George's Gem Number 3

'[on outdated models,] a disease, then, has substantive qualities, and the patient can be cured if the diseased part is removed. That this often proves to be the case, as attested to by the successes of surgery, is actually not evidence for the validity of such a point of view.' [12]

George's argument is that it is no more valid to attribute the entirety of a shift in human state to an isolated cell or tissue event than it is to isolate that cell or tissue and expect it, once removed, to generate the same signs or symptoms that were present before it was removed. This argument is even stronger now than it was then and underpins the preciousness of the biopsychosocial model to modern pain science. George might not have realised that developments across a range of scientific disciplines would back up this perspective time and time again – nor might those who brought his ideas into the pain field.

George spent time and energy pitching the biopsychosocial model *against* the biomedical model. Of his many scathing observations, for example that advocates of the biomedical model depend on a delusional premise that it is an adequate model for medical research or practice [13], the common theme is that the biomedical model has no place in health care. We share this view but we have a very important caveat: that disturbed state or function of particular tissues, for example because of injury, tissue overload, inflammation, aberrant activation of primary nociceptors, injury to nerves, altered response profiles of immunocompetent tissues all constitute valid and potentially major contributors to a pain state. This is not in question in the biopsychosocial model. In *The Explain Pain Handbook: Protectometer* [14], these things may be considered powerful evidence of 'Dangers In Me' (DIMs). There is therefore, real power in the diagnostic and clinical examinations that allow health professionals to identify just how influential a DIM may be, but we are convinced that this must be done in light of true scientific evidence (not dodgy pathoanatomical models) and within the wider context of the biopsychosocial model.

To iterate (because it is of fundamental importance to the rest of this book), the biopsychosocial model *does* reject the biomedical model because the biomedical model is not concerned with the person, but it does not reject the role of structural, biomechanical and functional disturbance of body tissue as potentially powerful DIMs that modulate an individual's wellbeing [15]. George's wisdom permeates much of this book. It is present throughout this section on theories, though you may not notice it, and you will clearly see its influence when we dig deeper into pain biology (Chapter 3), learn about Explain Pain evidence (Chapter 4), and conceptual change science (Chapter 5). For now let's just be clear on what exactly we are saying when we talk about the biopsychosocial model as it applies to pain.

The *Wikipedia* entry on the biopsychosocial model defines it and contrasts it with the biomedical model (herein called the Jurassic model) really nicely:

'The biopsychosocial model is a broad view that attributes disease causation or disease outcome to the intricate, variable interaction of biological factors (genetic, biochemical, etc), psychological factors (mood, personality, behavior, etc), and social factors (cultural, familial, socioeconomic, medical, etc). The biopsychosocial model counters the biomedical model, which attributes disease to roughly only biological factors, such as viruses, genes, or somatic abnormalities. The biopsychosocial model applies to disciplines ranging from medicine to psychology to sociology; its novelty, acceptance, and prevalence vary across disciplines and across cultures [16].'

Every clinician who trained in the last couple of decades will have been told about the biopsychosocial model and a few lucky ones – the occupational therapists, psychologists and students of enlightened professors – would have actually learnt about it. It didn't really reach the pain field until the indefatigable John Loeser introduced it in the 1980's [17] – presenting his now famous 'onion skin model' of pain and suffering (Figure 2.2).

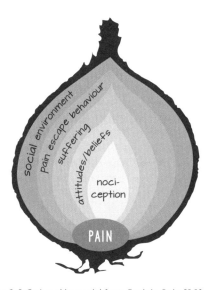

Figure 2.2 Onion skin model from Explain Pain [30]

Intriguingly however, its endorsement by the pain field seemed to be centred around its application to suffering rather than to pain. We think this is a clear case of being at least partially lost in translation and, as we have argued, reflects George Engel's own understanding of the biology of pain. Nonetheless, that the biopsychosocial model was about the suffering associated with pain, not pain itself, has cast a big shadow and it is a shadow that has frustrated both of us and we are sure many of you. We have no doubt that suffering is clearly the manifestation of biological, psychological and sociological processes, but we are mystified as to why pain is not! Here is our argument, one we will endeavour to ram home with gusto over the course of this book:

Pain involves the intricate, variable interaction of biological factors (genetic, biochemical, etc), psychological factors (mood, personality, behaviour etc.) and social factors (cultural, familial, socioeconomic, medical etc.).

Sound familiar? Well it should be because it is totally lifted from the *Wikipedia* entry defining the biopsychosocial model [16]. We would predict that, when you strap any card carrying pain scientist or clinician to the chair, hold that definition in their face, and ask for the truth or their life – '*do you believe it, punk?*', they are highly likely to say – '*yes*'. However, when the pain community talks of the biopsychosocial model, they seem to apply it liberally to how people *respond* to their pain and sparingly to *pain itself*. Let's change this. Let's hold high the flag of some of the pioneers of our field who really planted *'Pain 2.0'* decades ago – Pat Wall, Ron Melzack, Steve McMahon, John Loeser, John Bonica and Clifford Woolf among others. At risk of sounding repetitive and obstinate, we reckon the biopsychosocial model of pain was hijacked along the way because of the dominance and incredible pervasiveness of the idea that nociception and pain are much the same thing, which brings us to the Grand Poobah[7] Pain Theory.

---

7   'Pooh-bah' was coined by Gilbert and Sullivan in *The Mikado* [18]. There it was used in jest to describe someone who thought themselves the most important in the community. The literary genius of The Flintstones included the Grand Poobah as the leader of a secret society of which Fred and Barney were members. Happy Days carried on the theme and ultimately influenced us to use this term to convey the idea that this is the all-encompassing, most important theory related to *EP Supercharged*.

Theory One: The Grand Poobah Pain Theory (GPPT)

Anyone reading this book will likely not need to be told that *'nociception is neither sufficient nor necessary for pain'*, that *'pain is an output not an input'*, that *'pain is a feeling'*, nor indeed, that *'pain is an unpleasant sensory and emotional experience associated with actual or potential tissue damage or described in terms of such damage'* [19]. However, it would be remiss of us to not mention these things because they reflect, in essence, the Grand Poobah of all theories to do with pain. It is remarkable that these concepts are yet to be completely adopted within the pain science and clinical community.

The GPPT deniers

Here are our top four reasons that very clever and well meaning people might be GPPT deniers[8]:

1. The 'GPPT deniers' don't actually deny the GPPT but say they do because they think other people can't understand the concept. They might argue that being caught up on these issues is all about semantics and it is simpler to conflate nociception and pain to avoid confusion. After all, nociception can be measured in action potentials or electrical activity and noxious stimuli can be measured in Celsius[9] or pressure or chemical concentration. In contrast, pain can't really be measured at all – the closest and most valid we get is self-report, which is not without problems. The view that 'my patients won't understand' is wrong. They can and do understand [20] – we just need to be better at explaining it.

2. The GPPT deniers don't actually believe what they say but are frightened by the potential implications of admitting that there is more to pain than nociception. We are sympathetic to this one – coming from a background of manual therapy (DB) and motor control training (LM) – we understand that if one's identity is held in part by the conviction that he or she is a superb manual therapist or motor control trainer, then the notion that things are not that simple can be very confronting. Losing clinical mileage can hurt.

3. The GPPT deniers find the concepts too difficult to understand. We are also sympathetic to this one, but we know that most people including health professionals can understand these concepts [20].

4. The GPPT deniers are correct. There is a veritable mountain of evidence against this but we can't fully rule it out. GPPT deniers, climate change deniers, flat earth advocates unite!

Here are some statements that describe the GPPT in a nutshell:

- Pain is an unpleasant feeling that is felt somewhere in the body and urges us to protect that bodily location.

- Pain is one of many protective mechanisms. Others include movement, immune, cognitive, endocrine and autonomic.

- Pain is the only protective mechanism we are *necessarily aware* of and *compels us* to do something to protect the painful bit.

- Pain is modulated by any credible evidence that protection is warranted.

You might be reading this and thinking to yourself, *well that may be the case for the patients in this or that project, but I can tell you now, MY patients won't get it*. Well consider this: hundreds of health professionals were asked to estimate how well they thought 'the typical chronic pain patient' could understand modern pain biology; hundreds of 'typical chronic pain patients' were taught modern pain biology in a three hour seminar in groups of 10 to 40 people. There were two main findings: (i) health professionals of all shapes and sizes thought that patients wouldn't 'get it'; (ii) those health professionals were wrong – patients of all shapes and sizes got it! [20]

Pain report: is there a better way? The best method of assessing someone's pain is to ask them to tell us about it. This reality drives scientists and clinicians crazy because it is so open to reporting bias. Reporting bias is when people are inaccurate in their report because of some systematic influence; they don't want to offend the clinician so they say their pain is not as bad as it really is. Clinicians commonly assume their patient is over-rating their pain – it's called 'symptom exaggeration behaviour'. Think of what that term really implies – 'patient is lying'. A fuller understanding of modern pain biology might help those clinicians think twice before making this call. Assessing pain ultimately relies most on report because pain does not exist outside of consciousness – we can't see it on a scan, a blood test or a performance measure. That pain involves intricate, variable interaction of biological, psychological and social factors is exactly the point!

---

8 'GPPT denier' is a term we just made up and describes those who deny that pain is any different to nociception, which we take to reflect that they deny pain exists at all outside of nociception. We could also call them 'nociception deniers' or 'nociception=pain conflaters'.

9 Fahrenheit if you live in the USA. *When will y'all get with the programme (program)?*

To finalise our introduction to the Grand Poobah Theory of Pain, here are two tables.

Table 2.1 is a cheat sheet that covers some characteristics of pain that separate it from other protective mechanisms and from a noxious stimulus, or activity in the nociceptive system.

Table 2.2 is a list of nonsense terms that are still often used when people, even smart people, talk or write about pain, matched with terms that are accurate and matched with terms that mean the same thing but can easily be grasped by people with no health or biology training [20-24].

Animals and pain

It is difficult to determine whether or not an animal is experiencing pain because animals cannot describe to us what they are feeling. We rely on interpreting the behaviour of the animal, alongside our own knowledge of the condition of their body. The same difficulties occur when we contemplate pain in humans who cannot communicate it (eg. those with severe cognitive impairment, an infant or a foetus). Class debates on such topics are often fiery and emotional, but the discomfort the debate brings to some is outweighed by the merits of the exercise itself – it really does make us all think about what pain really is.

Characteristics of pain	Characteristics of nociception
Pain refers to a feeling, of which we are necessarily aware, that urges protection of the body part that hurts.	Nociception refers to activity in high threshold primary neurones and their central projections, most often (although not always) in response to a noxious stimulus
Pain is always felt somewhere	Nociception always occurs somewhere
Pain is always felt	Nociception is never felt
Pain can only occur in an alive animal	Nociception can occur in a single neurone removed from a frog
A painful stimulus is one that triggers pain	A noxious stimulus is one that activates nociceptors
We often fear pain	We can fear damage, but we cannot fear nociception because we neither feel nor see nociception

Table 2.1 Characteristics of pain versus nociception

Nonsense	Accurate	Lay term
Pain stimulus	Noxious stimulus OR painful stimulus	Dangerous stimulus OR painful stimulus
Pain receptor/pain endings	Nociceptor	Danger detector/danger receptor
Pain pathway	Nociceptive pathways/second order nociceptor/spinal nociceptor	Danger transmitter/danger messenger
Descending pain inhibition (control)	Descending antinociception/inhibition	Turning down the danger message
Descending pain facilitation	Descending pronociception/facilitation	Turning up the danger message

Table 2.2 Nonsense, accurate and lay terms related to pain

Child of Grand Poobah Pain Theory: The Protectometer

In 2015 we published a patient-dedicated handbook *The Explain Pain Handbook: Protectometer* [14] and the Protectometer App [59] that centres on a clinical tool called the 'Protectometer' which some of you more established Explain Painers might have heard about as a 'danger meter'.

The Protectometer (Figure 2.3) is a patient-targeted tool that encapsulates and is informed by the Grand Poobah Pain Theory. It aims to help people in pain identify potential contributors to their pain state and plan their road to recovery. Suffice here to state that the Protectometer takes the reader on a journey of reconceptualising pain from that of damage meter or nociception meter, to that of protector. It is in some ways like a pilgrimage to a more science based and a more helpful understanding of pain. By doing so, pilgrims are encouraged to 'act as their brain might act' and look for anything that their brain might see as credible evidence of 'Danger In Me' (DIMs).

Pilgrims are triggered to look not just at their activities (the things they do), but also at the things they say, think, hear and see, the people they spend time with, the things they think and believe, the places they go, and the things happening in their bodies. What is more, pilgrims are also encouraged to go looking for anything that their brains might see as credible evidence of 'safety in me' (SIMs[10]) and to look for them again among the things they do, say, think, hear and see, the people they spend time with, the things they think and believe, the places they go, and the things happening in their bodies (Figure 2.4).

We could summarise the essence of the Protectometer into the following formula:

You will have pain when your brain concludes that there is more credible evidence of danger in me (DIM) than there is credible evidence of safety in me (SIM). [14]

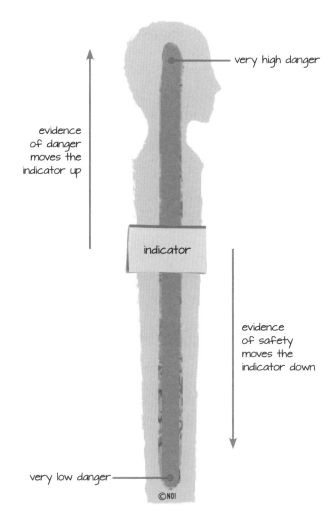

Figure 2.3 The Protectometer indicates the overall level of danger or safety in you [14]

---

10 Dim sims are also deep fried (occasionally steamed) dumplings filled with meat, vegetables and spices, very popular in Australia and New Zealand. For those of you outside of the two Great Southern Lands, you might expect some dumplings rather like dim sims at a traditional Chinese dim sum banquet.

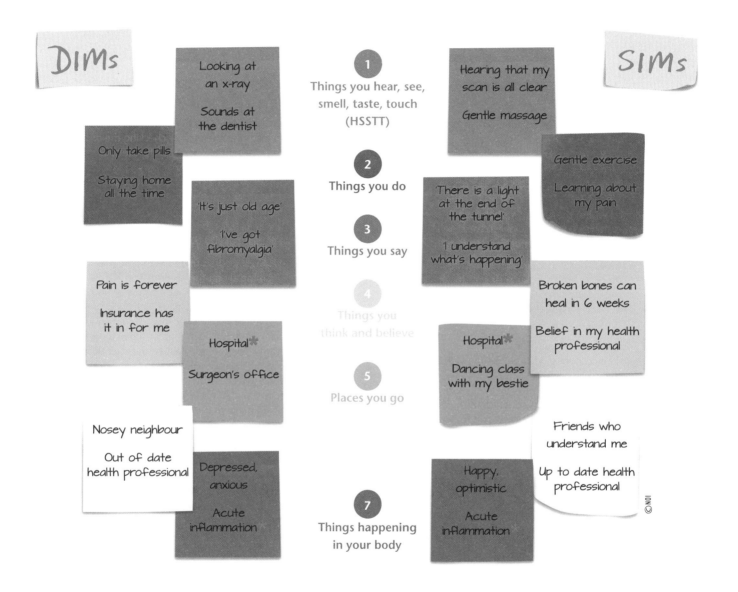

Figure 2.4 Categories and examples of DIMs and SIMs. Note that some* could be a DIM or a SIM depending on your knowledge [14].

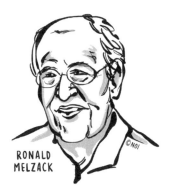

RONALD
MELZACK

Theory Two: Neurotags, collaboration and competition

Firmly embedded within the Grand Poobah Pain Theory are some conceptual frameworks that allow us to make sense of the massive amount of data that informs it. Here we provide an account of two other key theories that will arise throughout this book.

Lineage: Ron Melzack's neuromatrix and neurosignature

No-one yet knows how the brain works. However, the dominant *theories* incorporate what we do know about what the brain can achieve and what it is doing while it achieves those things. Those theories have much in common and perhaps their most shared characteristic is the idea of distributed processing. Distributed processing means that brain cells work in parallel and form networks that stretch across multiple brain areas.

This distributed processing idea clearly formed the platform for Ron Melzack's[11] very influential *neuromatrix theory (NMT)* [25]. In the NMT, the brain is considered a mass of neural networks that evoke outputs including motor output and pain. Melzack called the network of neurones that evoked a particular output the *'neurosignature'* of that output. Thus, there was a 'neurosignature' for pain, an idea and term also used by brain

imagers [26]. Melzack argued that this pain neurosignature 'bifurcates' to produce both a perception (pain) and a matching motor command (eg. bracing or guarding).

Melzack's idea was counter to what was developing in the pain and motor control community. That community, of which Lorimer was a bona fide member, was still stuck in the rather linear pursuit of how pain causes motor control changes and how motor control changes cause pain [eg. 27]. Melzack was at least one step ahead by identifying that if pain is felt and only felt, then the only way it would influence motor output was by conscious attempts to avoid or relieve pain or promote recovery (like making a call to the physiotherapist or checking the drug cabinet in the bathroom). We are now clearly in the Melzack camp on this issue [28-30], but there are many in the motor control community who still hold the view that pain is hierarchically differentiated from motor control, or who consider the issue simply semantic. More on that later but suffice now to say that Melzack's NMT was a clear trigger for changes in not only our understanding of pain but also our understanding of movement.

When the NMT was proposed there were some pretty frank criticisms [eg. 31], mostly on the grounds that the NMT did not propose a biological process that subserved this conceptual idea. However, the NMT seems to have withstood the test of time insofar as its fundamental concepts – that pain emerges once a particular set of brain cells is activated in a particular manner – appear widely endorsed across the scientific, clinical and lay community (too many citations to list). As we will discuss however, there are clear limitations of this idea of a neurosignature for pain, not least those posed by the massive *redundancy* in the brain.

Redundant brain! What the...? Okay, you had better accustom yourself to this term *'redundancy'* because it comes up time and time again in any discussion of biology. It does not mean something is useless or is about to be sacked. It means that there are many processes by which a stimulus can evoke the same response – or there are many means to the same end. In biological terms, you can think of a vast array of backup plans should one fail – the whole 'many ways to skin a cat' idea. That the brain is characterised by 'massive redundancy' means it can produce the same output in an infinite number of ways. It is a very good thing, not a bad thing.

Back to the NMT: we too count ourselves among those who find the NMT limited because of its highly conceptual nature and its separation from more fundamental matters of biology. This has led us to think more about the principles that might govern this neuromatrix. Despite extensive readings and strategic

---

11   Ron Melzack apparently struggled at university until he managed to get Donald ('neurones that fire together wire together') Hebb as his PhD supervisor. The moral here for researchers is to find the very best supervisor. Melzack was originally interested in animal behaviour, such as why dogs feared umbrellas opening, but always had an interest in phantom limb pain. He met Pat Wall at MIT in the early 1960s, and in 1965 the Gate Control Theory was published in Science. An earlier forgotten version was published in Brain in 1962. Ron Melzack – a true pain champion.

conversations, primarily within evolutionary biology, a growing literature on brain-computer interfaces and mathematical modelling of neuronal behaviours, we have not even begun to approach expert status. However, we will do our best to impart those aspects of the body of knowledge that seems most relevant to the understanding of pain, its prevention and treatment.

One of the fabulous things about working in the 'biology space' is how rapidly and sometimes completely things change. One can almost guarantee that in ten years some of the stuff we have written here will be 'out' and some other stuff will be 'in'. *At the moment* we tend to think of the brain as consisting of a heavily intertwined matrix of neuronal, immune and vascular cells that communicate with each other via a range of electrochemical and molecular mechanisms (Figure 2.5). For the vast majority of our lives the brain is losing connections, disbanding those that are not used at a staggering rate, up to millions of connections a day in infancy. Life itself seems to be a process of creating, buffing and modifying functional neuroimmune networks that are in a constant state of *competition and collaboration*. This is a rather Darwinian view of the brain – at each level of organisation it really does seem to be a case of *'survival of the fittest'* – the more a network is

'run', the stronger it becomes. The stronger it is, the more influential it becomes. Everything we have learnt about pain and rehabilitation seems to fit with this theory of the brain. Moreover it is, in a way, the 'theory inside the theories' of pain and it has fundamental implications for how we go about understanding pain's complexity.

Neurotags

Melzack's idea of a neurosignature for each given output made us think about how we would present this idea to the average punter on the street. We were chatting about this as we walked to Dave's favourite custard tart shop and noticed along the way the various 'tags' that had been sprayed by Adelaide's graffiti artists on the walls and doors en route. It struck us how similar some of these tags were to the squiggly lines that we had drawn over brains to conceptualise the idea of the distributed neuroimmune network that subserves pain. This is where the idea of a 'neurotag' was born – Loz reckons it was Dave's idea and Dave reckons it was Loz's. Regardless of its provenance, it seems to have stuck. Just to be clear – it is not an original idea, just an original name for one.

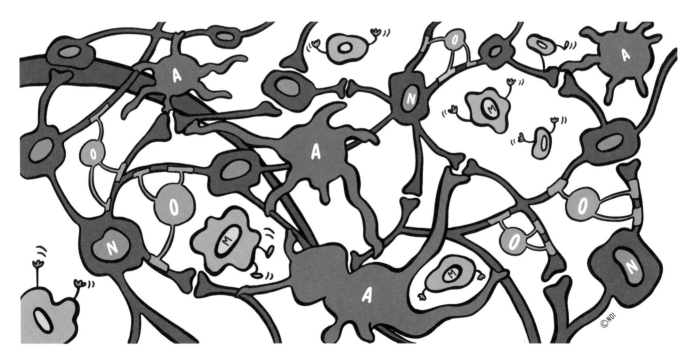

Figure 2.5 The neuroimmune mix: neurones (N), astrocytes (A), microglia (M), oligodendrocytes (O)

The brain as a mass of neurotags

We have previously suggested that the brain can be conceptualised as a mass of neurotags that are in a constant state of collaboration and competition, having influences over others and being influenced by others [32]. This conceptualisation provides a practical 'biological version' of the biopsychosocial model. In doing so, it provides a working framework by which the clinician can integrate the vast amount of data that underpin the biopsychosocial model and make predictions on the basis of it.

You can picture two broad categories of neurotags – those that have an influence only *within the brain* and those that have an influence that extends *beyond the brain*. We have recently proposed that this distinction be recognised by talking about 'primary neurotags' and 'secondary neurotags' [28]. However, in writing this book we have brought together several related but previously unhitched bodies of literature and schools of thought. In doing so we discovered a rather big problem with some of our previous terminology. It looks like this:

1. The vast literature on metaphors and their probable biological underpinnings bears an uncanny resemblance to the emerging literature on neurotags and their probable biological underpinnings. This is wonderful and corroborates the power of bringing them together – the two theoretical frameworks are superbly familiar to each other.

2. Metaphors, like neurotags, have been categorised as primary and secondary (see Chapter 7 for an introduction to the Malleable Magic of Metaphor), but they mean different, possibly opposite things in the two fields. The blame for this labelling discrepancy rests fairly and squarely on Lorimer's head. If only he had his head around the metaphor literature before he proposed the primary/secondary system of labelling neurotags.

We felt that sticking with the labelling system of primary and secondary neurotags we proposed in the peer-reviewed literature [28] would be really confusing. So, we are changing it. Everything stays the same – the wonderful, superb correlates remain – but the labels are different. Sorry.

The new nomenclature goes like this: Neurotags that exert an influence that extends beyond the brain can be thought of as *action neurotags* (the new language for 'primary neurotags'). Action neurotags might exert their influence on muscles (motor neurotags), on consciousness (thought or feeling neurotags), or on any of the output systems that can exert their effects outside

of brain matter [EP43, EPH27].[12] Action neurotags might also include secondary metaphors (see Chapter 7).

Other neurotags exert their influence only within the brain, so we can call them *modulation neurotags* (the new language for 'secondary neurotags'). Modulation neurotags might represent implicit concepts, unimodal sensory data (such as visual data), primary metaphors, spatial coordinates of body parts, length-tension relationships of muscles, characteristics of people or places, odours, previous exposures and so forth (see Table 2.3 and Figure 2.6). In short – modulation neurotags represent the things we know that we don't necessarily know we know [28].

Action neurotag	Modulation neurotags
Sight neurotag (what you see)	Visually encoded data, predicted visually encoded data, size of objects data
Movement neurotag	Proprioceptive encoded data, visually encoded data, state of the body

Table 2.3 Action and modulation neurotags

Take a person, let's call him Sven. Whether or not he is protected by pain, restricted movement or thoughts will depend on the relative influence of neurotags that subserve either protection or its opposite. There is no obvious opposite of protection, which is unfortunate because it would be most precise to talk of neurotags that serve to protect and those that serve to 'opposite of protect'. We have discussed this at some length with a reasonably large group of experts and each alternative has its problems. We have adopted the following approach: we call those neurotags that increase protection 'danger neurotags' and those neurotags that decrease protection 'safety neurotags', as discussed on page 17. We can categorise every cue that modulates danger or safety neurotags as either danger cues or safety cues.

> A cue, stimulus, input or event that provides credible evidence of Danger In Me = a 'DIM'. The neurotag that represents each DIM is a DIM neurotag.
>
> A cue, stimulus, input or event that provides credible evidence of Safety In Me = a 'SIM'. The neurotag that represents each SIM is a SIM neurotag.

---

12 Note: EP43 refers to *Explain Pain* page 43. EPH27 refers to *The Explain Pain Handbook: Protectometer* page 27.

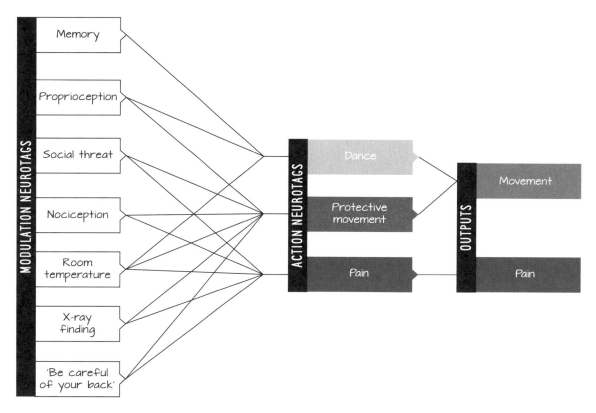

Figure 2.6 Influence of neurotags

Explaining Pain as a process of generating and reinforcing SIM neurotags

At the end of this book, there are practical examples of curricula[13] for explaining pain. In these, we focus on identifying *Target Concepts*. These are the concepts that a healthcare professional has reasoned are necessary to address in order to achieve behavioural change. The objective is to generate a neurotag that represents that concept and thereby influences the activation of protective outputs such as pain. So, the concept neurotag serves as a potentially powerful and long lasting SIM. There is a vast literature that demonstrates the power of concept neurotags – *Explain Pain's* amazing pain stories are mostly examples of this [30]. The remarkable effects of supposedly inert treatments that are incorrectly believed to be active (commonly called 'placebos') can be attributed to the engagement of concept neurotags as a result of contextual cues – the pill, the doctor, the setting.

When we establish an Explain Pain curriculum, our biological objective is to assist the learner's brain to make the critical connections so that each Target Concept becomes embedded in his or her brain, held by its own network of brain cells. In order to do this most effectively, we can draw on a rapidly growing body of research that investigates how neurotags form and what principles govern their operation and influence.

---

13 Don't freak out at the mention of curricula, the plural of curriculum. Curriculum is not a part of your digestive system. Curriculum is what we teach, how we teach it and why we teach it. Explaining anything to a patient or giving them any health related advice or instruction involves a curriculum.

Neurotags – Operation and Influence

There is a growing literature on the principles that govern the formation and influence of neurotags. In depth discussion of this literature is beyond the scope of this book and beyond our expertise. However, there are several principles that are worth thinking more about. They fall into two broad categories – operation (distributed coding, single cell insufficiency, multitasking) and influence (strength, precision).

Operation: Distributed coding

One of René Descartes' revolutionary ideas was that the pineal gland was the seat of the soul. His famous drawing of a fellow with his foot in the fire working a hydraulic system to ring a bell in his pineal gland really was an outstanding innovation (remember that at about this time the prevailing biological theories were centred on bodily humors – fire, water, black bile and white bile). However, Descartes' drawing is now beyond its use by date – it is troublingly misleading and no longer defensible, so we will do what few before us have managed to do: we will NOT include it in this book.

Descartes was not the only one to suggest that specific cells or nuclei in the brain subserve pain. Although we have known for centuries that the pineal gland is not the seat of pain,[14] each of the anterior cingulate cortex, the insula, the dorsolateral prefrontal cortex, the amygdala and the primary sensory cortex have had their time in the sun – proposed as being 'the pain centre' at one time or another. But the data have failed to back up these proposals - not surprisingly, because it seems that this is not how the brain works anyway. It is more likely that pain requires activation of a network of distributed brain cells. It is not just pain that requires distributed processing – it seems that everything does. Even the apparently simple process of sensing someone touching your arm involves processing across several brain areas, not just activation of a particular brain cell or cluster of brain cells in the primary sensory cortex.

Doh! I thought the sensory homunculus was the representation of touch! Well sort of, but not quite. Imagine there are two stimuli delivered to the skin. One is felt and the other is not. The activation in the primary sensory cortex (S1) is the same for both [33]. There goes the theory – if whether or not you feel doesn't relate to S1 activation, then S1 cannot be the representation of feeling touch. More on this in Chapter 3.

Operation: Single cell insufficiency

Implicit in the idea of distributed processing is the idea of single cell insufficiency. Single cell insufficiency means that a single brain cell can't really do anything on its own[15] – of course a brain on its own probably can't do much either.[16] Put a single brain cell in a bath of survival fluid and it will not be able to influence anything, nor collaborate with anything, nor 'see' your grandmother [34]. It is when these cells interact with other brain cells, when they collaborate to form neurotags, that they can exert an influence (Figure 2.7).

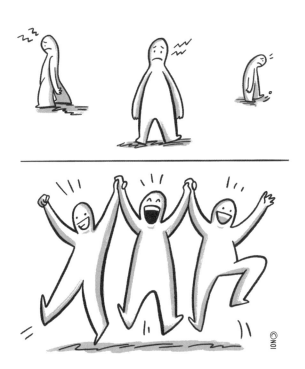

Figure 2.7 Single cell insufficiency – cells collaborate to form neurotags

---

14 Even René himself is said to have been fidgety about the necessary implication of his idea – that inside the little man in the pineal gland there must be a really little man and inside that really little man there must be a teeny weeny little man, etc. etc.

15 Lorimer fondly remembers a speech by a mate, affectionately known as Wasim, on the event of his 50th. He observed that meaning is instilled by the connections between things. He was talking about the connections between people but he could easily have been talking instead about brain cells – their power is in their connections.

16 Roald Dahl, in his short story 'William and Mary' captures this idea well as he describes William being 'saved' as a brain on a pillow in a bath of survival fluid, one eye connecting 'him' to the world. Needless to say the experiment as to whether William still existed was just that – a thought experiment – and one that is well worth a read.

Operation: Multitasking brain cells

Alongside single cell insufficiency is the property of multitasking. As it sounds, multitasking means that single brain cells, or single neuroimmune units (discussed later as tripartite synapses) can contribute to an infinite number of neurotags. As we discuss in the next section on the cortical body matrix, this has potentially profound implications for our understanding of the suite of dysfunctions that can accompany chronic pain and for our approach to rehabilitation. Both female and male brain cells are multitaskers!

Influence: Neuronal strength

Neuronal strength is determined by neuronal mass and synaptic efficacy. *Neuronal mass* refers to the size of a neurotag, or more correctly, how many cells it has. The general rule is that the higher the mass of a neurotag, the more influence it will have. Nociception (more of this in Chapter 3) activates a vast network of brain cells. That is, nociception neurotags have high mass. They will have a large influence and will be likely to compete well against other neurotags.

Nociception neurotags are always modulation neurotags, but they are powerful influencers of action neurotags such as pain, protective movements, gaze direction and certain spatial data.[17] Remember here of course that nociception is clearly not *sufficient* for pain – if it were we would have no explanation for the times when we sustain a clear injury that is pain free. In addition – nociception is not *necessary* for pain – if it were we would have no explanation for those times when a cognitive illusion evokes pain [35, 36].

The other contributor to the strength of a neurotag is *synaptic efficacy* (Figure 2.8). Synaptic efficacy refers to how rapidly and efficiently a post-synaptic cell is activated by pre-synaptic input and how quickly the synapse returns to a 'ripe' state. The concept was captured well by Hebbs' *cells that fire together wire together* [37], but also by *practice makes perfect* and *try, try and try again*. Together, neurotag mass and synaptic efficacy are powerful determinants of a neurotag's influence. It is no wonder then that as pain persists, allodynia and hyperalgesia increase: the influence of the pain neurotag becomes greater, via both increased synaptic efficacy and collaboration between neurotags, effectively increasing neurotag mass.

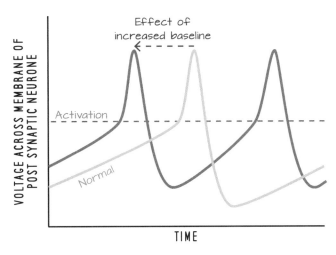

Figure 2.8 Synaptic efficacy – more bang for your buck

Influence: Neurotag precision

Neurotag precision can be a tricky concept to wrap your head around, at least in physiological terms. Clinically it is a very intuitive term – loss of precision in neurotags for movement will result in imprecise movements – but biologically it is not well understood. Precision reflects the likelihood of one brain cell being activated relative to the likelihood of its neighbouring cells being activated. For example, if one cell is 80% likely to fire and its neighbours are all <1% likely to fire, the neurotag would be very precise. On the other hand, if one cell is 80% likely to fire and all its neighbours are 70% likely to fire, the neurotag would be imprecise. Not too tricky right? (See Figure 3.12 page 76.) We call these relative likelihoods 'activation probability gradients'. The tricky bit is that the particular brain cell most likely to fire is not necessarily fixed, so these 'activation probability gradients' are modulated in real time by other neurotags, each with their own probability gradients, each of which is being modulated in real time by other neurotags, each with *their* own probability gradients, and so forth… you get the picture?

We have thought long and hard about going into this much detail about such fundamental concepts and we have carried out a large amount of 'market research', which involves asking people at courses, seminars, lectures and conferences whether it helps to understand neurotags at this level. The feedback has been overwhelmingly positive *yes! absolutely!* Perhaps this is because once the model 'sticks', the rest of our reflections on the current state of the science in chronic pain make very good sense.

---

17 Don't be put off by this reference to 'gaze direction and certain spatial data'. A noxious stimulus will cause you to look at the location of that stimulus; when a part of you is injured, a stimulus that occurs near the injury is much harder to ignore than an identical stimulus that occurs somewhere else. These things reflect increased influence over where we look and increased influence related to that location.

This 'tricky' bit results from the massive redundancy of the human brain. Remember that redundancy here refers to the many different ways the brain can evoke the same output. A terrific concrete example of this comes from the study of professional, elite shooters and amateur or novice shooters. When scientists compared body movements and muscle activations across the whole body, they found that in one group there was great variability within individuals in what their body parts did for each shot. In the other group there was far less variability. The surprising thing was that the highly variable group were the elite shooters and they hit the bullseye in the vast majority of trials. The relatively invariable group were the novices who hardly ever hit the target board. Expert shooters have multiple options for achieving a stable output, novices don't (see [38] for more on this concept). These multiple options are made possible by redundancy.

The implications for our understanding of pain are really significant here: although the pain might feel exactly the same one day to the next, it is highly likely that the contributors to that pain vary from day to day, potentially from moment to moment. In fact, it is also likely that there is a gradual shift over time in the contributors to a pain state.

Another quick word on Target Concepts

This stuff on the operation and influence of neurotags has clear implications not just for understanding someone's pain but also for providing a biological context for explaining pain. We go into this in some detail later in this book but for now, here are some implications:

How can we increase neuronal mass of Target Concept neurotags?

By helping the person in pain to generate several stories, a range of metaphors, sayings, self-explanations and examples all addressing a Target Concept,[18] we are bringing neurotags to collaborate. This increases the number of brain cells that represent that Target Concept, meaning greater mass and influence – a stronger SIM.[19] Having a range of neurotags associated with a Target Concept instils some of this glorious

---

18 Examples of Target Concepts include: *'We are bioplastic', 'Pain is one of many protective outputs'* and *'Pain depends on the balance of perceived danger and safety'* (see page 128).

19 Remember that concept SIMs (the things you think) are only one type of SIM – there are many others: the things you hear, see, smell, taste, touch, do, say; the places you go; the people in your life and things happening in your body.

redundancy. It is the redundancy and profound variability in neurotag influence that is thought to underpin experiential learning – the more varied the methods by which the brain can solve a problem, the more likely it is to find solutions to completely new problems. This strongly implies that the more varied the neurotags that hold Target Concepts, the more likely it is that the brain will continue creating new SIMs. Just take a moment to think how remarkable this opportunity really is – we don't just Explain Pain, we help the person to become a SIM self-generator!

How can we increase the synaptic efficacy of Target Concepts?

Well, no surprises here – Practice. Practice. Practice – in as many contexts as possible. This is why catchy slogans such as *'motion is lotion'* (Nugget 63) are better than awkward ones such as *'movement helps release the synovial fluid in your joints making them healthier'*. Critically of course, the catchy slogans must be meaningful so that they tap into a Target Concept – you must first explain *why* motion is lotion, but once they've taken it on board, the catchy phrase can be easily practised. This is also why we recommend sticky notes, or fridge magnets with Target Concepts written or drawn on them. For example, a note saying *'Don't flare up. But don't freak out if you do'* stuck on the fridge will increase the influence of this key concept neurotag when the opportunity to do so arises.

How can we increase the precision of Target Concepts?

This is really intuitive – to make a neurotag more precise, it needs to be differentiated from other neurotags. One very effective method of doing this is by using vision, which is a very precise sensory channel. This is one reason why drawing Target Concepts and using multimedia is so helpful. Reflect here on the artwork in *Explain Pain* – the drawings are quirky and striking for a reason – they provide several methods by which the visual system gains precise data. We know that colour, contour and character give important cues to differentiate similar pictures from each other (contrast this with the typical textbook and its homogenised 'textbooky' images devoid of character!). One implication for you, the teacher, is to draw things yourself to help explain concepts, or potentially even better – have the person in pain draw them!

Theory Three: The cortical body matrix theory

The cortical body matrix theory built on the neuromatrix theory, and is grounded in the principles that govern how neurotags form, collaborate and compete with each other. There is now a large body of literature concerning the cortical body matrix theory (see [39] for one review) so it is sufficient to cover just the basics here. In short, the cortical body matrix theory posits that there is a 'matrix' of thalamocortical neural loops that *subserve the protection and regulation of the body and the space around it, at both a physiological and perceptual level.* If you think that is a bit of a mouthful, we agree, so let's untangle it a little.

'... subserve the protection and regulation...'

You might argue that ultimately our entire biology subserves bodily protection as our highest priority and that bodily regulation is a day-to-day ongoing version of protection: for example, by maintaining normal blood pH we maintain protection against acidity or alkalinity, too much of which will damage tissue and disrupt function. Application, interrogation and discussion of the cortical body matrix concerns those processes that are driven or modulated by brain responses. Therefore, they are processes (outputs) that result from activation of action neurotags because they extend beyond the brain to the body (think muscles, immune responses, blood flow) or to consciousness (for example feelings of swelling, feelings of one's anatomical structure, that you own your body and of course, your pain).

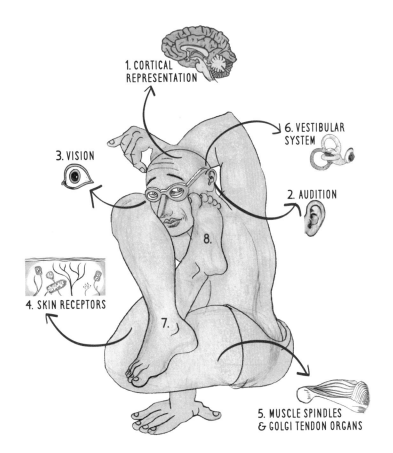

Figure 2.9 The cortical body matrix theory, adapted from [60]

(1) A widespread network of cortical brain areas are thought to be involved in body representation and, thus, in self-localisation. However, a major role is also played by audition (2) and vision (3). In order to locate one's body part both skin receptors (4), muscle spindles and Golgi tendon organs (5) are crucial. Together these cues contribute to create a unique and coherent percept of one's own body, well described with the concept of cortical body matrix. In particular, the innovative aspect is the body-centred representation of the body itself (instead of a body part-centred representation) such as the right leg (7) usually in the right side of the space (8) can occupy the left side of the peripersonal space simply crossing over in the space where the left leg usually is.

'... the body and the space around it...'

One aspect of the cortical body matrix that clearly differentiates it from previous ideas is the inclusion of space. In a way, we tend to 'own' the space that immediately surrounds us. Scientists call this space the peripersonal space and even now as you read, your brain is mapping out your peripersonal space (Novella 5 *Protecting your turf*). A fly is far more likely to trigger protective swipes or increased tactile input if it enters your peripersonal space. You will be immediately alerted should the fly land on your skin. Have you ever entered another person's peripersonal space and seen them withdraw without you even touching them? But how does the brain do this?

There are actually very clever people dedicated to finding this out. They have learnt that when our brain localises anything around us, it has a range of coordinate systems according to where the event is located. A coordinate system might be relative to our face (a face-centred coordinate system); it might be relative to our limb (limb-centred coordinate system); it might be relative to our body midline. The final localisation depends on all these systems integrating with each other. Here is another example of the wonderful redundancy in the system – if one coordinate system is unavailable, then the brain can use the others and still come reasonably close.

The point is that it is not just our body tissues that are regulated and protected in real time by physiological events and perceptions – it is also our peripersonal space. Who cares? Well we do, because as you will see, when the cortical body matrix gets disrupted, some of our physiological regulations are disrupted on the basis of these spatial coordinate systems – most obviously the body midline-centred coordinate system.

'... at both a physiological and perceptual level.'

This linkage between what happens physiologically and what happens perceptually is clearly a spin off from the neuromatrix theory's proposition that a single command bifurcates to yield a motor output and the experience that matches the motor output [25]. The cortical body matrix theory extends that idea by drawing on the neurotag based model outlined earlier and on a large number of research findings. Broadly speaking, this research speaks to the unity of the mind-body connection. We are both slightly nervous admitting that so early on in this book because we know it triggers rolling eyes and accusations of quackery and woolly thinking, but wait! What *we* mean by this mind-body unity is that we are one biological environment that is in a constant state of change, correction and, well, *life*.

Before we describe some of the specific research examples from Team Lorimer's laboratory and the labs of others, consider some of the things we have already argued here in *EP Supercharged* as well as some of the things we will cover in Chapter 3 which digs deeper into the biology.

- Action neurotag outputs can produce feelings (eg. pain), thoughts, worries, happiness, words (the ones you say *and* the ones you use to make sense of things) and movements – that is not all, but hopefully you get the picture!
- Action neurotags are under the influence of a massive range of modulation neurotags.
- All neurotags depend on, and are under the influence of their environment – the molecules that float around them, the molecules they release and to which they react, the immune cells that hug almost every synapse and supply it with conductive power – the real time state of the body.

There is already bucketloads of evidence that feelings and physiological reactions go together – when we are *feeling* frightened our heart beats faster and our face goes pale; when we are feeling *very* frightened we might scream or jump; when we are feeling *terrified* we might poo our pants. We know that when we are *feeling* sexually aroused, our reproductive organs change their size, shape or state.

It makes no sense that these physiological responses would occur in isolation – they usually co-exist. Neither would it make sense to feel such things without a physiological response. The cortical body matrix simply extends these highly intuitive connections to the full suite of bodily systems by drawing on some remarkable experiments and clinical findings that might surprise you – we are both like a garden and like a machine.[20]

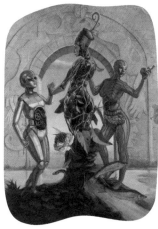

Figure 2.10 The body is like a garden and a machine

---

20 Prof Mark Hutchinson from Adelaide University introduced us to this idea of machine vs garden. The body is often thought of as a machine – pulleys, levers, electrical wiring and plumbing. However, we now know that a shift in function in one corner of the human can be accompanied by a shift in function in another corner. The immune system for example – distributed across almost all the tissues of the body and moving throughout the body not just via the blood but through extracellular space and cerebrospinal fluid – like bees pollinating far away plants.

Feeling or emotion? Same same or different?

We tend to use 'emotion' and 'feeling' interchangeably, but do they really mean the same thing? Biologists would argue not and some of the nicest theories about how we feel things would also argue not. Biologists would see emotions as physiological responses to stimuli, for example the increase in heart rate and redistribution of blood flow that you have from the visual input of a snake would be an emotion. That conscious experience that we might also have compelling us to escape would be called the feeling.

These concepts are at the heart of Damasio's Somatic Marker Hypothesis [40], which also provides the platform for a compelling model of how we learn to feel. The Somatic Marker Hypothesis, melded here with principles of neurotags, suggests that we have automatised protective reflexes to threatening stimuli.

That is, a threatening stimulus is highly influential over action neurotags for a given physiological response – which we call the emotion. The emotion triggers a bombardment of feedback that itself activates a range of modulation neurotags. Those neurotags influence action neurotags including the neurotag that produces a particular feeling. Coupling the stimulus with the ultimate feeling results in the stimulus being able to directly trigger the feeling.

There are critiques of the Somatic Marker Hypothesis that are reasonable, but differentiating feelings from physiological responses is valuable and as such, we will use 'feeling' to describe anything we 'feel'.

Put like that it is pretty sensible isn't it?

Movement and structure

It has long been believed that the repertoire of movements held by our brain reflects the biomechanical or anatomical constraints of our body [41, 42] – we do the things our body lets us do. Is this tight relationship between biomechanical constraints and movement repertoire hard wired into the brain, or does it simply reflect that we have never attempted to learn movements that are physiologically impossible? This may seem a pointless question, but consider this: seven upper limb amputees with intact phantom arms were encouraged to learn how to perform a movement of their phantom arm that would be impossible if the arm was still there [43]. Four of the amputees mastered the task in a couple of weeks. The scientists devised a couple of timed assessment tasks on which it is impossible to cheat and matched the results to the participants' reports. The results clearly showed that the four who said they could do the task were not lying – they had learnt to perform a movement that would be impossible to perform with a normal intact arm. But here are the really groovy bits:

1. All four reported that at the exact moment they learnt to perform the task, their phantom arm had a new anatomical structure that felt different from the former structure and different from their other (intact) arm.

2. All four reported that phantom limb movements they had previously found easy became difficult to perform. The scientists' cheat check tests clearly supported their report. Think how remarkable this is! The changes in felt structure and movement occurred simultaneously and they became less able to perform previously easy movements!

What does this study show? That the way our body feels to us relates closely to what we are able to make it do.

Ownership, blood flow and histamine

The rubber hand illusion is a compelling trick in which participants experience the illusion that their real hand has been 'replaced' by an artificial counterpart [44]. There are many studies that have used this illusion to investigate how the brain integrates other things into maps of the body. However, an alternative application of this illusion is to use it to determine what happens to the hand that has been 'replaced'. Studies that did exactly that revealed that blood flow to the 'replaced hand' is decreased [45] and histamine reactivity increased [46], but only in the hand that has been 'replaced'.

What do these studies show? The way our body feels to us relates closely to how the immune and autonomic systems regulate it.

Space, temperature and touch

Having demonstrated that the relationship between how our body feels and how it is regulated is a two-way street, the next question raised by clinical findings in people with pain in one hand is '*does regulation of our body depend on where in space the body part is?*' Suffice here to say that the answer to this question is '*yes, it does*'. How do we know? In those with a cold, painful hand associated with complex regional pain syndrome (CRPS), crossing their hand over the midline for 10 minutes warms it up and crossing the unaffected hand over the body midline cools it down; tactile stimuli from the unaffected hand are prioritised over identical stimuli from the affected hand unless the hands are crossed, in which case the reverse occurs (so there is a space-based prioritisation not a limb-based one). When patients wear prism glasses so that their visual field is shifted to one side, the changes in processing and temperature match where the limbs appear to be, not where they really are [47-50].

What do these studies show? That our brain's maps of space as well as our brain's maps of our body interact with blood flow and touch processing.

Thoughts, mood and protective bodily outputs

Reflections on the relationships between what we think, how we feel and how our system and the space around it is regulated, always arrive at the Chicken or the Egg problem. Are our heart rate and respiratory rate elevated because we are anxious or are we anxious because our heart rate and respiratory rate are elevated? The neurotag framework and the cortical body matrix would predict that, in adolescent and adult humans at least, it may well be that neither is chicken and neither is egg – they are both chicken and egg. They are outputs that serve the same purpose (or more accurately, 'have the same effect') – they modulate each other in a constant state of change.

It hurts to put your arm into a bucket of icy cold water. This task is widely used by pain researchers to assess pain tolerance and it is called the cold pressor test. In the blood, the concentration of pro-inflammatory cytokines – the workhorses of the immune system – is increased 30 minutes after the test. This increase occurs in response to other painful stimuli too [51]. What's more, the degree to which the noxious stimulus triggers a body-wide inflammatory response – sending out pro inflammatory mediators to the entire system via the blood stream – is not clearly related to the amount of pain people feel, showing that different protective systems can be recruited to different extents. And the more that participants endorse catastrophic thoughts about pain and injury, the bigger the

increase in inflammatory response, showing the influence of cognitive modulation neurotags on immune action neurotags.

> **Pain tolerance or pain threshold?**
>
> **Pain threshold** refers to the minimum intensity of a given stimulus at which one first feels pain. It is measured according to the units that describe the stimulus, for example temperature, pressure, concentration, deformation, energy level (in the case of laser stimuli). Pain threshold is highly variable between individuals and within individuals. This is not at all surprising because pain reflects the particular mix at a particular time of all the information available to the brain. On the basis of that the brain decides whether or not to protect.
>
> **Pain tolerance** refers to the maximum exposure to a painful stimulus that one will tolerate before aborting the test. Pain tolerance is also highly variable between individuals and within individuals, in part because it is influenced by everything that influences pain as well as the distraction and coping skills available to the participant. People commonly mix up pain threshold and pain tolerance and often think they are both reasonably stable. But they are not. Here are data from Team Lorimer's laboratory: the same individual, given exactly the same laser stimulus, to almost exactly the same location, in a white-walled, silent, highly sterile and standardised environment, with no one else in the room, will have a pain threshold to laser that changes from trial to trial by up to 30% [52]. How much more might pain threshold vary in the *real* world?

This link between thoughts and protective bodily outputs has also been shown with respect to movement. That is, when people are in pain, they move differently – no surprises there. However, when they expect to be in pain, they move differently too. If someone, let's say Wendy, with no history of back pain is given an injection of salty water into her back muscles, it hurts and it changes the way she uses her trunk muscles during walking [53] or during arm or leg movements [54, 55]. Perhaps this too is not surprising, although don't be suckered into concluding that it is the pain that is making the motor control change.[21] This conclusion can only be supported if you don't think pain is an output of the brain, if you are mistaking pain for nociception – remember the Grand Poobah Pain Theory.

---

21 This is a classic case of mistaking association or correlation for causation. It is the great clinical finding sucker punch. Don't fall for it.

A far more defensible conclusion is that both pain and altered muscle activations are outputs that serve to protect the back. We have written extensively on these things elsewhere [28, 57].

Now here is something to make you think '*what if these people with no history of back trouble are made to think that they are about to have back pain?*' Well, they do the same thing as people who have back pain associated with noxious experimental stimulation do – there are subtle changes in the way they use their trunk muscles. These subtle changes serve to limit movement of the area under potential threat, even during fairly benign limb movements [58].

There are other changes too that speak to a much more complex modification of all sorts of processes in the face of threat. For example, these same people lose the normal variability of movement [38] and some of them don't regain this normal variability even when the threat of noxious stimulation is removed. At this point you might be thinking '*what's different about the people who don't regain normal variability and those who do?*' Well we were thinking this and we now know that the degree to which someone believes that the human back is fragile, and the degree to which they endorse catastrophic thoughts about back pain, differentiates those who regain normal variability and return to a normal safety strategy from those who don't [38]!

We can make sense of this in terms of the neurotag conversations above: the modulation neurotags that represent cognitions (eg. the human back is fragile, back pain is a catastrophe) – the DIM neurotags – have become far more influential over the action neurotag – a movement strategy. They are not so influential so as to trigger pain, but they are clearly triggering protection when protection is not in fact required. These ideas are integrated deep within the Protectometer [14].

What do these studies show? That protective cognitive outputs such as thoughts and beliefs relate to the extent of protective bodily outputs such as systemic inflammation and movement.

The main thrust of the cortical body matrix literature and of the model itself is that we are a unified mind-body entity. Presuming that there is no major damage to the brain, we will have agency over our body; we will know it is ours; we feel our body; our body's regulation and protection is our number one priority. If we are to endorse these ideas, and we humbly suggest that the evidence to do so is very compelling, then we need to think seriously about the last line in the cortical body matrix statement above [39], which we paste again here:

'*… at both a physiological and perceptual level.*'

This idea of a single unified system pulling the strings on our survival by regulating bodily functions and our perceptions of our body has potentially profound implications for dealing with pain. Pain is a feeling but it will almost necessarily be accompanied by other protective outputs. In fact, one might predict that other protective outputs occur more readily and pain is only engaged when entire organism activation is required. That is, other protective outputs may well be triggered in line with cognitive outputs such as *my back is ruined*. Let's take a slightly different case – that of a patient one of us saw who described his back as his 'Roman ruins'.

Jamie was a 48 year old ex-builder with back and leg pain sufficiently intense and disabling to prevent him from working for the previous decade or so. Jamie described his back as his 'Roman ruins'. Clearly this was a metaphor for what he considered a crumbling, unstable, very old structure bearing little resemblance to its former glory. When asked about this label he explained that the idea came to him when discussing his MRI and x-ray reports with his physiotherapist and then it somehow just stuck. His wife would ask him '*how are the Roman ruins today?*' He would put clinical appointments in his diary as 'Roman ruins appointment'. He had a photo of The Forum in Rome on his wall and his dream was to one day travel to Rome to see the 'real Roman ruins' for himself. We can make sense of Jamie's prolific use of a highly dangerous sounding metaphor in terms of neurotags and the cortical body matrix.

Roman ruins and the principles that govern the influence of neurotags

We can consider that Jamie has a neurotag that represents the metaphor of Roman ruins. Let's call it 'the Roman ruins neurotag'. We would predict that the Roman ruins neurotag has very high synaptic efficacy because it is activated many times daily. We might also predict that there is some redundancy[22] in his brain when it comes to Roman ruins because 'Roman ruins' has penetrated the things he says, the things he hears, the things he sees (diary entries, photo on wall, imagined holiday to Rome), the people he is with (clinicians who are themselves attending to the Roman ruins; his wife and friends who associate him with his Roman ruins). Finally, we would predict that the Roman ruins neurotag(s) is rather precise because it involves visual components (from the radiology reports, the photo of The Forum on his wall, and the visualisation of his dream-trip to Rome). All these characteristics make for a highly influential neurotag. As such, it will serve as a powerful DIM and contribute to any number of protective (action) neurotags and their outputs – back pain, muscular guarding, endocrine, immune and autonomic. Remarkably Jamie changed his name to Julius and began wearing a toga and sandals.[23]

Roman ruins and the cortical body matrix

We know that purely cognitive or perceptual manipulations can change immune regulation [46], blood flow [45], motor output [55] and perceived bodily structure [43] in remarkably refined ways. The cortical body matrix theory would predict that the more Jamie runs the Roman ruins neurotag, the more likely it is that the physiological regulation of his back will fall in line with the cognitive/perceptual manipulation. So if we are to accept the cortical body matrix theory, we must be open to the possibility that 'running the neurotag' of the highly influential Roman ruins metaphor over and over and over will trigger immune, endocrine and motor responses consistent with a crumbling, unstable and very old anatomical structure. We know that descending facilitation can trigger peptide release in the tissues; we know that one of those peptides called CGRP is a powerful facilitator of bone formation and remodeling (see Chapter 3); we know that far more subtle perceptual outputs like those induced by the rubber hand illusion can modulate histamine and blood flow in gross ways. Therefore we have a *feasible* biological pathway by which Jamie's continual activation of 'Roman ruins neurotags' might contribute to changes at a tissue level.

Roman ruins is but one metaphor from one patient. Chapter 7 focuses on the wide range of metaphors that pervade the pain field. There is an entire research field in the classification and understanding of metaphors and *EP Supercharged* may well

represent the coming together of two major bodies of work, in a manner that should make us all think twice before we *let another metaphor go*.

Brace yourself for the next chapter...

Well that is theories done and dusted – phew! Obviously there are many good theories related to pain that we have not touched on. That is because our objective was not to give you a comprehensive list of current theories in the pain field. Our objective was to give you the scaffolding on which to stick all the juicy biology that is coming in the next chapter. Hang on to your hat, it's going to be fun!

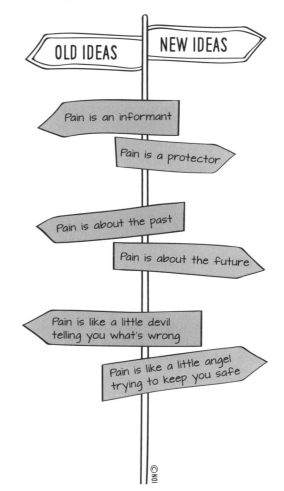

Figure 2.11 Signpost of old ideas versus new ideas

---

22 Remember that here 'redundancy' refers to the capacity of the brain to find numerous combinations of brain cells to produce the given output. In a sense, there are numerous Roman ruins neurotags

23 Okay, so we made this last bit up.

References

1. Popper KR (1959) The logic of scientific discovery. Hutchinson: London.

2. Chalmers AF (1976) What is this thing called science?: An assessment of the nature and status of science and its methods. University of Queensland Press: Queeensland.

3. Wang L, et al. (2011) Why do woodpeckers resist head impact injury: a biomechanical investigation. PLoS One 6: e26490.

4. May PR, et al. (1976) Woodpeckers and head injury. The Lancet 307: 454-455.

5. Kuhn TS (1962) The structure of scientific revolutions. University of Chicago Press: Chicago.

6. Williams MT, Gerlach Y & Moseley GL (2012) The 'survival perceptions': time to put some Bacon on our plates? J Physiother 58: 73-75.

7. Taleb NN (2012) Antifragile: Things That Gain from Disorder. Random House: New York.

8. Clark A (2015) Surfing Uncertainty: Prediction, Action, and the Embodied Mind. Oxford University Press: Oxford.

9. Lotze M & Moseley GL (2015) Theoretical Considerations for Chronic Pain Rehabilitation. Phys Ther 95: 1316-1320.

10. de Botton A (2016) The Course of Love. Penguin Books: London.

11. Engel GL (1977) The need for a new medical model: a challenge for biomedicine. Science 196: 129-136.

12. Engel GL (1960) A unified concept of health and disease. Perspect Biol Med 3: 459-485.

13. Engel GL (1980) The clinical application of the biopsychosocial model. Am J Psychiatry 137: 535-544.

14. Moseley GL & Butler DS (2015) The Explain Pain Handbook: Protectometer. Noigroup Publications: Adelaide.

15. Moseley GL & Butler DS (2015) Fifteen Years of Explaining Pain: The Past, Present, and Future. J Pain 16: 807-813.

16. Biopsychosocial model, in Wikipedia. Viewed 24 January 2017: https://en.wikipedia.org/wiki/Biopsychosocial_model.

17. Loeser J (1982) Concepts of pain, in Chronic Low-back Pain, Stanton-Hicks M & Boas R Eds. Raven Press: New York.

18. Sullivan A & Gilvert WS (1885) The Mikado. Savoy Theatre: London.

19. Merskey H & Bogduk N (1994) Classification of Chronic Pain. 2nd Edn. IASP Press: Seattle.

20. Moseley GL (2003) Unravelling the barriers to reconceptualisation of the problem in chronic pain: the actual and perceived ability of patients and health professionals to understand the neurophysiology. J Pain 4: 184-189.

21. Moseley GL (2002) Combined physiotherapy and education is efficacious for chronic low back pain. Aust J Physiother 48: 297-302.

22. Moseley GL (2003) Joining forces - combining cognition-targeted motor control training with group or individual pain physiology education: a successful treatment for chronic low back pain. J Man Manip Therap 11: 88-94.

23. Moseley GL, Hodges PW & Nicholas MK (2004) A randomized controlled trial of intensive neurophysiology education in chronic low back pain. Clin J Pain 20: 324-330.

24. Moseley GL (2004) Evidence for a direct relationship between cognitive and physical change during an education intervention in people with chronic low back pain. Eur J Pain 8: 39-45.

25. Melzack R (1990) Phantom limbs and the concept of a neuromatrix. Trends Neurosci 13: 88-92.

26. Tracey I & Mantyh PW (2007) The cerebral signature for pain perception and its modulation. Neuron 55: 377-391.

27. Jull GA & Richardson CA (2000) Motor control problems in patients with spinal pain: a new direction for therapeutic exercise. J Manipulative Physiol Ther 23: 115-117.

28. Wallwork SB, et al. (2015) Neural representations and the cortical body matrix: implications for sports medicine and future directions. Br J Sports Med. Dec 2015. doi:10.1136/bjsports-2015-095356.

29. Rio E, et al. (2014) The pain of tendinopathy: physiological or pathophysiological? Sports Med 44: 9-23.

30. Butler DS & Moseley GL (2013) Explain Pain. 2nd Edn. Noigroup Publications: Adelaide.

31. Keefe FJ, Lefebvre JC & Starr KR (1996) From the gate control theory to the neuromatrix: Revolution or evolution? Pain Forum 5: 143-146.

32. Moseley GL & Vlaeyen JW (2015) Beyond nociception: the imprecision hypothesis of chronic pain. Pain, 156: 35-38.

33. Schubert D, et al. (2006) Morphology, electrophysiology and functional input connectivity of pyramidal neurons characterizes a genuine layer va in the primary somatosensory cortex. Cereb Cortex 16: 223-236.

34. Gross CG (2002) Genealogy of the "grandmother cell". Neuroscientist 8: 512-518.

35. Bayer TL, Baer PE & Early C (1991) Situational and psychophysiological factors in psychologically induced pain. Pain 44: 45-50.

36. Acerra NE & Moseley GL (2005) Dysynchiria: watching the mirror image of the unaffected limb elicits pain on the affected side. Neurology 65: 751-753.

37. Hebb DO (1949) The Organization of Behaviour: A Neuropsychological Theory. Wiley: New York.

38. Moseley GL & Hodges PW (2006) Reduced variability of postural strategy prevents normalization of motor changes induced by back pain: a risk factor for chronic trouble? Behav Neurosci 120: 474-476.

39. Moseley GL, Gallace A & Spence C (2012) Bodily illusions in health and disease: physiological and clincial perspectives and the concept of a "cortical body matrix". Neurosci Biobehav Rev 36: 34-46.

40. Damasio AR (1996) The somatic marker hypothesis and the possible functions of the prefrontal cortex. Philos Trans R Soc Lond B Biol Sci 351: 1413-1420.

41. Wolpert DM & Ghahramani Z (2000) Computational principles of movement neuroscience. Nat Neurosci 3: 1212-1217.

42. McIntyre J, et al. (2001) Does the brain model Newton's laws? Nat Neurosci 4: 693-694.

43. Moseley GL & Brugger P (2009) Independence of movement and anatomy persists when amputees learn a physiologically impossible movement of their phantom limb. Proc Natl Acad Sci USA 106: 18798-18802.

44. Botvinick M & Cohen J (1998) Rubber hands 'feel' touch that eyes see. Nature 391: 756.

45. Moseley GM, et al. (2008) Psychologically induced cooling of a specific body part caused by the illusory ownership of an artificial counterpart. Proc Natl Acad Sci USA 105: 13169-13173.

46. Barnsley N, et al. (2011) The rubber hand illusion increases histamine reactivity in the real arm. Curr Biol 21: R945-946.

47. Moseley GL, et al. (2013) Limb-specific autonomic dysfunction in complex regional pain syndrome modulated by wearing prism glasses. Pain 154: 2463-2468.

48. Moseley GL, Gallace A & Iannetti GD (2012) Spatially defined modulation of skin temperature and hand ownership of both hands in patients with unilateral complex regional pain syndrome. Brain 135: 3676-3686.

49. Moseley GL, Gallace A & Spence C (2009) Space-based, but not arm-based, shift in tactile processing in complex regional pain syndrome and its relationship to cooling of the affected limb. Brain 132: 3142-3151.

50. Reid E, et al. (2016) A New Kind of Spatial Inattention Associated With Chronic Limb Pain? Ann Neurol 79: 701-704.

51. Edwards RR, et al. (2008) Association of catastrophizing with interleukin-6 responses to acute pain. Pain 140: 135-144.

52. Madden VJ, et al. (2016) The effect of repeated laser stimuli to ink-marked skin on skin temperature–recommendations for a safe experimental protocol in humans. PeerJ 4:e1577.

53. Lamoth CJ, et al. (2004) Effects of experimentally induced pain and fear of pain on trunk coordination and back muscle activity during walking. Clin Biomech 19: 551-563.

54. Hodges PW, et al. (2003) Experimental muscle pain changes feedforward postural responses of the trunk muscles. Exp Brain Res 151: 262-271.

55. Moseley GL, Nicholas MK & Hodges PW (2004) Pain differs from non-painful attention-demanding or stressful tasks in its effect on postural control patterns of trunk muscles. Exp Brain Res 156: 64-71.

56. Moseley GL & Hodges PW (2005) Are the changes in postural control associated with low back pain caused by pain interference? Clin J Pain 21: 323-329.

57. Moseley GL, Nicholas MK & Hodges PW (2004) Does anticipation of back pain predispose to back trouble? Brain 127: 2339-2347.

58. Moseley GL, et al. (2008) Thinking about movement hurts: the effect of motor imagery on pain and swelling in people with chronic arm pain. Arthritis Rheum 59: 623-631.

59. The Protectometer App (2016) available to download via iTunes.

60. Bellan V, et al. (2016). Where am I? Integrating modern concepts of self-localisation and proprioception with movement performance. J Dance Med Sci: in press.

Notes...

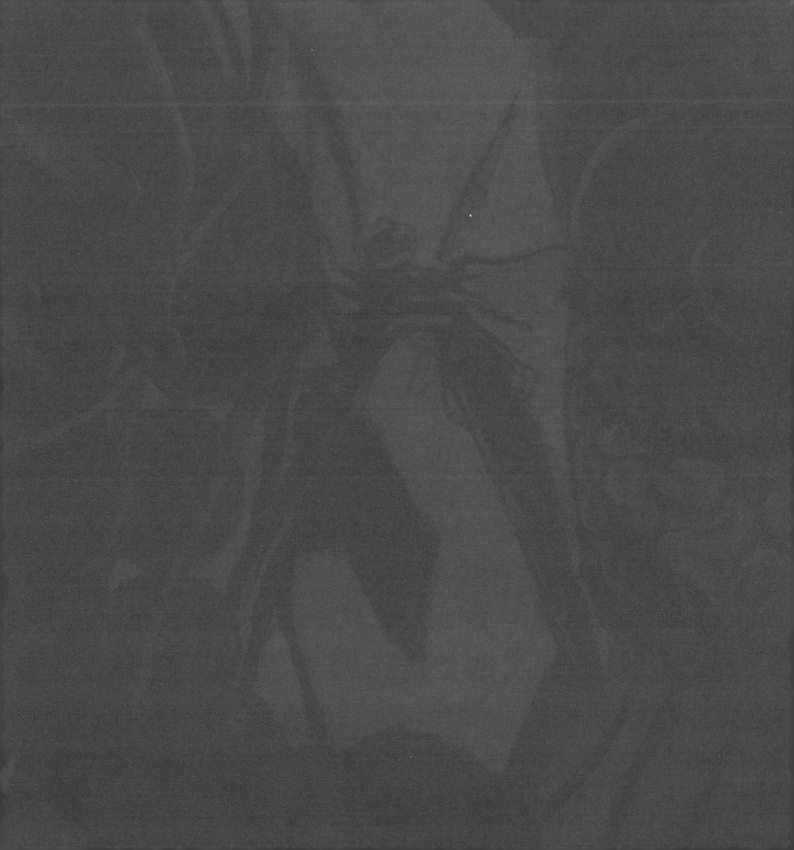

3

Supercharge your pain biology

This chapter contains some pretty hardcore biology and some brand new ways of making sense of it. If you are anything like us, you might have thought *'wouldn't it be nice if we could just stick with what we all think we know and add the new bits like some supernuts in your favourite salad'*. Alas, science doesn't always work like that.

We know that this chapter will be tough going and hard reading for everyone (Dave has read it five times and almost gets it!). Be brave as you take this on and realise that to really integrate this amazing stuff, you will need to put in time and effort.

We suggest that you take your time – read it section by section. Stop and think about the clinical nuggets and the implications that are highlighted along the way.

You might need to read it a few times, write notes in the margins, explain it to yourself and others. That's okay. That's learning.

We remember Mick Thacker's insightful advice to a group of pain clinicians – *'If we are to accept the immense privilege of helping people understand their pain and how they can recover from it, then we are absolutely obliged to know what it is we are talking about and if that requires some serious work, then so be it.'* We agree, Mick.

Part A

Digging deeper into the relationships between damage, nociception and pain

The Grand Poobah Pain Theory, which pertains to *EP Supercharged*, clearly tells us that pain is distinct from nociception and is a feeling that compels us, the sentient being with agency over our body, to protect a body part. Integral to this are the relationships between true danger to the body, nociception, and pain. In *Explain Pain* [1] we introduced the reader to some of the evidence that shows these relationships to be variable and to be progressively more tenuous as pain persists. We urge you to remember too that the biopsychosocial model declares that:

'Pain involves the intricate, variable interaction of biological factors (genetic, biochemical, etc), psychological factors (mood, personality, behaviour etc) and social factors (cultural, familial, socioeconomic, medical etc).' [1]

The unfortunate trivialisation

Patrick Wall, arguably the most influential pain scientist of the modern age, a committed anarchist and proficient trouble maker perhaps because of his remarkable intellect and foresight, often lamented the disconnect between what the biology of pain was saying and what the clinical community was doing. For both of us the abiding memory of Pat was being dragged away from conferences to share numerous beers and talk about 'the real issues'. About 30 years ago, Pat and his PhD student at the time, Steve McMahon (now rightly considered a giant of the field), wrote a paper on the relationship between pain and action potentials in primary nociceptors. It was a very important paper and caused a bit of a storm. To demonstrate its remaining pertinence, let's revisit the first paragraph:

---

1   The second mention of this critical idea!

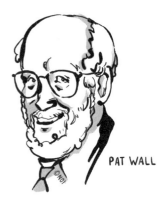

PAT WALL

©NOI

'The word nociceptor is a purely physiological term meaning a nerve fibre that responds to stimuli that damage tissue or would damage tissue if they were prolonged. The word pain is a purely psychological term defined as 'an unpleasant sensory and emotional experience associated with actual or potential tissue damage or described in terms of such damage'. [2]

The pivotal experiments that laid the platform for what was then a new understanding of nociception and pain are now pretty old, but they are more than useful. Here are some of the pivotal discoveries. We suggest you lock these discoveries away and put them somewhere precious inside your memory bank.[2]

1. Recordings from Aδ and C fibres during the application of sharp, hot or cold stimuli clearly show that they become active well in advance of pain. For example, heat-sensitive C fibres become active when the skin reaches about 41°C [3], but data from hundreds of participants in labs around the world, including Team Lorimer's, show that pain thresholds are seldom below 44°C and can be as high as 52°C.
    Clearly the point at which nociceptors are activated does not match the point at which a stimulus triggers pain.

2. If a sharp pin is pushed into the skin the response in nociceptors depends on the temperature of the pin. Nociceptors fire at about once every two seconds (frequency = 0.5Hz) when the pin is at room temperature and about 10 times a second (10Hz) when the pin is hot [4]. However, people can't differentiate between the two stimuli – they are equally painful and are not qualitatively different.
    Clearly the firing rate of nociceptors does not match pain.

3. There is another aspect of the above study [4] that sometimes slides under the radar of the naive reader – in neither scenario does the pin actually penetrate the skin – there is no tissue damage, yet the nociceptor response is highly variable.
    Clearly the amount of damage does not determine the firing rate of nociceptors.

4. A noxious warm stimulus of about 45°C triggers different feelings depending on the size of the stimulus: when the probe is 1mm wide the feeling is usually described as a 'pricking pain'; when it is 4mm wide it is described as a 'stinging pain'; when it is 20mm wide it can be described as 'pleasant strong warmth' [4]. Think about that – the wider the probe, the more nociceptors are activated, yet the less painful the stimulus.
    Clearly the number of nociceptors activated does not match pain.

5. During a 15 second painfully hot or pinching stimulus, primary nociceptors go berserk initially but then rapidly quieten down, sometimes all the way back to silence, even though the stimulus is still in place. In fact, the pain continues to rise after the primary nociceptors start to quieten down [5].
    Clearly the time course of pain does not match the time course of nociceptor firing.

We do not mean to preach against the very important role of nociception in pain, nor the very important role of potential or actual tissue damage in both nociception and pain. However, we do mean to remind you that things are not as simple as they may seem (although read on because in some ways pain really is simple even if its underlying biology is highly complex).

When you really dig into the relationship between injury, nociception and pain, it becomes blatantly obvious that the entire system is all about protection and not about conveying an accurate indication of the state of the tissues. The changes that occur within both the peripheral and central nervous systems when nociception or pain or both persist, mean that protection increases. Such is our fearfully and wonderfully complex biology, the tissues themselves become affected by the very mechanisms that normally subserve protection!

The key point here? ***Pain is all about protection.*** In fact, the purpose of this preamble to a wider section on the biology of pain is to paint a clear picture that, to engage with the biology of pain is to let go of the erroneous notions that pain is a measure of nociception and that nociception is a measure of tissue damage. Even in highly controlled experiments the notion of tissue damage = nociception = pain *does not apply*. You may

---

2   We call this information *declarative knowledge.* You may not need to pass this onto a patient, but it is the foundation of *functional Explain Pain knowledge –* more of this in Chapter 6, but can you see how this fits on the iceberg in Figure 1.1 (page 1).

need convincing of this. However, it is possible that somewhere deep in your belly you think that in the simplest of acute painful experiences, where psychosocial complexities don't intrude and the system is 'true', not yet sensitised or corrupted by cognitive manipulations or systemic modulations, that pain = nociception = tissue damage? If you hold up the mirror and can say honestly, that this is not you, then you are well and truly ahead of the pack. You are completely consistent with the massive amount of research on this, and sadly but understandably you are still in the minority – it sure can be a lonely place!

To come full circle, we have chosen to rely again on the astute commentary of Wall and McMahon [2] which reminds us that this stuff is not new, just not very easily accepted:

'[these are] normal volunteers who are trained and attentive and subject to brief harmless stimuli. If even they cannot sense the painfulness of a stimulus as encoded in a special set of afferents, it is not surprising that the slings and arrows of the real world produce pain by mechanisms that require more factors for their explanation than the firing of a specific type of afferent. At one extreme, 90% of patients with brachial root avulsions suffer severe pain in the absence of afferents let alone impulses in afferents. At the other extreme, 40% of patients admitted to a civil accident hospital suffered no pain at the time of their injury in spite of being fully aware that they were severely injured … [clearly] pain is an integrated package of analysed results related to meaning, significance and imperative action.' [2]

And finally, to bring home the point with some gusto – again from Wall and McMahon from *three decades ago*:

'The labelling of nociceptors as pain fibres was not an admirable simplification but an unfortunate trivialization. The writers of textbooks will continue to purvey trivialization under the guise of simplification. The experimental results show that the final analysis that produces the perception of pain is not monopolized by the peripheral receptor properties of nociceptors. The response of nociceptors is one of the factors incorporated into the central analytic mechanisms that can generate many perceptual syndromes including pain.' [2]

We can honestly say, with hands on our hearts, that we have NOT purveyed trivialisation under the guise of simplification. We know it is complex and we know that people can understand it. Take you for example.

Begin supercharging at the surface – detecting tissue based events

If we are to understand how our brain is alerted to the presence of a potentially damaging situation, we need a basic understanding of the somatosensory system, not just the C fibres and Aδ fibres and their projections. The somatosensory system serves three functions:

1. *Exteroception*: detecting, encoding and transmitting news of external stimuli that we encounter.

2. *Interoception*: detecting, encoding and transmitting news of internal events occurring within the tissues of our body.

3. *Proprioception*: detecting, encoding and transmitting biomechanical data, for example joint angles, muscle stretch, tendon tension, skin stretch.

The first step in any somatosensory perception is usually activation of a primary sensory neurone,[3] which has its cell body in the dorsal root ganglion (or the trigeminal equivalent). Perhaps the most important function of the somatosensory system is to keep us safe – to protect us from danger – so not surprisingly, a significant proportion of the primary somatosensory system contributes to this end. This is one reason we can't really consider only Aδ and C fibres when we are thinking about danger detection. We now know that a range of fibres contribute to the detection and processing of noxious events, which is why we need to think about the whole kit and caboodle.

The vast majority of research in this area has looked at how we detect potentially dangerous events happening to us, not *within* us. That is, the research investigates what happens in the system when danger detectors are triggered by a known stimulus, delivered by a researcher. This contrasts with the vast majority of clinical situations, which are almost always triggered by, or associated with, potentially dangerous events happening *within* us, not *to* us. That is, we don't know exactly what the stimulus is – its magnitude, timing or exact location. Notwithstanding that limitation, let's take a quick tour of what is currently known about the somatosensory system.

---

3 If our brain has any forewarning at all of an impending stimulus, the very first thing that happens is a top-down tuning of the somatosensory pathways most likely to be activated. This tuning can extend at least as far as the spinal neurotag (more on this later) and there are plausible mechanisms by which tuning may extend as far as the primary sensory neurone.

The detectors themselves

Nearly all the tissues of our body are served by a range of sensory neurones, which respond to a *change* in tissue environment. Tissue changes might include, for example mechanical deformation or a slight shift in temperature or a slight change in molecular profile. Such changes are called stimuli when they have been imparted by something else, for example a poke or prod or something hot or cold.

Our tissue environment changes constantly and these changes are sampled by a range of clever and sometimes very specialised *detectors* or *sensors*, often called receptors. We have found that the term detector is more easily understood and Explain Pain friendly. In this book we use the terms interchangeably to suit the moment.

Sensory neurones take messages *towards*[4] the spinal cord, so they are also called 'afferents'. Primary afferents are the first neurones to carry information towards the brain. These 'primary sensory afferents' can be classified in many different ways. If you've had the usual training in this stuff, then you will be most familiar with their categorisation according to either:

* how fat they are and whether or not they are myelinated – this gives a Roman numerals categorisation – Groups I (fattest) to V (thinnest), or

* how fast they conduct their message – this gives them a letter (Type A or C) and a Greek symbol. Aα (alpha) are the fastest and serve proprioceptive functions from the muscle spindle and the Golgi tendon organ; Aβ (beta) are next fastest and serve the deciphering of safe and dangerous[5] mechanical and thermal events; Aδ (delta) are the slowest of the myelinated primary afferents and detect hair follicle deflection and dangerous mechanical events; C are unmyelinated, slow as watching a kettle boil on a winter's morning, and serve safe[5] and dangerous mechanical, thermal and chemical events.

So that's already a bit more than what we covered in *Explain Pain* and is about all most Neurophysiology 101 courses cover. However, it is worth digging a little deeper here because:

* several classes of primary sensory afferents, not just Aδ and C fibres are 'nociceptively competent'.

* the range of nociceptively competent neurones increases in the presence of inflammation or central sensitisation.

* aspects of modern treatments such as tactile discrimination training depend on the different properties of different types of sensory neurones.

* Aδ and C fibres are important in deciphering a range of inputs, not just those that are potentially dangerous.

* it is probably more helpful to think about primary afferents according to their *optimal stimulus* and how quickly they stop responding to repeated stimuli because those things are what determines what triggers them and how long they have an immediate influence and, ultimately, it is all about *influence* (see Chapter 2 pages 23-25).

* the redundancy in the detection system increases in line with the magnitude and rate of change in the tissues. That is, the more dangerous a change in tissue state, the more potential pathways we have to detect it and influence the central nervous system.

Perhaps we've been a bit too Aδ and C fibre-centric in the past…

The optimal stimulus

First up, get your head around this. Many primary sensory afferents can be activated by several sensory modalities but that doesn't mean that we necessarily consider them as 'multimodal'. Instead, primary sensory afferents are labelled in terms of what is known as 'the adequate stimulus' [6] or 'the optimal stimulus' [7]. We prefer optimal stimulus and will refer to it from now on. **A neurone's optimal stimulus is the kind that best activates that neurone.** It is dependent in most cases on the specialised receptors that sit on the neuronal terminal. Importantly, there might be other stimuli that can activate the neurone and the relative sensitivity to different kinds of stimuli can change in accordance with the *state of the neurone* (think here of peripheral sensitisation in which mechanosensitive neurones can become particularly sensitive to increases in temperature).

---

4 Afferent means 'carry towards', from the Latin *affere*. Efferent means 'carry out' from the Latin, *effere*.

5 Yes, you read this correctly. Read on!

Detecting mechanical deformation of the tissues

The vast majority of what we know about detecting mechanical deformation of tissues comes from research using stimuli delivered to the skin (tactile stimuli). Critical here are specialised receptors that wrap around the base of hairs and different but equally specialised receptors that sit in the skin itself. Tactile function is not only about detecting *external* stimuli. Much of what we do deforms the skin somewhere – think for example of some skin being squashed a little and other skin stretched a little whenever we move.

Touch-based therapies are commonly used to treat people in pain. It is therefore helpful to understand the basics of how we detect mechanical deformation. Here are what we think are the essential basics:

Sensory Scenario 1: Passive spinal mobilisation by a manual therapist

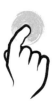

Picture in your mind's eye, skin being deformed under a therapist's finger. This indents the skin – the boundaries are gentle, not sharp – as long as the therapist keeps her nails short! The pressure also stretches the skin a little and if the thumb remains in place for long enough the temperature underneath the therapist's thumb increases. Let's presume the force being applied is quite small, just enough to blanch the skin a little.

The deformation pulls on collagen fibres that are attached to detectors, activating those detectors and making the neurone that innervates them just a little more excited. These particular detectors are called Ruffini corpuscles, named after the Italian chap who first described them [8].

Ruffini corpuscles are cylindrical stretch receptors [9] rather like Golgi tendon organs. Each Ruffini corpuscle is innervated by a single Aβ slowly adapting neurone (see Figure 3.1 response properties). The receptive field[6] of a single Ruffini corpuscle is in the order of 15mm diameter in the hand and probably over 50mm in the back, where receptive fields of single Ruffini corpuscles can extend across several dermatomes.

---

6 Receptive field refers to the volume of body tissue served by a particular neurone or neuronal structure.

This slow adapting Aβ neurone gives off two branches – one has numerous targets over several centimetres of the dorsal horn. The other skips the dorsal horn and heads straight to the brain. The slow adapting Aβ neurones that are activated by Ruffini corpuscles are probably the main driver of competitive anti-nociception effects (ie. you rub the sore spot) at the dorsal horn – effects that inspired the gate control theory [10] and remain very relevant to our new understanding of nociceptive processing in the spinal cord.

Think of the implications of this for understanding manual therapy and pain. If we are indeed contributing to analgesia because Ruffini corpuscles trigger anti-nociception effects at the spinal cord, then we must concede that precise placement of our hands and direction of our forces is not an important requirement for analgesia. The *functional* receptive field, taking into consideration both the receptive field size of a single Ruffini and the divergence of the Aβ neurone in the spinal cord may well cover one side of the entire low back. We can also conclude that other 'manual therapy' techniques applied somewhere in that broad area could also induce analgesia via the same anti-nociceptive mechanism. There is a critical caveat here, however: that manual therapy induces analgesia does not mean this anti-nociceptive mechanism is the only one at play, nor indeed the most important. On appraisal of the available scientific evidence, we would expect powerful safety cues (think here your clean room and your dethreatening explanation) that are delivered alongside the manual therapy are likely to be more potent analgesic triggers.

Sensory Scenario 2: Tactile discrimination training using location and object discrimination

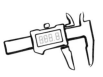

The array of specialised receptors that reside in our skin gives us a remarkable ability to decipher different kinds of mechanical stimuli [7]. You may recognise the names of most of them – you've already met Ruffini, but there's also Meissner, Merkel, and Pacinian. These receptors sit on the ends of low threshold neurones, so they are sensitive but they do not respond any differently to dangerously large deformations, which is why they are not considered nociceptive. Some receptors respond to an indentation; some respond to a moving stimulus by triggering a barrage of messages at both the application and release of the stimulus.

Some adapt very quickly – they stop firing immediately after the stimulus is applied even though it may still be in place – and others adapt slowly – they remain active even after the stimulus has been removed (see response properties in Figure 3.1).

This biology becomes very relevant for people with persistent pain – for example those for whom sustained mechanical stimuli are more painful than transient stimuli; those for whom slow moving stimuli are more painful than stationary stimuli; or those for whom their tactile detection threshold is normal but their two point discrimination threshold is abnormal.

To gain a better understanding of what happens during tactile discrimination training, or indeed when we do anything that requires high level processing of tactile input, it will help to first understand the basics of these mechanical detectors, what activates them and what effect they have on primary sensory neurones. Here is the bare minimum of info:

Merkel cells are important in detecting static tactile stimuli. They were named by the German fellow who first described one – although Herr Merkel knew nothing of what it did [11]. The ratio of Merkel cells to sensory neurones matches very closely the tactile precision of the area. In the back, for example, one neurone might innervate 15 Merkel cells; whereas in the lip or fingertip, several neurones might innervate one Merkel cell (1:15 in the back – low precision – and 5:1 in the lip – very high precision). Having one Merkel cell innervated by several neurones means we have tactile precision that is not limited by the receptive field of individual neurones [12]. This in itself reminds us of what Bob Coghill, Professor and Chair of Pain Research at Cincinnati Children's Hospital describes as *'massive computational capacity of the spinal cord'*. Think how remarkable this really is – it's all about *timing*. A single stimulus activates several Merkel cells each innervated by several neurones and because the message from each arrives at slightly different times, the spinal cord is able to precisely locate the stimulus – außergewöhnlich Herr Merkel!

Meissner corpuscles[7] respond primarily to low frequency vibrations [13] – the initial indentation of the corpuscle causes a transient barrage of action potentials and the release of the

indentation does the same. Progression of this double barrage of action potentials across adjacent receptive fields is how we detect a moving stimulus. The receptive fields are larger than those for the Merkel cells – up to 80 Meissner corpuscles can be innervated by a single sensory neurone [14].

Pacinian corpuscles respond to high frequency vibrations and are exquisitely sensitive to small amplitudes (how small? nanometers! [15]). For our purposes, they don't seem as interesting as Meissner corpuscles, but they are no less remarkable. In fact, the unique response properties of the Pacinian corpuscles allow us to discriminate vibration information almost as well as our auditory system can discriminate sound waves [16] – now that is truly impressive! Fun fact: Pacinian corpuscles are present in peripheral nerve sheaths [17]. Could this be part of an extra layer of protection for our precious nerves?

Are you keeping up? If not, read back over those paragraphs and we'll let you draw some pictures in the margin of your book… go on – you know you want to.

Now, back to tactile discrimination training. The astounding computational capacity of the spinal cord is matched and indeed upped by that of the brain. When a patient presents with tactile problems it may be helpful to determine whether they involve static or moving stimuli, or both. So, a patient may perform normally on tests of tactile detection but not on two-point discrimination; a patient may perform well on two point discrimination of sharp edged stimuli, which would be detected mainly by Merkel cells, but not on two point discrimination of moving stimuli, which would be detected mainly by Meissner corpuscles.

Intuitively, these two presentations would imply distinct tactile training, but this implication has not, to our knowledge, been tested. We can, however, use this powerful biology to engage the patient in conceptual change (Nugget 11 *The orchestra in the tissues*).

---

7   Here is some physiology trivia for you: Meissner was a PhD student under the supervision of a guy called Wagner. Meissner came across a new kind of receptor. Prof Wagner, so excited by this discovery, suggested to Meissner that it might be best if *Wagner himself* led this paper to give it the impact it deserved. He humbly referred to the new receptor as 'Wagner's Corpuscle'. Meanwhile, Meissner's PhD thesis had been snail mailed to the key scientists in the field. On reading the thesis, the scientists realised that Wagner had been rather opportunistic. They condemned his poor form and officially renamed the discovery 'Meissner's Corpuscle'. A fifty year disagreement ensued until Wagner's retirement when, presumably fatigued and resigned to his student's relative notoriety, he too conceded credit to Meissner. Some things never change…

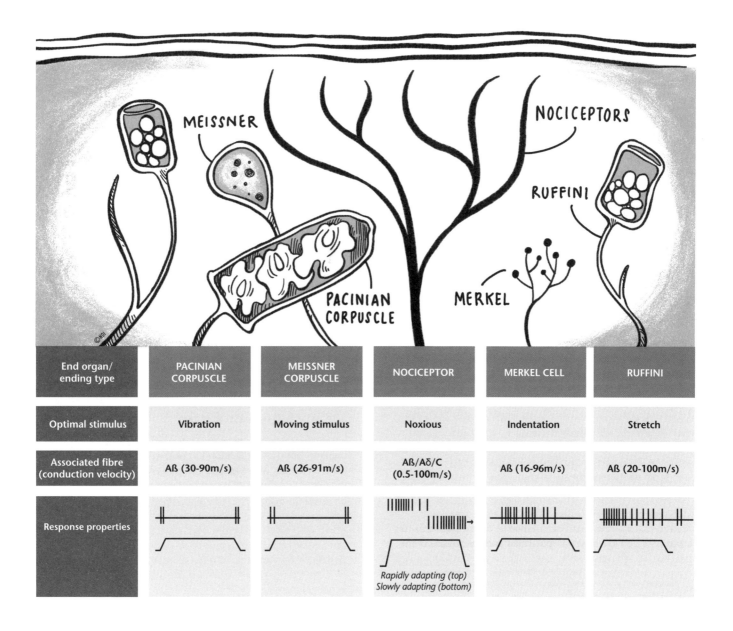

End organ/ ending type	PACINIAN CORPUSCLE	MEISSNER CORPUSCLE	NOCICEPTOR	MERKEL CELL	RUFFINI
Optimal stimulus	Vibration	Moving stimulus	Noxious	Indentation	Stretch
Associated fibre (conduction velocity)	Aß (30-90m/s)	Aß (26-91m/s)	Aß/Aδ/C (0.5-100m/s)	Aß (16-96m/s)	Aß (20-100m/s)
Response properties			*Rapidly adapting (top) Slowly adapting (bottom)*		

Figure 3.1 *The properties of different types of sensory neurones in the skin, adapted from [7]*

Sensory Scenario 3: Gentle caresses

Mammals standout from the wider animal crowd by our rather liberal covering of hair – even though we have toned it down a bit over the evolutionary generations, the vast majority of our skin has hair on it (more for some than others!). Hairy skin is critical for protection, body temperature regulation, and also for detecting, transforming and transmitting external stimuli. As we comb deeper into hairy skin, it becomes more and more obvious that our conventional ideas about Aδ and C fibres, nociception and pain are overly simplistic.

Let's return to a couple of fundamentals. The critical connectors between the external stimulus and the detectors in hairy skin are the hair follicles. There are three kinds of hair follicles, each with a different detector mix. All the detectors respond to movement of the hair follicle they are hugging. There is a vast amount of literature on the detectors that hug hair follicles, their massive morphological and molecular diversity, and their interconnections. It is sufficiently remarkable for those in the know to now see hairy skin as a highly specialised sensory and thermoregulatory organ [7].

Think twice before you pay the waxing price!
Hairy skin offers thermoregulatory function and tactile performance simply not obtainable in glabrous skin. Remove the hair – reduce these functions. It is not unreasonable to suggest that the less hairy skin you have, the less capacity you have for potentially powerful C fibre mediated sensual touch SIMs!
PS – From our editor: all those hairless body beautifuls should really know this – that in fact they are *reducing* their sensual capacity by making themselves look sleek and hairless, which they think makes them look sexier!

Almost all the information now available, as fascinating as it is (and it really is!), is way beyond what you will need when dealing with all but the very unusual pain presentation. If you are particularly turned on by incredible biology and haven't contemplated hairy skin before now, or if you are just a very keen bean, here are a few key studies to suss out [18-22]. For the rest of you, here are the most relevant bits.

The optimal stimulus of most of these detectors is some sort of movement of the hair on which they sit. However, they are also highly responsive to rapid cooling of the skin and completely unresponsive to rapid heating of the skin [20].

Test the claim that hairy skin is a sensory organ of remarkable precision. Try this little experiment:
Find a partner (or a hobbit) with a hairy hand. With their eyes closed, use the blunt end of a pin to gently flick one hair and then a neighbouring hair – make sure you only disturb one hair at a time. Ask him whether you flicked the same hair twice or two different hairs. Now turn his hand over and use the pin to touch two points of skin the same distance apart as the two hairs were. Ask him to tell you if you touched the same point or a different one. If you're really careful with this experiment, you will see that our sense of touch is more precise on hairy skin than it is on non-hairy skin. This is important when it comes to clinical presentations where sensory acuity is lost for non-hairy skin but maintained for hairy skin in the same body region, or vice versa. Such a presentation is more consistent with problems at a tissue level than problems in the central nervous system.

Hair follicles are innervated by fast conducting Aβ neurones and slower C neurones. This reminds us that C fibres are not necessarily nociceptors. Indeed, the optimal stimulus for these C fibre receptors is a mechanical stimulus that moves across receptive fields – from hair to adjacent hair. These C fibres have a reputation as the generators of 'emotional touch' or 'sensual touch' [23] and are often called 'caress receptors' [7] – so we're going to cleverly refer to them as C(aress) fibres. There is some evidence that C(aress) fibres have less direct projections to sensory brain areas and more direct connections to brain areas traditionally associated with affective processing (such as the insular cortex). This implies that these fibres don't help much with *locating* the stimulus but are still very informative as to what *kind* of stimulus it is. In the very small number of people who by genetic lottery are lacking A fibres, activation of these C(aress) fibres evokes a pleasant feeling that is very vaguely located.

It looks like there might be a catch to the C(aress) fibres, however. Although it is not settled just yet, there is a building argument that they stop their lovey-doveyness after local injury and instead contribute to localised mechanical hypersensitivity, or tactile allodynia [24, 25].

The implications of C(aress) fibres

The characteristics of these fibres have clear implications for our interpretation of brush-evoked tactile allodynia, something we attribute to central sensitisation (Version 1) and the consequent triggering of spinal nociceptors by Aβ input. This observation is considered by many as diagnostic of neuropathic pain. That C(aress) fibres become more conventional nociceptors in the presence of injury reminds us to consider the entire sensory and clinical picture when contemplating the mechanisms underpinning someone's pain. Put simply: don't conclude central sensitisation caused by peripheral nerve damage on the basis of brush-evoked tactile allodynia alone.

The so what? factor

Aδ and C fibres play such important non-nociceptive roles in hairy skin that we want to reiterate this: Aδ and C fibres are not solely concerned with the detection and transmission of dangerous or potentially dangerous events. Therefore, the idea that they are 'primary nociceptors' needs to change. It is more reasonable to conceptualise nociceptors as neurones for which the *optimal stimulus* is a noxious one. In this way, nociceptors become true to their name – 'noxious (stimulus) receptors' – and they no longer confine themselves to thin, myelinated or thinly myelinated neurones. This is also relevant to the nociceptive function of Aβ neurones, but that is jumping the gun – read on!

A new look at primary nociception

The previous section focused on touch because (i) there is a large body of research on touch from which we extrapolate other stuff – a process with obvious problems but also one with clear relevance to understanding the detectors that 'feed' the cortical body matrix, and (ii) there are clear implications for our assessment and treatment of people in pain. So let's continue the theme and start digging deeper into nociception via the skin.

First things first – Aδ and C fibres

 The most studied and most prevalent nociceptors are the free nerve endings of Aδ and C fibres, but as we have just said, not all Aδ and C fibres are nociceptors. Moreover, and probably more significantly, not all nociceptors are Aδ and C fibres. 'Free nerve endings' mean that the neurones do not innervate specialised receptors such as those discovered by Meissner, Merkel, Golgi and the like (Figure 3.1).

Nociceptive Aδ and C fibres are mostly high threshold mechanoreceptors. The optimal stimulus of these nociceptors is a high intensity mechanical stimulus. Tug on a nasal hair and you've got a few going! There are two types – those that also respond to noxious heat and those that also respond to noxious cold. These are called bimodal heat/mechanoreceptor or bimodal cold/mechanoreceptor nociceptors and most of these bimodal nociceptors are Aδ free nerve endings.

C fibre high threshold mechanoreceptors are more specific. They do not respond to thermal stimuli (hot or cold) when they are in their normal state, but things change drastically in the presence of inflammation – more on that later.

There are pros and cons of having 'free nerve endings' instead of 'specialised detectors'. Pros include a distinct advantage when it comes to detecting and responding to danger – the neurone itself is capable of generating action potentials rather than relying on a specialised detector at its terminal, such that the stimulus detection zone extends proximally. This characteristic is also considered a con because it cannot provide clear information about the location of the stimulus. This is one reason given for pain felt distally when the nociceptor is being triggered proximally (some referred pains). However, there are better explanations for that sort of thing. Think about this – that nociceptors are necessarily imprecise encoders of spatial location implies they are probably never the main providers of spatial data concerning a stimulus. This is demonstrated in the laboratory by occluding blood supply at the thigh, wait for the touch function to be lost (this means the wide diameter Aβ neurones are no longer working) and then place an ice cube on the knee. It will hurt, but the pain will be vague and poorly located because the only functioning neurones are the C fibres and they can't encode where its happening. Professor Allan Basbaum demonstrates this phenomenon in a lovely YouTube video clip... Google it.

So, how do we normally know with such precision where a dangerous event is occurring? Well, it turns out that we rely on the vast array of peripheral receptors that accurately and precisely encode location even if they do not encode danger. Referred pain then seems more likely to reflect problems with spatial encoding in non-nociceptive processing than in nociceptive processing itself.

Notions of first pain and second pain have historically been attributed to activation of Aδ and C neurones respectively. This attribution was based on two apparently aligned discoveries:

1. that Aδ and C neurones respond to noxious stimuli and have different conduction velocities, and

2. when we deliver a highly controlled noxious stimulus to a reasonably naïve volunteer, they report an initial sharp prick (the first pain) and then a subsequent deeper, vaguer burning pain (the second pain).

There are problems with this explanation. For example, the extensive processing of all nociceptive inputs at the dorsal horn and the discrepancy between the delay between first and second pain and the hypothesised delay between Aδ and C neurone impulses arriving at the dorsal horn. The explanation that is winning friends in the pain science community is that Aβ nociceptors and non-nociceptive neurones are more important than Aδ neurones in triggering the first pain. The neuroimaging data that are available are more consistent with this explanation [28].

In short: it is, as ever, not as simple as it may have once seemed!

Now for something really new – Aβ

Aβ high threshold mechanoreceptors – the surprise packet. We tend to associate Aβ neurones with everything lovely – touch, warmth, vibration and proprioception – we don't ever think of them as being involved in nociception. However, when Aβ neurones don't supply a specialised detector, they too are free nerve endings and they respond to mechanical stimuli including those in the noxious range. Are you realising that it's time to let go of some of your previous Aβ preconceptions? Some of them also respond to noxious heat [26] and are likely to be critical in the short loop withdrawal reflex that occurs during the infamous 'hand on the stove' example. Perhaps the most remarkable thing about Aβ nociceptors is that scientists have actually known about this for half a century, yet Aβ nociceptors rarely find their way into textbooks on neurophysiology, nociception and pain [27]. Some of these Aβ nociceptors are 'wide dynamic range' primary nociceptors because they respond to stimuli over a range of intensities.

Just so you know – classifying nociceptors

Nociceptors can be classified in ways other than by their conduction speed. One way is by trophic factors – the molecules that keep them alive and communicate with their neighbouring cells. Trophic refers simply to 'feeding and nutrition', but for the more melodramatic neurophysiologists, it means 'survival'. You might have heard of some of them such as the famous nerve growth factor (NGF). We don't think it's important to know what they are all called and what differentiates the nociceptors that depend on NGF from those that depend on, for example, TrkA, because it has no obvious clinical relevance that we can see *and* because the nice and neat differentiations go out the window in the presence of inflammation and sensitisation anyway [29, 30]. As far as applying this to the real world, adding a section on categorising nociceptors according to their trophic factors would waste your time and ours.

We ummed and aahhed about sticking that paragraph in – but if you dig deeper into the scientific literature (for example, you'll come across terms such as 'purinergic' – see even the word makes you feel sick) that categorisation is assumed knowledge. Indeed, most scientific books about sensory neurophysiology will start with an account of trophic categorisations and we don't want people thinking we are naïve to that information – we just think that most of those accounts are as turgid, foetid and dense as they are probably accurate.

So that's the end of trophic classifications of nociceptors from us. Amen!

Building the bottom of the iceberg – what makes primary nociceptors fire?

Let's recap – we have established that primary nociceptors can be Aβ, Aδ or C fibres; we have established that all this really means is that they can be very fast conducting, not very fast conducting or slow conducting; we have established that most of what we know about primary nociceptors is based on those that innervate the skin; we have identified specialised touch and other receptors that have no known nociceptive function and can also be innervated by Aβ, Aδ or C fibres. All of this tells us that we need to let go of the idea that all primary nociceptors are slow conducting and all small diameter fibres are nociceptive.

Now it's time to understand how these primary nociceptors work and explore their interaction with injury and inflammation.

The mystery of the ion channel

Although we often take it for granted, it is no small miracle that stimuli can be detected in the first place. How lucky we are to have this nociceptive capacity almost everywhere – we're so well protected. Of course, different tissues of the body have different degrees of nociceptive competence, ready to detect trouble – Figure 3.2 provides a rough guide.

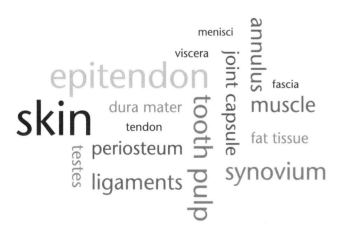

Figure 3.2 Nociceptive competence of different body tissues. The larger the type, the higher the nociceptive density.

The specialised detectors that sit on the end of Aβ neurones have been well studied and they make for lovely drawings (take Figure 3.1 for example). However, nociceptors have been a relative mystery because they do not have such detectors. How then are they triggered into action? As it happens, it all comes down to ion channels – fancy pants proteins that sit in the cell wall.

Most neuroscience discoveries have tended to be named for and by their discoverer (Merkel, Meissner, Golgi and Luschka hang your heads in embarrassment). There are exceptions to this rule and the ion channels that stand between us and potentially lethal naivety to tissue danger are fine examples. These are named instead according to what they do, or what they let through the channel, or the order in which they were discovered. For example, the $Na_v1.7$, lets sodium (atomic symbol 'Na') into the nociceptor, is activated by a change in voltage ('v') across the membrane and is the seventh such channel to be discovered.

Thermal and chemical sensitive ion channels

Several ion channels have been identified within nociceptors, but our favourites are the TRPs – 'transient receptor potential' ion channels. TRPs respond to stimuli by opening their doors to sodium (Na^+) or calcium (Ca^{2+}) ions, which rush into the neurone, rapidly depolarising it – changing the voltage so that the inside becomes less negatively charged than the outside. In nociceptors, such a depolarisation is usually not sufficient to trigger an action potential – that job is done by voltage-gated channels, most famously the $Na_v1.7$. More of that later.

 As mentioned above, the scientists discovering these ion channels called the first one they discovered 'TRPV1'[8] and the subsequent discoveries followed suit – TRPV2, 3, 4, 5 etc. The TRPV1 ion channel is now thought to be critical in detecting fluctuations in tissue temperature – more specifically *increases* in temperature. TRPV1 is not simply about nociception, which is one reason drugs that have been developed to block it have hit problems with body temperature regulation. That is, TRPV1 is thought to be tonically active in the viscera and perhaps elsewhere and is now more often considered a 'body temperature maintainer' – triggering messages that themselves trigger bodily cooling.

The TRPV1 is also activated by acidic conditions and is thought to be the danger detector most sensitive to acid build up in

---

8   The 'V' refers to 'vanilloid', which is a class of proteins that contain a special bit called vanillyl.

the tissues (think lactic acid here and think of the potential value of flushing out your tissues with a bit of movement – see Nugget 63 *Motion is lotion*). But the role of TRPV1 doesn't stop there – it is, as it turns out, a rather promiscuous customer: in the periphery, TRPV1 is activated by metabolites (by-products) of some polyunsaturated fatty acids, which themselves have been linked to exaggerated responses to noxious stimuli in rats [31]. And here is an unexpected one that might make the prescribers stop and think – TRPV1 is activated by a by-product of paracetamol (or acetaminophen for our North American readers) [32].

The TRPV class of ion channels might be the most famous, but there are other TRPs that are also important for detecting dangerous events in our body. The next cab off the rank is the TRPM class of ion channels. The M stands for 'melastatin' but we reckon it is easier to understand if you make it stand for Menthol. These ion channels (so far there are eight that we know about: TRPM1 – 8) are activated by menthol; they are mainly found on nociceptors that are activated by temperatures below 25°C, and are most obviously associated with that cold feeling you get in your mouth when you suck on a peppermint. However, TRPMs are not just on nociceptors – for example TRPM5 channels on the tongue are thought to be important in taste.

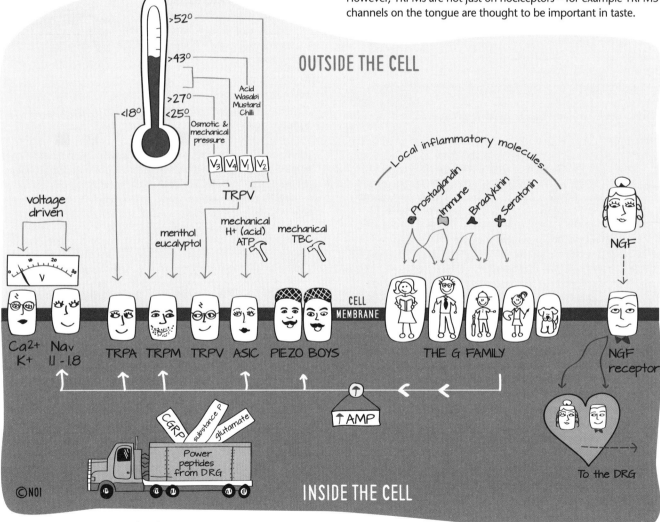

Figure 3.3 Basic components of nociceptors

Then come the TRPA class, which are more sensitive to colder temperatures than the TRPM class (<15°C); they are spice lovers – mustard, cinnamon, wasabi, and both menthol and icilin (a synthetic uber menthol) all activate TRPA ion channels. They are also activated by nicotine and formalin, possibly causing the skin itch that some people report with nicotine patches [33]. They might be suppressed by caffeine [34] and they are thought to have an anti-nociceptive response to paracetamol, possibly explaining in part paracetamol's analgesic effect [35]. But here is the tricky thing about the TRPA class – they are more associated with a burning sensation than a cold type pain and they may be, at least during temperatures between 0°C and 15°C, a bit redundant – mice that don't have TRPA receptors (thanks to some scientists messing with their genes) have completely normal nociceptive responses until the temperature sinks below zero [36]. Finally, TRPA receptors are also thought to be involved in some way in mechanically induced nociceptive responses, but this is where it all gets a bit murky and the scientists are dragging the chain!

Mechanically sensitive ion channels

The transduction of mechanical noxious stimuli into nociceptor activity is not anywhere near as well understood as the transduction of thermal and chemical stimuli is. This is a bummer for those of us in the pain rehabilitation space because the vast majority of our clinical presentations at least *seem* to be associated with mechanical stimuli (although perhaps we are underestimating the role of inflammation-mediated nociception here). There was some excitement, however, when scientists discovered particular kinds of Acid Sensing Ion Channels (ASICs) on mechanosensitive nociceptors in drosophila flies.

These flies have been studied to bits (both literally and metaphorically) in laboratories all over the world – not because they are particularly complex or critical for the survival of our ecosystem, but because they are one of the most stupid animals with a nervous system that is still a bit like ours. Once something is settled in these flies, scientists usually take it the next step to mice or frogs and then eventually to humans. This process can be called the 'Fly2Human translation'. In this particular instance, the Fly2Human translation of mechanosensitive nociceptors progressed as far as rats – but the rats bred without ASICs seemed pretty much normal in their responses to mechanical noxious stimuli. Back to the drawing board…

The Fly2Human translation has begun again with the discovery of the 'Piezo Boys'[9] – receptors that have been isolated in the drosophila flies and seem to only respond to noxious mechanical stimuli. The scientists have now engineered drosophila flies without the Piezo Boys. Last we heard, there was some excitement because the flies that were engineered without the Piezo Boys had completely normal responses to thermal and chemical stimuli and to non-noxious mechanical stimuli, *but* they were not responsive to noxious mechanical stimuli. Not surprisingly, the scientists working on the Piezo Boys are excited that the Fly2Human translation will yield something worthwhile – hopefully an important discovery about human mechanical nociception. Only time will tell.

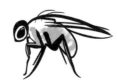

The more you learn about primary nociceptor function and properties, the more complexities arise. For example, some nociceptors are thought to be triggered not by depolarisation but by hyper-polarisation. That is, whereas most nociceptors are activated by opening Na^+ and Ca^{2+} channels, some seem to be activated by closing K^+ channels. This has profound implications for the design of molecules that aim to modulate nociceptor activity. By binding with different ion channels or manipulating different biological cascades, what turns one nociceptor down may well turn another one up.[10]

The mighty $Na_v1.7$ and $Na_v1.8$

Sodium channels are either voltage-gated or ligand-gated. This means that they are either driven by changes in voltage (the difference in charge across the membrane) or by particular molecules called ligands (like acetylcholine). We introduced $Na_v1.7$ earlier. $Na_v1.7$ are found on many nociceptors, which is why they are a target for drug development. The challenge facing the drug developers however, is finding a molecule that blocks $Na_v1.7$ but does not block $Na_v1.4$, found in muscle (clearly blocking these would be a problem!) or $Na_v1.6$ found in smooth muscle (blocking these would also be a problem!) or anything else. Such a molecule would be

---

9   They are not really boys. We just couldn't resist how much *Piezo* seems to fit with *Boys*. Good name for a pizza delivery service.

10   Another reminder that our biology has a huge number of checks and balances and different mechanisms by which our bodies are protected – known as redundancy.

called a 'selective Na$_v$1.7 blocker'. Professor Glenn King and his buddies at the University of Queensland's Institute of Molecular Biosciences are looking for such molecules in venomous animals – spiders, snakes and sea snails. They have had some success, for example finding a Na$_v$1.1 blocker in the poison of a West African Tarantula that is so big it is described as 'the ornamental baboon'! But Na$_v$1.7 is seen as the holy grail because it is critical to propagation of danger messages in nociceptors. We are presently aware of a potentially exciting and reasonably selective Na$_v$1.7 blocker that has been discovered in the poison of a sea snail. The decade long Rat2Human translation now begins, so we hope that in the second edition of this book we can report that a safe selective Na$_v$1.7 blocker has been tested in clinical trials and provides significant analgesia in acute pain with no side effects. Time will tell...

The critical role of Na$_v$1.7 has been demonstrated in animals that are bred to not have Na$_v$1.7, and in people with a mutation of the genes that express Na$_v$1.7. Animals that don't have Na$_v$1.7 show reduced responses to noxious mechanical stimuli and inflammatory chemicals. People who don't have Na$_v$1.7 because of genetic mutation present in three different ways, and this difference reinforces the incredible complexity of our nociceptive system. Some people develop spontaneous attacks of burning pain in their feet and hands, warm and red skin – a condition called erythromelalgia (or 'redness and pain'). Other people develop severe sensitivity to noxious stimuli of all types and other people still (well three Pakistani families at least) develop marked insensitivity to noxious stimuli such that they have almost no sensible protective function.

Another Na$_v$ – Na$_v$1.8 – is also expressed in the primary nociceptor, particularly in the dorsal root ganglion where it plays an important role in the development of hyperalgesia due to peripheral sensitisation. It is also thought to be critical for the unique capacity of nociceptors to remain responsive to noxious stimuli at very cold temperatures – when the other receptors are rendered useless, the Na$_v$1.8 keeps on keeping on.

Inflammation sensitive receptors and peripheral sensitisation

Inflammation

First up, let's be clear on the difference between a systemic inflammatory response and a local one. A *systemic response* involves a shift in the ongoing balance between pro-inflammatory and anti-inflammatory molecules. We can talk about a shift in one direction putting our body into a pro-inflammatory 'state'; we can

talk about anything that has a pro-inflammatory effect as exerting a pro-inflammatory 'load'.

For now, we are focusing on primary nociceptors, so we will focus on the *local inflammatory response*. Nociceptors are reactive to the molecules released by damaged tissue and inflammatory mediators causing an increase in sensitivity to other stimuli. This is called peripheral sensitisation. As we learn more about the complex and tight interactions between neurones and immune cells, the term 'inflammatory mediator' is becoming more and more ambiguous because in effect, it means 'something that releases molecules that cause inflammation' and we are realising that a vast number and array of human cells can do this. We call these cells 'immunocompetent' and muscle, blood vessel, tendon, meninges, synovium and blood cells have all now been shown to be immunocompetent, at least to some extent.

When tissue is injured the first immunological response is the release of molecules that are pro-inflammatory. Usually the first cabs off the rank are TNFα and interleukin 1 (IL-1). They don't last long in the midst of the battle – the half life of TNFα is about 20 minutes and IL-1 is a measly 6 minutes [37]. In that time however, they can have a pretty major impact – they trigger nearby cells to release other pro-inflammatory cytokines [38], most notably IL-6 and IL-8. IL-6 can be detected in the bloodstream within an hour of significant tissue trauma and is considered an important biomarker of the immune response to damage [39].

It is not all pro pro pro, however, TNFα and IL-1 also trigger the start of an *anti-inflammatory* response, the most significant molecule of which is IL-10 [40], but there are others. IL-6 also triggers the production of soluble TNFα receptors (like absorbent paper mopping up excess TNFα) [41] and IL-1 receptor antagonists – reducing the pro-inflammatory effect of IL-1 within hours of its release [42].

Complicated huh? Table 3.1 provides a brief summary of the main players but remember, it is nowhere near this simple and the redundancy in the system is profound. To reiterate, we have drawn the line at this level of complexity because it provides a good balance between needing to know enough to handle all but the most tricky of questions, but not digging so deep as to get stuck in the content mud.

The effect of local inflammation on nociceptors

A couple of inflammatory mediators can directly activate ion channels – ATP and protons are the most obvious ones. To be harsh, ATP and protons, which clearly activate ASICs, are hardly heavy hitters in the inflammation space and are also by-products of normal everyday activity. To be fair, they have their role, but we find more interesting the mechanisms that relate to the famous inflammatory mediators, such as bradykinin, prostaglandin, nitrous oxide and serotonin. Unlike ATP and protons, these mediators don't directly activate ion channels, but this doesn't mean that they don't pack a punch. Far from it – these mediators are seriously big punch packers and they do it via specialised immune receptors that sit in the nociceptor's cell wall.

There are two broad types of immune receptor that sit in the wall of nociceptors – the G protein coupled receptors, which we like to call 'The G Family', and the mediator-specific receptors, tailor made[11] for one mediator only.

The G Family of inflammation receptors

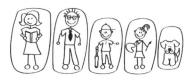

Different members of the G Family receptors work in different ways. For example, they might change the level of AMP[12] within the neurone. All you need to know here about AMP is that it changes the sensitivity of all the other ion channels on the nociceptor – it amps it up! (see Figure 3.3). One G receptor stimulates an enzyme that changes AMP level and another G receptor inhibits that same enzyme. Other members of the G family are activated by, let's say, prostaglandin, and ramp up local sensitivity by 'exciting' the internal operations of the nociceptor. Still other members of the G Family can change the internal environment of the nociceptor through specific effects on the TRPV1 channels, ASICs and even the Piezo Boys. (Nugget 20 *Security guards on Red Bull*)

---

11 We intentionally removed any reference in this book to our biology having been 'designed' because neither of us think it was. This would imply also that things can't be 'tailor-made', but we don't mean someone made it, especially not a tailor. We just mean they are uber-selective for specific molecules.

12 We have drawn a line at naming the enzymes and spelling out the acronyms such as AMP (pronounced ayempee) because we know that adding the full terms takes up brain space with minimal benefit. If you want to drill down further than this, you'll have to go to the primary literature. Be brave – it is not for the faint hearted.

Molecule	Trigger	Effect
IL-1(β)	Macrophage/tissue trauma (6 minute half-life)	Pro-inflammatory, sensitise nociceptors via mediator-specific channels and G family, triggers IL-6 and IL-8 release
TNF-α	Tissue trauma	Induces secretion of IL-6 and 8
IL-4	Tissue trauma	Anti-inflammatory
IL-6	IL-1β TNF-α (20 minute half-life)	Pro-inflammatory – sensitise nociceptors via G family, trigger a systemic response via extensive neural and glial receptors in CNS, induce fever, change mood. Anti-inflammatory – IL-1 receptor antagonist, TNF-α mop-up
IL-8	IL-1 (β)	Pro-inflammatory – attracts monocytes, fibroblasts. Prolongs half-life of leukocytes
IL-10	Prostoglandin	Anti-inflammatory
IFN-γ	Tissue trauma	Pro-inflammatory

Table 3.1 Triggers and effects of inflammatory mediators, adapted from [43]

The G family is one large and connected family! Their potential impact on nociceptive functioning in response to a wide range of inflammatory mediators is potent. An important take home message here is that the G Family don't directly influence the flow of Na⁺, Ca²⁺, K⁺ into the nociceptor, but they change the sensitivity and efficiency of the ion channels that do.

Mediator-specific inflammation receptors

 There are several inflammatory mediators that are actually important for the survival of neurones. We mentioned them in passing when we justified not spending lots of time on categorisation of nociceptors according to their trophic factors. These inflammatory mediators have two ways to change activity of nociceptors: (i) they can cause a very rapid internal cascade similar in method to that used by the G Family but using different molecules or, (ii) they can cause a rather slow process by which the mediator (let's say NGF) and the receptor join together in their very own protective capsule and slowly make their way up the nociceptor to the cell body, which is in the dorsal root ganglion (DRG). Once they arrive, they break up. They turn on genetic switches that change the mix of ion channels being produced within the DRG and the rate at which they're produced. These new ion channels travel back down inside the neurone to the site of the original disturbance. Voilà! Sensitivity increased. This entire process might take a week if the involved nociceptor innervates your big toe (the longest primary nociceptor). What is more, because the DRG is a rather open environment, it might also increase the sensitivity of nearby nociceptors. Just think about how remarkable this really is – the nociceptor has some mechanism of knowing where to send the new ion channels – they are transported to the site of the original disturbance! As far as we can find out, there is no human who knows for sure how this is coded. Amazing eh!

Romance gone wrong

The process by which neurotrophins, for example NGF and NGF receptor, cause peripheral sensitisation is a bit like this: a young couple meet in the countryside. One is NGF and one is NGF receptor. They fall in love and head off, hand in hand, on the long road to the city – DRG. When they arrive, they are blown away by the manic pulse of DRG, molecules of all shapes and sizes whizzing past, shady deals in dark synapses, dizzy lights, beautiful cells everywhere. Oh the endless opportunities! Oh the wonderful distractions! It is all too much for them and their relationship ends, a rather violent and irreconcilable separation. NGF causes such a stir that the DRG sends out all kinds of receptors to the countryside. NGF receptor quickly fades into obscurity, so affected by the experience that it becomes another molecule altogether. Note that it actually does become a different molecule altogether, but that might best be left for the sequel.

Another adaptation that occurs within the primary nociceptor in the presence of inflammation is the expression of opioid receptors [44]. This response is thought to take a few days, which means that in the vast majority of cases, inflammation subsides before this response is triggered. The ecological value of expressing opioid receptors in the sustained presence of inflammation is not clear. However, a good guess is that this evolved because it offered a pain relief advantage via anti-nociceptive effects when endogenous opioid systems are activated. This situation has clinical relevance because it means that, in the presence of sustained inflammation, local administration of opioids via patches over the painful area may offer analgesic benefit while minimising the pro-nociceptive effect that exogenous opioids have on CNS nociception, something we discuss soon.

Remember here of course that there are always many influences on a nociceptor including descending control (later in this chapter). It is quite possible that other influences will cancel out the slow effect depicted by our NGF-NGF receptor romance, particularly if inflammation dies down quickly and noxious stimuli abate. However, reflect on what this process would look like clinically and how many days later might symptomatic sensitivity arise. It could be a week or more.

Two way traffic – efferent function of nociceptors

Nociceptors tend to be thought of as largely negative, pessimistic, kill-joys. However, we should let go of this one sided perspective because nociceptors are not just about sending 'danger messages' – they are also about facilitating growth, healing and recovery (Nugget 18 *Danger detectors – the great givers of life!*). There are at least three molecules that are released by nociceptors and that are important in healing and health. We call them the 'Power Peptides' because they power up protection and healing. This is why we are prepared to spell them out for you: Calcitonin Gene Related Peptide (CGRP), substance P[13] and glutamate.

> **Nociceptors nurture us.** This is actually a potentially powerful piece of biological nuggetry! By activating nociceptors at some level, we actually facilitate the release of those 'trophic' factors that help tissues heal and in some tissues keep them alive. This is one good reason to conclude that a little pain might be a sign that tissues are being nudged toward positive adaptation – a SIM for sure. Of course remember here the Grand Poobah Pain Theory – that nociception and pain are different and we can have one without the other.

CGRP is a facilitator of bone formation and resorption, both of which are key to keeping our bones strong, healthy and biomechanically ready for the forces of life [45]. All three of the Power Peptides are critical for kickstarting the healing process after injury. CGRP and substance P, released at the terminals of nociceptors, increase blood flow (vasodilation) and mobilise immune cells – white blood cells, monocytes and T cells (extravasation, ie. swelling and maybe bruising) [46]. How is it then that these Power Peptides come to be released? Well at the time of writing, there were four different mechanisms that had been discussed in the literature, but two of them (inter- and intra-axonal coupling) are either thought to be very rare, or too confusing for even the molecular scientists to untangle, so we will skip them here and focus on the other two, which are both thought to be common and are relatively well understood.

The axonal reflex

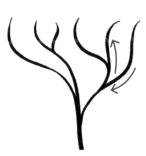

Action potentials generated in one branch of a nociceptor travel proximally. Wherever other branches of the nociceptor join the first branch, the action potential simultaneously runs distally to the terminals of the other branches. Once there, they have nowhere to go, but they have all this electrical energy they simply have to use (remember that energy cannot be created or destroyed – thanks Isaac[14]). It is this energy that causes the release of the Power Peptides. The peptidergic inflammation generated by the axonal reflex has potentially profound implications because it tells us that any nociceptor that is active will generate its own inflammatory state.

Considering that the Power Peptides also sensitise nociceptors to heat, it follows that tissue in which nociceptors are active will become sensitive to mechanical *and* hot thermal stimuli.

> **Try this.** Run your fingernail along the palm of your other hand with enough pressure for it to hurt a bit. You have just activated nociceptors in the palm of your hand with receptive fields about 1-2mm wide. The action potentials travelled to your spinal cord. The action potentials also travelled down each of the branches they came across en route. When the action potentials reached the end of the other branches of your neurones they caused the release of CGRP and substance P. These peptides caused vasodilation which is why you now have a red line emerging across the palm of your hand. You are seeing protection at work – peptidergic inflammation!

---

13 The P stands for 'preparation' or 'powder' which sounds rather boring, so we just say substance P!

14 The provenance of this idea is actually very contentious – every scientist and his or her dog can be linked to it.

Antidromic activation

Action potentials can be generated anywhere along a nociceptor – such is the pro (or con) of 'free nerve ending' status. In a *normal* state, action potentials will only be generated where there are the ion channels we discussed earlier; and in a normal state these ion channels are primarily located on the distal ends of the nociceptors.

However, action potentials can also be generated in the DRG or in the dorsal horn (at the nociceptor's proximal terminal) *even in a normal* state. Remember that once an action potential is generated it will go wherever the neurone goes – just like a dominoes trail. Clearly this means that action potentials can start 'upstream', travel 'backwards' and arrive at the distal terminals. Here, they have to do something with that energy, so they release the Power Peptides, *just as they do for the axonal reflex.* This process is enhanced when there is ectopic impulse production mid axon as may occur in an entrapment neuropathy.

Generating action potentials at the proximal end of primary nociceptors where they reside in the dorsal horn of the spinal cord, will also result in release of the power peptides in the tissues, but how can an action potential be generated right up there?!? Descending facilitation is the most obvious mechanism. Remember from EP that if the brain concludes that the tissue is in more danger than the spinal nociceptors suggest it is, then the brain will upregulate the spinal nociceptor via descending facilitation. Projection fibres from midbrain nuclei (eg. the periaqueductal grey) that terminate at the dorsal horn release excitatory neurotransmitters. Sufficient excitement of dorsal horn neurones can depolarise the proximal terminals of primary nociceptors, generating an action potential.

Protection in response to entirely cognitive cues
Lorimer had a remarkable experience discussing a particularly gruesome operation with someone who had, unbeknown to him, previously undergone this same operation. As they were talking, she developed a clear flare (mediated by vasodilation) neatly extending about half a centimetre either side of her very old and very faint scar.

What an incredible but biologically understandable response!

Part B

Time for neuroimmune coupling – hang on to your hats!

Systemic inflammation – don't shoot the messenger!

Whenever we talk of inflammation we tend to think of it as bad. This is shifting a bit and there is real therapeutic power in recognising the glorious healing power of inflammation. One of us is becoming quite famous for his enthusiastic appraisal of a big swollen joint after injury (Nugget 15 *Well done you old self-healer*). But remember – there is local inflammation and systemic inflammation. There is a great deal of overlap and interaction between them, but there are also differences. At a systemic level, we are in a constant state of 'inflammation' and it is the balance between pro and anti-inflammatory influences around an ideal set point that is critical.

Let's mine this even deeper. We are starting this section on systemic inflammation in a new way. We want to delay the usual hard line critique of why inflammation makes pain worse (which it does) because we want to be slow to shoot the messenger: in the context of injury and pain, inflammatory molecules are spreading the word that we are under threat. We are starting elsewhere because we want to celebrate how critical inflammatory molecules are for making us clever and adaptable. We suggest that it may indeed be in the adaptability of our cells and systems that life itself is captured – might then the messenger we have spent so long trying to shoot also be the messiah?[15]

Inflammatory balance, learning and plasticity

A common way to investigate what role particular cells play is to genetically engineer an animal that doesn't have those cells. Mice are the usual suckers. Mice can be 'bred' to have no T cells (T cells have a critical role in immunity. They are otherwise known as T lymphocytes,[16] white blood cells that are produced primarily in the thymus – hence the 'T'). Mice without T cells find it harder to get around a maze and perform other spatial

working memory tasks than 'normal' mice do [47, 48]. These mice are not dodgy at spatial tasks because they have been sick most of their lives. We know this because other mice that have their immune systems obliterated by irradiation, lose their ability to negotiate the maze but regain it when they have a bone marrow transplant [48]. We also know that mice that have been engineered to have excess T cells are water maze experts [49]. **So, T cells make mice smarter.**

Thinking makes T cells. That is, performing cognitive tasks increases the stocks of T cells, particularly those that express interleukin 4 (IL-4) an anti-inflammatory cytokine. Mice that are bred to be IL-4 deficient are no good at water mazes and normal mice transplanted with IL-4 deficient bone marrow see their formally good water maze times go out the window. In contrast, when IL-4 deficient mice get a blast of T cells, their water maze times drastically improve [50]. **So, IL-4 makes mice smarter.**

How would humans perform in a water maze? Ethics committees the world over will be reluctant to let us engineer T cell or IL-4 deficient humans and make them swim through Venice. However, there are correlational data – diminished T cell activity correlates with cognitive impairment in HIV infection, chemotherapy, schizophrenia and with ageing [47, 51] and we know that physical exercise and restricting calorie intake both improve cognitive performance and increase T cell counts [52] (Nugget 56 *Make your own anti-inflammatories*).

Intuitively we would predict that a similar relationship would be observed in people with chronic pain. With regard to T cell expression in the bits that matter, there doesn't seem to be much evidence either way. There is an increase in T cell expression in the periphery, DRG and spinal cord in animal models of neuropathic pain [53], but we don't know about the brain, specifically the meninges, which is where it seems to matter in the mice studies. IL-4 however, is a different story – studies tell us that IL-4 is reduced in people with chronic pain in a range of conditions [eg. 54] and that people with chronic pain perform worse on spatial working memory tasks than people without chronic pain [eg. 55].

The problem with any study of cognitive performance in people with pain is that their pain requires a good chunk of brain processing resources. Patients with chronic pain certainly report that they have problems thinking and performing spatial tasks, for example remembering how to get somewhere. It is reasonable to predict that IL-4 and cognitive performance would be related in people in much the same way that they are related in mice and that if IL-4 levels are low in chronic pain then that may contribute to disrupted cognitive performance.

---

15 We realise this mainly tongue in cheek stuff might be a bit provocative or perhaps annoying, but that is the point – it is a blatant strategy to help you remember.

16 Lorimer once met an oncologist who described himself as a *lymphomaniac*. Classy.

Inflammatory cytokines and cognitive performance

What might pro-inflammatory cytokines (in particular IL-1, IL-6 and TNFα) do to cognitive performance? First, IL-1. The story is similar to that of T cell-derived IL-4. Think about this experiment: take a normal mouse out of its home, put it in a different place, let's say Donald's Place, give it a noxious shock and then put it back home again. The mouse learns that Donald's Place is not a good place to be, so that when it is put back in Donald's Place, it freezes even without a shock – 'no movement except for respiration' is the official definition of a freeze.
(Nugget 56 *Make your own anti-inflammatories*)

This is one of the most common animal studies in behavioural neuroscience – the contextual fear conditioning paradigm. Anyway, put a normal mouse through this and a day later, his IL-1 gene expression is elevated. Here is the interesting bit. If you then shock the mouse in its nice, usually-safe home cage (not at Donald's), IL-1 gene expression is not affected. So, it's the learning of the association between Donald's place and shocks that triggers IL-1 expression, not the shock itself [56]. The process of associating danger with the places you go increases manufacture of the pro-inflammatory cytokine IL-1. It seems that learning in a fear paradigm induces an inflammatory-like process, at least in the hippocampus.

> **What if?** These are mouse studies but what they imply is that the creation of a DIM is a pro-inflammatory event. Jeepers! It makes total sense that creating a SIM is an anti-inflammatory event. If that doesn't excite you we just don't know what will!

But don't go bagging out IL-1 just yet, because it can also facilitate learning. Give a mouse a shot of IL-1 immediately after a learning task [57], or immediately before it [58] and it has better memory of the task a week later. It's not just about fear either – giving a mouse IL-1 just before it does a water maze improves its performance on that too and if you block IL-1 signalling, or breed a mouse that can't make IL-1, spatial memory is impaired [58]. Critically, all of the data on IL-1 involves spatial memory tasks, for which the hippocampus is critical – very similar tasks that do not rely on the hippocampus are unaffected by dosing up on IL-1, nor are they affected by knocking out the gene that signals IL-1. The hippocampus is known to be important in spatial navigation – London cabbies have big hippocampi and the longer they have been cabbies the bigger their hippocampi [59]! Anyway, IL-1 manufacture seems to increase spatial learning and memory.

> **How might IL-1, a pro-inflammatory cytokine, relate to the coalface?** One speculative, but by no means outrageous implication is that there may be extra merit in doing spatial and localisation training in the presence of mild inflammation. Of course we have no human data to support this, but here lies a great little educational opportunity: explaining to the patient that there are molecules that are both contributing to their inflammation and giving them a temporary boost in spatial learning and memory. Perhaps suggest that now might be a good time to get stuck into left/right discrimination (*Recognise*) or tactile discrimination training.

Interleukin-6, or IL-6, can be anti-inflammatory or pro-inflammatory. It is perhaps not surprising then, that this 'swinging voter' can enhance or impair cognitive function. Lo and behold, there is actually a relevant human study looking at IL-6 administration to people with chronic fatigue syndrome just before they performed a range of cognitive tests [60]. Nothing happened. Disappointing! However, other studies measured IL-6 levels in plasma taken from patients with lupus [61] or post-laparoscopic surgery [62] and found that the higher the IL-6 count the better the cognitive retention. So, more IL-6 production seems to be associated with improved memory. By the way, TNFα probably has a similar effect [52].

Finally, prostaglandins, surprise surprise, enhance spatial learning. Prostaglandins are mainly made via rather famous enzymes called COX-1 and COX-2, which are expressed in neurones, glia and endothelial cells [52]. The COX brothers are defined according to where they have their effects – COX-1 is responsible for maintenance and protection of the gastrointestinal tract and COX-2 is, for us, more famous – it contributes to inflammation and thereby pain. COX-2 inhibitors impair memory and performance on spatial tasks, although, intriguingly, mice with genetically impaired COX-2 expression are just as good as their mates at learning to freeze at George's place [52].

Do you take ibuprofen? Do you feel as smart as you were before you started taking it? Okay – this is slightly tongue in cheek. There is actually no evidence we can find that COX-2 inhibitors impair spatial memory in humans but it's not an outrageous suggestion.

Cytokines, long term potentiation and neuroplasticity

As a finale for this section, let's try to wrap our heads around the role of cytokines in facilitating long term potentiation (LTP) and nurturing neuroplasticity.

LTP means a sustained effect on the post-synaptic neurone such that it is more easily activated by a pre-synaptic activity – a process that Hebb described as 'neurones that fire together wire together' [63]. The key work in this field [64] showed for the first time (to our knowledge at least) an inflammatory-like process – the secretion of pro-inflammatory cytokine IL-1 – occurring in key brain areas in association with LTP. Other researchers have shown a relationship between LTP and IL-1 levels, shown no LTP when IL-1 antagonist is injected, and shown no LTP in mutant mice without the IL-1 manufacturing gene [52]. Here is where the story becomes a bit juicier because the role of IL-1 is not just limited to the hippocampus and to spatial and related memory formations. For example, IL-1 expression is associated with LTP in the dorsal horn of the spinal cord at the level of the spinal nociceptors.

IL-6, our swinging voter, sometimes anti-inflammatory sometimes pro-inflammatory, might have an important role in turning LTP off. That is, IL-6 is upregulated 4-8 hours after high-frequency stimulation of a mouse's hippocampus, but if IL-6 is blocked by anti-IL-6 antibodies, then LTP persists for longer [65]. So, IL-1 seems to be particularly important in establishing LTP and IL-6 seems to be particularly important in turning it off. Extrapolating now to things we do not want to potentiate, one wonders if augmenting IL-6 might reduce the likelihood of LTP in the nociceptive system after acute injury, or in the circuits that subserve post traumatic stress. It would be very difficult to change IL-1 expression because it happens so quickly, but we have 6 hours to change IL-6 expression. That seems possible. The potential power of scientifically based reassurance in the acute phase after injury may well act via this mechanism [116].

IL-1 and IL-6 are involved in LTP in the acute setting, but TNFα saves itself for later. In mice with impaired TNF signalling, early learning progresses normally, but the dendritic pruning and synaptogenesis that characterises later learning does not occur [66]. This has clear implications – we know that the brains of people with chronic pain or post traumatic stress are different from those of healthy controls and it seems possible that abnormal TNFα regulation might contribute to these differences.

Finally, we return to prostaglandins. The usual experiments have shown that prostaglandins have a role in LTP. Again, this might have a direct application to us in the pain world. Selective COX-2 inhibitors impair LTP in the mouse hippocampus, which raises the possibility, not completely outrageous or remote, that taking a bit of ibuprofen impairs the LTP that contributes to chronic pain. We know that COX-2 inhibitors are proposed to limit the development of chronic pain in several ways, but this mechanism doesn't get much press. We tend to think of anti-inflammatories acting solely at a peripheral level, but clearly they also act centrally.

Okay, now for the messenger: The immune set point, TLR4 and why you should care

We have spent some time reminding you that the neural system is clearly under immune-mediated modulatory influence. Now it is time to talk about how the immune system is under neurally-mediated modulatory influence. Right up until the current millennium, the prevailing view of the immune system was of a stand-alone protective army that operated independantly, answerable just to itself and going about its business in a reasonably private sort of way. Discovery and characterisation of the *inflammatory reflex* and the *immune set point* changed all that [67].

The inflammatory reflex

Conventionally, reflexes are thought of as automated responses triggered by certain stimuli. That holds true at least to some extent, although we are quickly gathering evidence that reflexes themselves are under potentially potent descending control [68]. Many clinicians are familiar with simple motor arcs – tapping on a tendon triggers a brief contraction in the appropriate muscle: specialised receptors detect the mechanical effect of the tap and an efferent motor output contracts the muscle. The inflammatory reflex is remarkably similar. It works like this: molecular products of an injury, inflammation or infection are detected and an efferent output modulates the immune response [69]. For example, really important research in animals showed that the vagus nerve transmits news of abdominal tissue inflammation to the brain and that this news results in fever [70] and probably some of the 'feelings' of being sick (see the cortical body matrix section page 26). The question then became – so how are these molecular products of injury, inflammation or infection detected?

The amazing Christiane Nüsslein-Volhard and toll-like receptors

Christiane Nüsslein-Volhard is a German biologist whose science career was taking off around the same time that George Engel began laying into the biomedical model in earnest. Like George, Christiane has gone on to be one of the most influential people in her field. George intentionally coined the term 'biopsychosocial'. Christiane, unintentionally coined the term 'toll' when she observed some odd aspects of fruit fly lava and exclaimed *'Das ist ja toll!'*, which means *'That is amazing!'* Clearly, this moment was rather amusing as 'toll' was adopted as the name of a

particular group of genes that were important for the fruit fly's development. Her influence went completely out of control and beyond her own field when a completely different group of researchers discovered a particular protein that sat in the cell membrane of a range of cells and responded to bacteria by triggering an immune response. The protein receptor looked quite similar to the toll genes so they called it a 'toll-like receptor' (TLR). Needless to say the name stuck.

Found in a range of cells, TLRs are critical for protection against pathogens and as such are mediators of acquired immunity. Once activated, they trigger a cascade of events that ultimately leads to upregulation or downregulation of genes that cause inflammation, phagocytosis of bacteria or pathogens, or death of invader viruses. Most relevant of these immune responses to *EP Supercharged* are the inflammatory effects because it is those effects that have an immediate modulatory influence over the neuroimmune complexes that subserve nociception and pain.

A key characteristic of the TLRs is that they 'remember' what a dangerous event 'looks like'. What they actually do is detect molecules that are associated with different types of dangerous events, of which there are five broad types [71]:

1. **Pathogen-associated molecular patterns (PAMPs)**
   PAMPs are exactly as they seem to be – molecular patterns that are associated with bacteria, viruses and other disease-causing microorganisms. The particular PAMP varies according to the pathogen involved, but they all have pretty dangerous sounding names (Table 3.2).

2. **Damage-associated molecular patterns (DAMPs)**
   When body tissue is damaged in some way, whether it be through injury or ischaemia, a range of molecules including cytokines, 'heat shock proteins', ATP, uric and lactic acid are released. Collectively these molecules form DAMPs, which are detected not just by TLR but also by other equally oddly-named receptors called NOD-like receptors. NOD-like receptors are also located on immune cells and on endothelial tissue.

3. **Xenobiotic-associated molecular patterns (XAMPs)**
   A xenobiotic molecule is one that is not normally found in a particular biological environment. The most obvious of these are pharmacological agents that are not naturally found inside our body. The most relevant of these agents to *EP Supercharged* is exogenous morphine. Exogenous morphine is a XAMP.

4. Read on for **BAMPs**

5. and **CAMPs**…

Endoxin	The poisonous insides of bacteria
Exotoxin	Poison released by the outside of bacteria
Lipopeptides	Molecules consisting of a lipid connected to a peptide (amazing huh!) expressed by some bacteria (some antibiotics are lipopeptides)
Glycopeptides	Molecules consisting of sugar connected to a peptide. Many antibiotics are glycopeptides

Table 3.2 PAMP types

The TLR that has attracted the most attention with respect to pain is TLR4. TLR4 has been described by Professor Mark Hutchinson as the 'most moronic' of the TLRs, because once TLR4 has 'remembered' an insult, it will respond rather indiscriminately to anything that resembles it in any way.

Prof Mark Hutchinson professes to be 'just a pharmaconeuroimmunologist', but he demonstrates a sufficiently acute insight into the human condition and empathy for people in pain that we suspect he might be either a closet clinician or just a remarkably nice person. Either way, his perspectives on TLR4 are rather unflattering.

Mark's analogy is this: TLR4 is sufficiently focused on the detection of that which doesn't belong, that it will be activated, with equal vigour, by both the locomotive that is crashing through your living room wall and the train driver's hat that blows in through an open window. The key thing is that it remembers both. Clearly both are not 'equally dangerous', but it seems both can evoke a similarly protective response. Obviously this is presuming that all other things are equal, which they never are, but even still, the principle applies – TLR4 can be a rather over-reactive little pest.

The AMP gang and us

The effects of PAMPs, DAMPs and XAMPs[17] on TLR4 that are most relevant to us in the *EP Supercharged* world is the trigger of pathways that lead directly to increased expression of pro-inflammatory cytokines and the direct access that these pathways have on nociception. These pathways are critical for survival and are just one part of a highly complex balancing act that protects us from pathogens, cell stress and injury and foreign molecules. The magnitude of our protective responses has been honed by a very long evolutionary process.

The potential impact of XAMPs on our nociceptive system is substantial when it comes to opioids. Think about this for a moment – opioids are effective analgesics in the case of acute pain, but they are also XAMPs, which means that they will probably have two simultaneous and opposing actions – one via opioid receptors in anti-nociceptive pathways (taking the Protectometer down) and one via TLRs in pro-inflammatory pathways (taking the Protectometer up). However, with long term use the anti-nociceptive effect loses steam while the pro-inflammatory XAMP-mediated effect does not (or does so much more slowly), which means the net effect on the Protectometer is to gradually push it up, ie. sensitivity increases. Although it is not the only mechanism, this seems like one mechanism that may explain why pain can gradually worsen even though one is taking more and more synthetic morphine. (Nuggets 41 *You are more powerful than pills* and 57 *Morphine madness.*)

This XAMP-effect of exogenous, synthetic opioids might be reduced by using patches instead of pills. Patches have a stronger local effect that will act on local opioid receptors which are expressed in the sustained presence of inflammation – something we mentioned back on page 52.

Prof Hutchinson suggests that there is one more molecular pattern that will probably prove to be more important as discoveries continue – BAMPS or 'behaviour-associated molecular patterns'. This idea is resonant with physiological models of how we feel anything, most notably captured by the Somatic Marker Hypothesis [72] (see also Chapter 2 page 28).

In short and in the language of *EP Supercharged*, let's apply the Somatic Marker Hypothesis to a feeling such as fear:

- An external stimulus, let's say vision of a snake, triggers an automatic neural response, mediated by primitive (in an evolutionary and developmental sense) mechanisms.

17 These AMPs are different to the AMP (ayempee) we discussed earlier (page 51).

- This causes a rapid shift in the molecular profile within the tissues of the body. We can call this shift the BAMP.[18]

- This BAMP is detected by a wide range of receptors (here we might call them 'interoceptors', a term used a lot by others in this space [eg. 73]. These receptors include the TLRs on immune competent cells that are integrated in neuroimmune synaptic complexes in the danger transmission system and the brain.

- Upregulated danger transmission systems are activated sending 'tissue danger' messages to the brain. Meanwhile, news of the shift in molecular profile arrives back to the brain via interoceptive pathways and activates a suite of modulation neurotags such as increased heart rate, pupil dilation, blood flow redistribution.

- Quite possibly, the modulation neurotags exert sufficient influence on the action neurotag of 'fear' and voilà! The person feels frightened.

The speculative bit: what about Cognition Associated Molecular Patterns (CAMPs)?

The cortical body matrix model proposes that there are very tight connections within thalamocortical loops that subserve the protection and regulation of the body and the space around it, at both a physiological and perceptual level [74]. We know that during the amazing rubber hand illusion, in which one's hand is 'replaced' by an artificial one, autonomic and inflammatory responses occur in the real hand [75, 76]. We know that recounting an episode of being bullied increases the blood's level of pro-inflammatory cytokine induced by submersing one arm in an ice bath.[19] These findings provide compelling evidence that cognitive processes can become associated with certain molecular patterns and that these molecular patterns are not inherently any different from the DAMPs, XAMPs, PAMPs and BAMPs. On these grounds, we would predict that CAMPs will have similar effects. This is, at this stage, speculative but entirely reasonable. The implications are not novel but they are important – our thoughts and beliefs should be able to upregulate danger transmission at the spinal cord and brain through the TLR4 receptors on glial cells.

The immune set point

The set point of the immune system determines the size of the inflammatory response to a given PAMP, DAMP, XAMP or BAMP. Normally, scientists will use a stimulus-response curve to represent this. The 'normal' set point concerns the relationship between threat and immune response when the system is optimally balanced. The system is optimally balanced when pro and anti-inflammatory influences are roughly even, or perhaps ideal for survival (see Figure 3.4). As you look at the curve remember that nociceptive detection, transmission and processing is all influenced by the immune set point.

---

18 'Shift the BAMP' sounds like a groovy new dance move – Ed.

19 This experiment has been done by Dr Tasha Stanton, one of the most outstanding early career pain researchers on the planet (or at least that is what the International Association for the Study of Pain, the Australian Pain Society and the National Top 5 under 40 scientists panel think. So we are not just saying it because she is nice…) but Tasha has not published it yet.

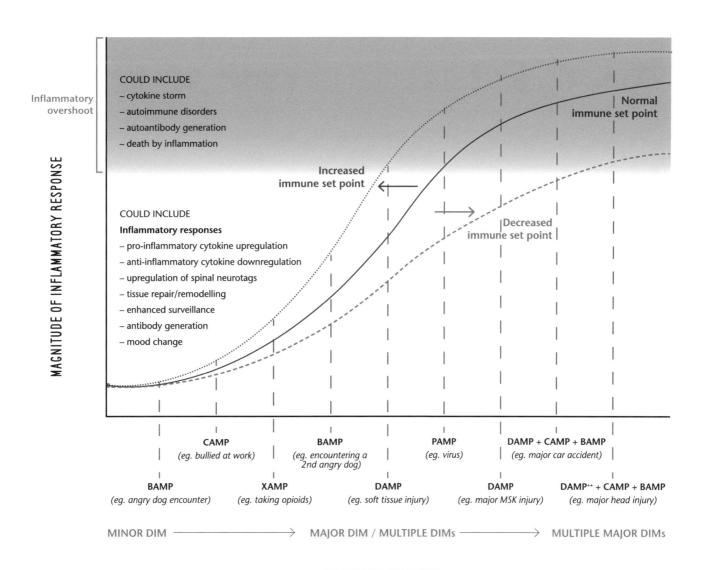

COULD INCLUDE
– cytokine storm
– autoimmune disorders
– autoantibody generation
– death by inflammation

Inflammatory
overshoot

COULD INCLUDE
Inflammatory responses
– pro-inflammatory cytokine upregulation
– anti-inflammatory cytokine downregulation
– upregulation of spinal neurotags
– tissue repair/remodelling
– enhanced surveillance
– antibody generation
– mood change

Increased
immune set point

Normal
immune set point

Decreased
immune set point

MAGNITUDE OF INFLAMMATORY RESPONSE

CAMP
(eg. bullied at work)

BAMP
(eg. encountering a
2nd angry dog)

PAMP
(eg. virus)

DAMP + CAMP + BAMP
(eg. major car accident)

BAMP
(eg. angry dog encounter)

XAMP
(eg. taking opioids)

DAMP
(eg. soft tissue injury)

DAMP
(eg. major MSK injury)

DAMP++ + CAMP + BAMP
(eg. major head injury)

MINOR DIM ⟶ MAJOR DIM / MULTIPLE DIMs ⟶ MULTIPLE MAJOR DIMs

MAGNITUDE OF THREAT

Figure 3.4 The immune set point affects inflammatory responses.

At a normal set point the inflammatory response 'fits the threat'.

If the immune set point is increased the curve shifts to the left (red line) and the same threat causes a bigger inflammatory response – the system is overprotective.

If the immune set point shifts to the right (green line – for example taking immunosuppressants) the same threat causes a smaller response – the system is underprotective.

Most people, even clever people with substantial health training, find stimulus-response curves difficult to decipher [77], so it is easier to integrate this immune set point into the Protectometer (Figure 3.5) (Nugget 39 *Getting sick is a pain in the neck*). Remembering that the Protectometer is modulated by the biological state of the tissues, an increase in the immune set point will have two effects:

1. The Protectometer level will be higher. Simple. An increased set point can also be thought of as a 'pro-inflammatory state'. Because of the upregulatory effect of a pro-inflammatory state on danger detection, danger transmission and pain production, the Protectometer will necessarily be upregulated.

2. The effect of any stimulus that evokes a response in the danger detection and transmission system will be larger – more bang for your buck. In classic clinical terms, this scenario will manifest as allodynia and hyperalgesia.

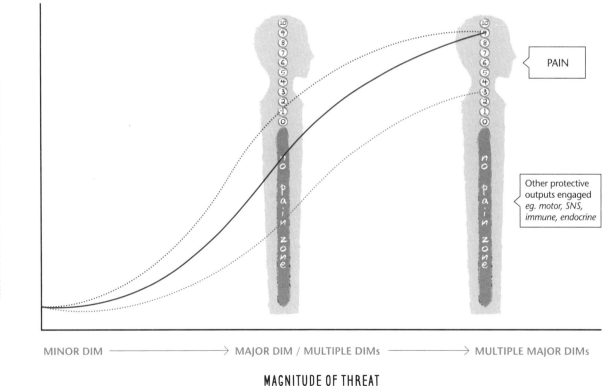

Figure 3.5 The immune set point and the Protectometer

Part C

The dorsal horn – time for a rethink

Bob Coghill is a very fine neurophysiologist currently plying his trade at Cincinnati Children's Hospital. He is a perfectionist and a researcher of the utmost integrity. We credit him with our reignited fascination with what he describes as *the massive computational capacity of the dorsal horn*. We will return to that, but first let's quickly review the bits and pieces we are talking about here.

There is now a huge amount of literature on the circuitry of the spinal cord, including (but not limited to) nociceptive circuitry. We now know a fair amount about how this circuitry develops, when it develops and what implications there might be for injury, stress and inflammation at different stages of development. Some of it might be just a little bit surprising.

Take this for example: during development nociceptors are the last of all the primary sensory neurones to enter the dorsal horn. This means that although dangerous events can be detected in the tissues from well before birth, the mechanisms by which they trigger a nociceptive signal to the brain don't fully develop until after birth [78]. In the first weeks of life, noxious stimuli trigger body-wide protective responses, some of which have no sensible protective value [79] – it seems that we need to learn what is the best response and we need to *learn* what in fact the brain needs to know. It is not surprising then that injuries that often result in severe chronic pain in adults – such as brachial plexus avulsion – do not have this result if they occur before or very shortly after birth [80]. The growing body of research suggests that the way in which the spinal cord develops the capacity to send data to the brain is very dependent on exposure and experience after birth.

EP Supercharged is all about digging deeper into the biology of pain and then using this deeper understanding to provide people in pain with the resources to master their situation. Well, the deeper we dig into the way the spinal cord works, the more it starts to look like the brain; the more we need to rethink those neat drawings of primary nociceptors synapsing with spinal nociceptors, under the influence of an inhibitory interneurone or two (as depicted in the gate control theory [10]). Perhaps, if you are close to the cutting edge of nociceptive neurophysiology, you will also include a couple of descending projection neurones that come primarily from the brainstem as we did in EP.

Our neurophysiological drawings are usually simplified to demonstrate the key points. However, there are some things we draw so often that we slip into the illusion that things are indeed that simple. Here are three examples that have fundamental relevance to how we understand nociception and that glorious privilege – movement.

1. Rethinking the connection between a primary nociceptor and its spinal nociceptor

The way we draw the connection between a primary nociceptor and its spinal nociceptor projection usually looks a bit like Figure 3.6a (overleaf). A primary nociceptor, denoted as such by an alarm bell on the tissue end, synapses with a spinal nociceptor. This synapse is also influenced by a branch from an Aβ neurone, a descending inhibitory projection (-ve) and a descending facilitatory projection (+ve).

The picture on the right shows it a little more realistically – the primary nociceptor has many synapses in the spinal cord. These synapses spread out in all directions such that there are synapses up to two levels higher and lower. Most of the synapses are with interneurones – over 95% of the neurones in the grey matter of the spinal cord are interneurones – and there are hundreds of descending inhibitory and facilitatory projections.

This incredible complexity underpins what Bob Coghill calls *the massive computational capacity of the spinal cord* and is one justification for what we are calling 'spinal neurotags'.

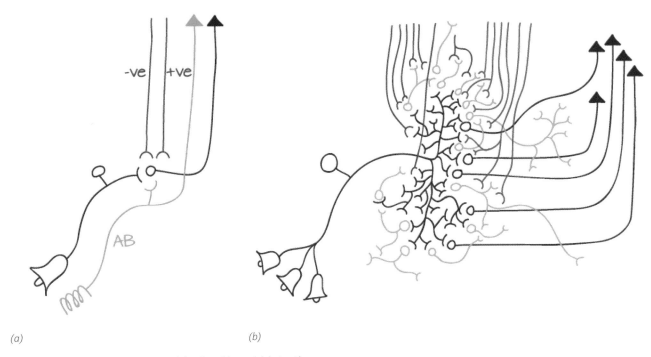

(a)   (b)

Figure 3.6 The primary nociceptor and the dorsal horn, (a) being the traditional view and (b) being the (still very simplified) more realistic view.

2. Rethinking alpha motor neurone drive

The contrast between how we tend to draw the motor system – a primary motor cortex cell (green dot on the left Figure, 3.7a) driving an alpha motor neurone, and what we now know – an alpha motor neurone receives input from many descending neurones. Projections to the alpha motor neurone come from all over the brain (green dots on the right, Figure 3.7b), not just from the primary motor cortex. Movement is the result of many brain neurotags exerting their influence, not just one.

3. Rethinking the ventral horn

We often tend to draw and think of an alpha motor neurone being driven by a single descending motor fibre (see the single circled synapse in Figure 3.8a). However, the alpha motor neurone cell body has a very large number of synapses in the ventral horn (see all those orange bits in Figure 3.8b).

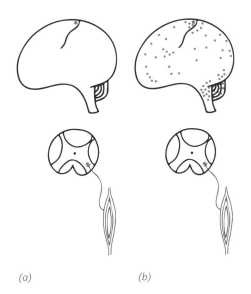

(a)   (b)

Figure 3.7 Rethinking alpha motor neurone drive (a) the traditional view, (b) the more realistic view

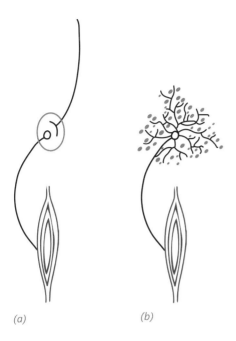

(a)   *(b)*

Figure 3.8 Rethinking alpha motor neurone drive (a) the traditional view, (b) the more realistic view

Recap the main players in the dorsal horn

Primary nociceptors terminate in the dorsal horn at the level they enter and up to two levels up or down. The dorsal horn can be divided into several layers or laminae, the details of which are not that important here. What is important is the immense and sophisticated network of interneurones that modulate inputs from ascending neurones (primary nociceptors and non-nociceptive input from the periphery), descending neurones (from the brainstem, thalamus and cortex) and intraspinal neurones (from, for example, the ventral horn or 'intra-dorsal horn' neurones). What's more, all of these neurones are dwarfed by a massive population of glial cells that modulate the neurones and are themselves critical in signal processing.

To give you a feel for just how complex this really is, take another look at the connection between the primary nociceptor and it's spinal nociceptor (see Figure 3.6b). Most of the primary nociceptors terminate in the most superficial layers of the dorsal horn and these layers also have the highest density of spinal nociceptors (that is, the danger transmission neurones that exert their influence up in the thalamus). However, even in these layers supposedly dedicated to the transmission of primary nociception

to spinal nociception, interneurones still make up over 90% of the cells and there are as many non-neuronal cells as well. It really is more like a neuroimmune matrix full of overlapping networks. These networks *collaborate* and *compete* for influence.[20]

You can also see a good number of descending neurones that have pro-nociceptive functions (blue) or anti-nociceptive functions (red). A large proportion of these descending neurones project from the brainstem – not just from the periaqueductal grey – the show pony of the brainstem – but from several nuclei in that area. A significant proportion come from other brain areas, for example motor areas, frontal and prefrontal cortex, association cortices, insular and cingulate cortices and amygdala. More on the fabulous anti and pro nociceptive implications of that later. This much you would have understood, at least to some extent from *Explain Pain*, but let's dig deeper because this is where the real excitement starts.

The spinal cord is not like a stack of neuroimmune blocks

We tend to think of the spinal cord as consisting of segments, each with dorsal horns and roots, ventral horns and roots, and surrounded by the projection fibres that make up the white matter. Learning dermatomes and myotomes, while of some use, promotes this segmental thinking. We tend to think about the spinal cord in the same way it is usually drawn – as a cross sectional plate of neurones, communicating in a rather linear fashion. We tend to think that each little section of the spinal cord sends outputs up and out, and receives inputs from above and from outside. It is seductive to think about it like this because there are clearly certain entry and exist points (dorsal and ventral roots) and we know that the vertebral column looks like a stack of boney blocks (BEWARE! Remember that it is not really like that either – visit [EP54] to see how firmly enmeshed the vertebrae and the LAFTs really are). However, there really are no segments in the spinal cord – it is not a stack of neuroimmune blocks – it is actually a continuous neuroimmune complex. Incoming neurones branch in all directions, the interneurones run up, down and sideways and can be long enough to traverse many spinal 'levels', cross the spinal cord, run from the front to the back. There is no doubt in our minds that the grey matter of the spinal cord is much more like brain than it is like a stack of neuroimmune dinner plates! And like a brain, it is full of neuroimmune networks competing and collaborating for influence. No wonder Bob reckons it has massive computational capacity!

---

20 It is about now that somewhere in your mind you might hear the whisper – *'have I read this before, earlier in the book?'* Don't worry – just keep reading.

Goodbye nociceptive 'pathways' – hello 'spinal neurotags'

We have planted a couple of footnotes that refer to the whispering in your mind that you might have read all this stuff earlier in the book. Take note of these words: neuroimmune complexes, neural networks, competition, collaboration, influence and output. Now turn back to Chapter 2 on cortical neurotags and the principles that govern them. See the same words there? You can see the link and probably where we are going here. We are asking you to take on a radical new idea.

The radical new idea

The spinal cord works much more like a brain than it does like a relay station and the concepts of neurotags, influence and outputs help to make sense of the vast array of stimulus-response relationships that are readily observed in animals and humans.

To build up your new version of the spinal cord a bit more, just imagine that it was formed like this (Warning! It wasn't formed like this): To optimise function, the human needs a method of sending messages quickly over long distances. The spinal cord provides the freeways along which these messages can travel at speed. The neurones in these freeways are myelinated for speed, which makes them white. This is the white matter of the spinal cord. These freeways form a kind of cylinder and the empty space in the middle of the cylinder (grey matter) looks like a butterfly from above. Now imagine that there is simply not enough room inside the skull to fit all the thinking stuff – the masses of neuroimmune complexes that we call neurotags, which exist in a constant state of collaboration and competition. In order to optimise our thinking/processing capacity, the cylinder of the spinal cord is filled up with more brain – billions of neural and immune cells grow along the length of the spinal cord and, just like the brain, form neurotags that proceed to collaborate and compete for influence.

Again, we can think of *Action Neurotags*, which exert their influence on ascending neurones that take a message upwards (to the thalamus for example) or outwards (to muscles for example), and *Modulation Neurotags* that exert their influence locally. This new conceptualisation of the spinal cord means we can rethink the dorsal horn in terms of spinal neurotags (Nugget 58 *Flush your spinal neurotags*).

Hang in there! A range of neurones transmit data that enter the 'spinal neuromatrix' at each dorsal root. Many of these neurones are responsive only in the non-noxious range and project straight to the brain, bypassing the spinal neuromatrix while also sending collaterals into the spinal neuromatrix to exert their own influence. The gate control theory captures this functionality by summarising non-nociceptive fibre (usually Aβ) input as inhibiting nociceptive fibre input. All of the inputs that penetrate the spinal neuromatrix branch and diverge and exert their influence on networks of interneurones – networks we can call 'spinal neurotags'. Descending projection neurones also have many access points to the spinal neuromatrix and they exert their own influences on spinal neurotags. Perhaps the most significant outputs of the spinal neuromatrix are those that alert higher centres to danger and the need to protect, and those that influence activity of alpha motor neurones (the ones that modulate movement).

We can now think about Wall and Melzack's gate control theory [10] in terms of spinal neurotags, which is a more accurate way to think about it than the original drawings, as revolutionary as they were (and as legend has it, drawn on a napkin over much whisky and claret).

- Wide-diameter neurones (eg. Aβ) exert an influence over spinal neurotags that reduce the likelihood of activating spinal nociceptors.

- Small-diameter neurones (eg. Aδ) exert an influence over spinal neurotags that increase the likelihood of activating spinal nociceptors.

- Descending neurones also influence these neurotags and, based on the anatomical characteristics of descending projection neurones, it is highly likely that both pro-nociceptive and anti-nociceptive influences are active at once.

Let's keep going! Grab a drink! We can now think about *spatial summation*[21] according to the principles that govern neurotags (Chapter 2 page 23). Remember that neurotags collaborate and compete. Remember that influence depends on mass (the number of cells involved) and precision (the relative probability that member cells will fire and non-member cells will not). By delivering two noxious stimuli next to each other, we increase the influence over protective spinal neurotags because we are recruiting more spinal cells in synchrony (an increase in mass). As a result, the pain evoked is likely to be worse [81].

---

21 Spatial summation is the phenomenon in which two stimuli of equal intensity evoke more intense pain if they are close to each other than if they are a long way apart. There are two 'types' of spatial summation – area based (the larger area or volume of body tissue that is stimulated, the more intense the pain) and distance based (pain intensity increases in line with the distance between two stimuli, up to a point at which it decreases again) [81, 82].

Do we need this new spinal neurotag understanding?

How might this 'radical new idea' (which is actually not that radical when you consider that we have known about it for decades – we just haven't admitted knowing about it!) actually affect clinical practice? Is there any implication other than demonstrating why a cut spinal cord is so hard to put back together? We think so.

The spinal cord itself can induce significant adaptations to increase protection, for example vast increases in receptive field of the spinal nociceptor (eg. a noxious stimulus at the knee makes your ankle hurt); recruitment of extra spinal nociceptors nearby active ones (eg. stimulation of your painful ankle makes your whole leg hurt); the potential influence of descending inhibition and facilitation is way beyond upregulation and downregulation of the active spinal nociceptors.

Check out the cheat sheet on page 79 for clinical signs that point to spinal cord adaptations contributing to a pain state.

Digging deeper into the spinal neurotag

Take a step or two even further by honing in on the bits that make up a spinal neurotag. We have focused in particular on one of the neuroimmune complexes – a typical tripartite synapse.

We have taken the image from Chapter 2 (Figure 2.5 page 20) that shows the tangle of neurones and glial cells that make up the spinal neuromatrix and have magnified one of the tripartite synapses.

Here, you can see a TLR4 receptor – the surveillance camera (a) – sitting on the astrocyte cell (b) that is hugging the two neurones. TLR4 detects the presence of the DAMPs, PAMPs, XAMPs, BAMPs and CAMPs (the circle with an X on it) and triggers a release of molecules into the synapse (c). These molecules are detected by receptors on the post-synaptic neurone (d) and trigger a cascade of events (e) inside that increase the responsiveness of that neurone. Voilà! Sensitivity of danger transmission increased!

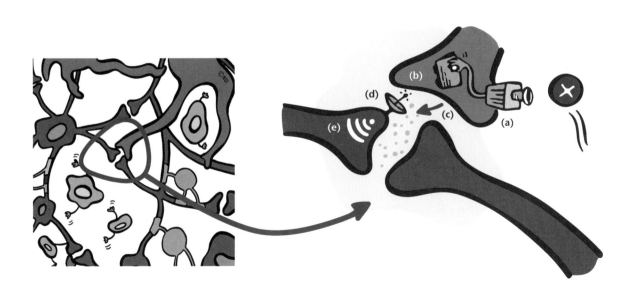

Figure 3.9 Tripartite synapse action as described in the text

More on the immune components of the tripartite synapse

There are three main players: a pre-synaptic neurone, a post-synaptic neurone and an astrocyte – that's why we call it a 'tripartite synapse'. Some synapses have other glial cells, for example microglia, involved and so are called 'tetrapartite' (4 players) or 'pentapartite' (5 players). Remove the glial cells and the synapse is rendered kaput – it is functionally dead! Mess with the glial cells and you mess directly with synaptic efficacy and therefore the potential influence of that spinal neurotag on ascending danger messages and efferent motor outputs.

There are so many molecules and mechanisms that are involved in operating this tripartite neuroimmune synaptic complex that even the most switched on molecular biologist is quickly bamboozled by their names, specific functions, interdependence and redundancy. We prefer a functional approach: the responsiveness of the post-synaptic neurone to neurotransmitters in the synapse depends on the status of the immune cell that hugs it. Turn back quickly to the section on the immune set point, the TLR and the AMP gang – DAMPs, PAMPs, BAMPs, XAMPs and CAMPs. Go on – turn back and re-read that …

Well done.

Welcome back.

Remember that on every immune cell there are detectors, including the famous TLR4, which works like a low-quality surveillance camera with a very long memory. It will respond to the AMP gang. We can think of these immune cells as having their own set point. Move the set point to the left and the post-synaptic neurone becomes more responsive to the same input. Move the immune set point to the right and it becomes less responsive (see Figure 3.4 page 61). In other words, activate the TLR4 and it triggers a cascade within the immune cells that results in upregulation of the release of pro-inflammatory molecules into the synapse. These molecules are detected by both neurones of the synapse, which increases the efficiency of the synapse. Through this mechanism, the influence of an incoming danger message will be enhanced in the presence of any of the AMP gang.

Bringing it back to the real world

TLR4 is a Protectometer shifter. In the presence of a DIM, for example the flu (a PAMP) or someone telling you that *'your back's out'* (a CAMP), TLR4 on glial cells recognises the molecular patterns associated with the DIM. For those glial cells that are hugging the synapse between the primary nociceptor and the spinal neurotags, TLR4 activation causes release of pro-inflammatory cytokines into that synapse. This increases the influence of that primary nociceptor on the spinal

Action potentials in the primary nociceptors	When a message (an action potential) arrives at the proximal terminal of a primary nociceptor, the electrical energy has to do something (remember that energy cannot be created or destroyed) so it causes the release of neurotransmitters into the synapse. These neurotransmitters are excitatory to spinal neurotags that are nociceptive.
Action potentials in the descending anti-nociceptive neurones	As above, when a message arrives at the distal end of these projection neurones, it releases neurotransmitters into the synapse. These neurotransmitters are *inhibitory* for spinal neurotags that are nociceptive, ie. the message is dampened.
Action potentials in the descending pro-nociceptive neurones	As above, when a message arrives at the distal end of these projection neurones, it releases neurotransmitters into the synapse. These neurotransmitters are *excitatory* for spinal neurotags that are nociceptive, ie. the message is ramped up.
Local immune set point of immune cells in the spinal neuromatrix	All DIMs and SIMs can influence the spinal neurotags. Individual immune cells can become sensitive to all the AMP gang, which means broad threats become *excitatory* for spinal neurotags.
Systemic immune set point	Remember that the immune cell is part of an immune system that recognises a range of molecular patterns and yet is still under some neural influence as well. So a single immune cell's inflammatory set point reflects both the general set point and local processes.

Table 3.3 Things that modulate the frequency of danger messages which are generated in the spinal nociceptor and ultimately sent to the brain.

neurotags. This in turn increases the frequency of messages in danger transmission nerves that project to the brain. Increased nociception arriving at the brain probably moves the Protectometer level up.

You're almost there – the finale here is that exactly the same process will occur at every tripartite synapse within the spinal neuromatrix. Each tripartite synapse can influence a million or more others (Nugget 14 *Astrocytes, more popular than the Kardashians*). Therefore, DIMs stand to influence not just incoming nociception, but also descending pro-nociceptive influences (descending facilitation). The broad range of factors that will ultimately determine the danger message that is sent to the brain can be broadly grouped according to Table 3.3.

The vast array of mechanisms that influence the spinal neurotag are further evidence of interdependence and redundancy. The really important implications for any intervention that involves adding something to the biological pot are:

(i) you can't alter how one system works without being sure there won't be a carry-on effect on another system (interdependence), and

(ii) even if you remove one contributor, for instance nociception, to an outcome, there will almost certainly be other contributors that can evoke the same outcome (redundancy).

These things also make it very difficult to reverse one problem, the whole problem and nothing but the problem in any situation that is biologically complex – for example chronic pain.

Part D

Central sensitisation

A quick background: There are three important mechanisms by which nociceptive neurotags are more readily activated by noxious tissue based events. These are (i) enhanced sensitivity of danger detection, (ii) ectopic pacemakers in primary nociceptors, and (iii) enhanced sensitivity of danger transmission.

Sensitised danger detection equates to peripheral sensitisation, which is discussed earlier in this chapter. Just as an ectopic pregnancy is pregnancy in the wrong place, an ectopic pacemaker is impulse generation in the wrong place – the middle of the axon. Ectopic pacemakers have been identified in animal and human studies and they are exactly as they sound – malfunctioning primary nociceptors (perhaps through injury) that continually trigger action potentials in the absence of any change in tissue environment. There was a flurry of research on ectopic pacemakers in the 1980's and 90's, and as a result there is quite a volume of heavy reading on them for those of you who are keen [83-87]. Whether or not ectopic pacemakers play a major role in human pain states has not really been determined although there is some evidence to suggest they might [88]. What is certain however, is that an ectopic pacemaker in a primary nociceptor is neither sufficient nor necessary for pain.

Central Sensitisation (Version 1)

Enhanced sensitivity of danger transmission in the central nervous system is called central sensitisation. It might mean two different things. Lets start with Version 1. Much of what we learnt about central sensitisation came from the research group of a fellow called Sir Clifford Woolf.[22] Woolf is a South African by birth; he has medical and research degrees from 'Wits' University and he did a good chunk of his research training under the Uber Grand Daddy Sir Patrick Wall.[23] Woolf led the research that first recorded altered response profiles in the dorsal horn neurones of animals and ultimately showed that opioids can nullify central sensitisation – pre-operative analgesia is a clinical practice pretty much attributable to Woolf. His work in animals showing that the spinal nociceptor undergoes functional changes to become

---

22 We are not the only ones who think Prof Woolf should be a Sir, but the people who can actually bestow such titles haven't quite come to the party just yet.

23 Patrick Wall was offered Sir status three times and turned them all down – a rather committed anarchist and anti-monarchist.

more responsive to excitatory neurotransmitters emerged several decades ago [89, 90], but it didn't impact the clinical world in a big way until the current millennium.

There are a couple of crucial bits of biology here. First, when we talk about the bioplasticity of danger transmission, we think about the shift that occurs in the stimulus-response profile of the spinal nociceptor. So, the more or longer a spinal nociceptor is active, the bigger the response to the same stimulus (or the same response to a smaller stimulus). We can label the shift in stimulus-response profile in a more friendly way – *'responsiveness'* or *'sensitivity'*.

Second, the mechanisms by which this happens are astoundingly diverse and, like everything else in biology, there is a lot of redundancy. Each of these mechanisms can be categorised into one of three broadly sequential types of processes.

Increasing baseline voltage across the membrane

Neurones normally have a baseline voltage. It doesn't matter if you don't remember what the voltage is – it's not important. However, remembering that there is a normal baseline is important.

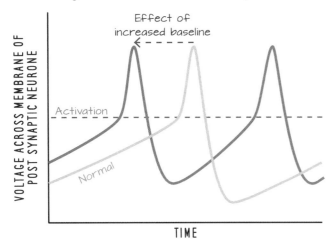

Once the spinal nociceptor becomes active, it starts to become more efficient. This might involve:

- activation of pumps that remove by-products of depolarisation, reducing the risk of 'message fatigue'
- activation of pumps that remove negative ions, bringing the voltage up a little
- internal molecular cascades that convert molecules into new versions that are easier to eject from the neurone. This increases the efficiency of repolarisation.

There are many other processes and it is beyond this book (and us!) to reel them all off. The key message is that they can all increase the baseline voltage making the spinal nociceptor quicker to fire because there is less depolarising to do. This adaptation is quick, common and easily reversed.

Increasing the efficiency of the ion channels

Remember that the primary nociceptor has many different kinds of ion channels. So does the spinal nociceptor. These ion channels can become more efficient. Perhaps the grooviest of all of the mechanisms is what we call 'the door stop effect' or the 'velcro team'.

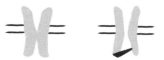

This is when the spinal nociceptor makes a small protein that inserts itself onto the back of the ion channels that are driven by excitatory neurotransmitters. When the ion channel opens, this protein slips into the gap and literally holds it open – just like a door stop. This mechanical effect means that the ion channel stays open longer than normal, allowing more ions to rush in, thus depolarising the spinal nociceptor more quickly. Cool huh? This type of adaptation is a bit slower than the first and more tricky to reverse, but still reversible.

Genetic switches

All of the ion channels that sit in the cell wall of the spinal nociceptor are made in the cell body of the neurone. This is always happening – right now, you have millions of tiny ion channels travelling in the 'Great Axoplasmic Current', inserting themselves into synapses. You are also losing these ion channels at about the same rate as you are making them. The result: you maintain a reasonably constant level of ion channels sitting in the synapse. However, if you increase the rate of manufacture but not the rate of loss, then you clearly have a gradual increase in the density of ion channels in the cell wall – this is the third type of adaptation. It is much slower than the first and much more tricky to reverse.[24]

This understanding of 'Central Sensitisation Version 1' is focused on the spinal nociceptors that serve the painful area. It explains mechanical sensitivity (to external stimuli and to movement) in

---

24 We are always asked *'How long does it take for these adaptations to occur?'* And the answer is always *'It depends'*. And it does depend on many, many things. In short, though – the more active the spinal nociceptor, the quicker the adaptation occurs.

the area surrounding the initial nociceptive event. The research in this area and the experimental findings from humans who volunteered for pain experiments[25] was so compelling that the phrase 'central sensitisation' has now become embedded within our clinical lexicon. Indeed, its profile still seems to be expanding.

Stimulus response patterns

So what does Central Sensitisation Version 1 actually look like? Well, let's walk through a typical scenario that would evoke it. In fact, let's walk through two – an unrealistic but repeatable scenario from the research laboratory and then a more realistic but shaded in uncertainty scenario from the clinic.

Example One: In the lab

Step 1: We place a hot thermode on the skin of a willing and fully informed consenting adult volunteer. This thermode causes a small burn about the size of a pea.

Step 2: We wait.

Step 3: The damaged area of skin may be spontaneously painful. The pain may have a throbbing quality, which reflects changes in temperature or mechanical stimuli associated with fluctuations in blood pressure caused by one's pulse. We then see a small area of redness that extends beyond the burn site. The extent of the redness will reflect the density of peptidergic nociceptors in the area (this is neurogenic inflammation at work). The area of skin that is red will be both heat-sensitive and mechanically sensitive. This sensitivity is caused by peripheral sensitisation.

Step 4: A couple of hours later, by gently running a (clean) toothbrush across the skin, we can map the boundaries of a slightly larger area – let's say about the size of a date – inside of which the brushing evokes low level pain, or at least a clearly more intense, less comfortable sensation. This sensitivity is caused by the first phase of Central Sensitisation Version 1.

Step 5: Between 6 and 12 hours later again, we test the sensitivity to a pinprick. This time, we can map an even larger area, about the size of a small mandarin, inside of which the stimulus evokes a clearly more intense pain. This sensitivity is caused by the second phase of Central Sensitisation Version 1.

Step 6: Somewhere in the next 12 or so hours, careful testing of pin prick responses on the corresponding location on the

opposite side of the body, reveals another area, about the size of a fig, that is sensitive. This sensitivity is *not* caused by Central Sensitisation Version 1, and this discovery, some time ago, should have alerted us early on to a problem with taking Central Sensitisation Version 1 into the real world of clinical practice.

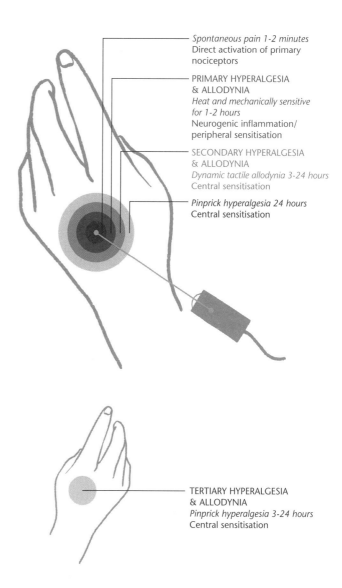

Figure 3.10 Central sensitisation in the lab

---

25 These humans who volunteer for pain experiments are probably not normal people – they are, after all, volunteering for pain experiments, however, we are very grateful for their support.

Example Two: In the real world

We can repeat the above in a real world situation. Take the scenario of a twisted ankle.

Step 1: Injury occurs. Unlike the experimental situation, we don't know exactly what stimulus has been delivered.

Step 2: We don't necessarily see any redness because the injury is not in the skin. However, we have peptidergic nociceptors in the area, therefore the area around the damage (roughly the size of a date) becomes heat and mechanically sensitive. Clinically we could heat the ankle (not that we would!), or poke it, and this date-sized area of sensitivity would be 'mappable' if you wanted to draw on the ankle.

Step 3: We see the area of mechanical sensitivity increase over the following hours. The area of heat sensitivity does not increase much – peripheral sensitisation is determined by how far the inflammatory mediators travel, and by the density of peptidergic nociceptors in the area. As Central Sensitisation Version 1 trundles on, the area of mechanical sensitivity might become as big as a fig, for example.

Step 4: The next day, careful testing might reveal that the opposite ankle is mechanically sensitive too. This sensitivity is NOT caused by Central Sensitisation Version 1. *This discovery well over a decade ago, should have alerted us early on to a problem with taking Central Sensitisation Version 1 into the real world of clinical practice* (Nugget 34 *Mirror pains*).

Problems with Central Sensitisation Version 1

So, what's the problem with Central Sensitisation Version 1? Well, not long after it became mainstream (there was a time not too long ago when central sensitisation was more popular in some circles than a banana in a monkey shop), we hit a problem: it does not actually explain the vast majority of persistent pain states [91, 92]. In fact, it became clear that in most people with persistent pain, the sensitivity to noxious and non-noxious stimuli extends well beyond the area of the body that is served by the spinal nociceptors that were originally involved. The sensitivity can spread across half the body [93, 94] or, more often, across the entire body [95]. In response, Sir Clifford Woolf, shifted the field again by suggesting that central sensitisation be used to describe any sensitivity that is not explained by peripheral sensitisation [96]. This new revised version of central sensitisation can be summarised like this:

Central sensitisation refers to reduced pain thresholds to non-noxious stimuli and increased pain evoked by noxious stimuli in tissues not affected by peripheral sensitisation.

Central Sensitisation (Version 2)

Central Sensitisation Version 2 does not allude to mechanism. It now encompasses everything that is *not* peripheral sensitisation, whereas before it referred to an adaptation in very specific neurones. We suspect that many well-meaning clinicians and scientists haven't realised this yet and are still equating broad based changes in nociceptive sensitivity to sensitisation of a small number of spinal nociceptors. But, this new understanding is completely in line with the Grand Poobah Pain Theory and very much supportive of the biopsychosociality of pain. Persistent pain is characterised by a multitude of mechanisms aside from peripheral sensitisation and these mechanisms involve spinal, brain, neural, immune, endocrine, cognitive, behavioural, perceptual and autonomic processes among others. This is completely in line with the Explain Pain revolution.

What would a pain state explained by peripheral sensitisation look like? Geronimo presents with a three-year history of pain in a reasonably confined anatomical distribution. The tissue is mechanically sensitive – particular movements are painful and the nature of painful movements has not changed since onset. The pain is increased by warmth – when asked whether a hot pack feels nice or nasty, his answer is a rapid *'nasty'*. The painful area throbs and has not spread or moved since onset.

This sort of presentation is pretty uncommon huh? Sure enough, there are conditions that can involve peripheral sensitisation alongside other mechanisms – inflammatory joint disease flare-ups are one example – but it is not often that peripheral sensitisation will be the obvious and potent explanation for someone's persistent pain state. Sensitisation of the spinal nociceptor doesn't explain many persistent pain states either because they have patterns of sensitivity that extend well beyond the area of the body that is served by the relevant spinal nociceptors.

However, our new appreciation of the complexity of the dorsal horn means we can conceptualise central sensitisation according to the principles that govern neurotags (Chapter 2). That is, repeated activation of a spinal neurotag leads to increased synaptic efficacy between its constituent cells (neuro-neural, neuro-glial and glio-glial). Increased efficacy of these connections increases their influence on other cells and spinal neurotags. Ultimately, these influences are exerted on the spinal nociceptor.

At a cell-to-cell level, we can think about it in terms of *probability gradients* – how much more is one cell likely to be activated than another cell? Sound confusing? Check out

Figure 3.11, which depicts this situation and the following text will walk you through what we mean.

Note below the spinal neurotag arising from the dorsal horn of the spinal cord, the output of which is to exert an excitatory influence on a spinal nociceptor. That cell can be considered a 'member cell' (orange) and its neighbours are 'non-member cells' (black). On the bottom panels each of the columns depict the probability that each of the cells above will fire.

- In a **normal state**, an excitatory influence on that member cell (orange) has a set chance of activating it. The excitatory influence might be a primary nociceptor. The likelihood that *that* primary nociceptor will activate its target member cell might be 50%, and the likelihood it will activate the non-member cells ranges from 15% down.

- In a **sensitised state**, where synaptic efficacy between the primary nociceptor and the spinal neurotag is enhanced, the relative probability of activating the member cell is increased, perhaps to 90%, whereas the likelihood of activating non-member cells is unaffected. This means that the primary nociceptive input is more influential. In this case, the pain will become worse (hyperalgesia) or require less primary nociceptive input (allodynia).

- In the presence of **descending facilitative**, or pro-nociceptive input (blue) on a non-member cell, which itself is a member cell of a different spinal neurotag, which itself exerts its influence on a nearby spinal nociceptor, the probabilities might change again. Here, the primary nociceptor still has a 50% chance of activating its target member cell but also a 50% chance of activating the other 'primed' cell. In this case, pain will spread.

- In the presence of **descending inhibitory**, or anti-nociceptive input (red), the probabilities are all reduced. This will result in analgesia. See flat probability graph below.

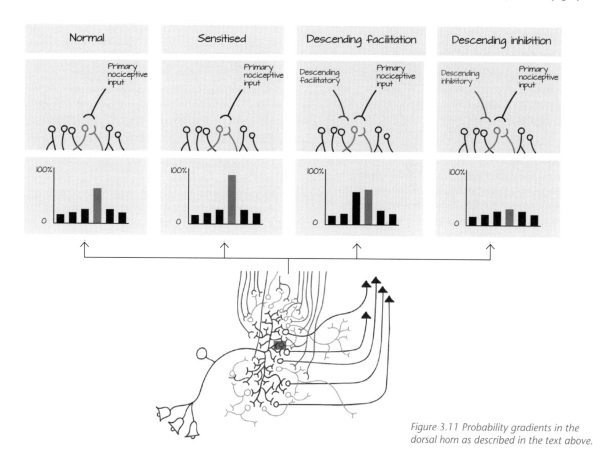

Figure 3.11 Probability gradients in the dorsal horn as described in the text above.

The beauty of bioplasticity

We have a saying in the *Explain Pain Handbook: Protectometer*, which resonates really well with people in pain. It goes like this:

'Bioplasticity got you into this mess and bioplasticity can get you out again.' [26] [97]

The fearful and wonderful complexity of the spinal cord should leave us thinking about it in the same way we think about the brain – a mass of neurotags collaborating and competing for influence. Bioplasticity means that those neurotags that are active become more influential by virtue of changes in the stimulus-response profile of their member cells. The processes that occur are versions of those processes that have been identified in Central Sensitisation Version 1 (page 69).

Let's travel up the danger transmission system into the brain. The location is different but the biological mechanisms are broadly the same – the more that neurotags are active, the more responsive they become to any excitatory input.

Increased responsiveness of protective neurotags

The functional impact of increased responsiveness of any neurotag will depend on the influence of that neurotag, and whether that neurotag is an action neurotag or a modulation neurotag. Let's take an action neurotag such as that which produces pain. There are no surprises here – increased responsiveness of the pain neurotag will mean that pain occurs when things are less dangerous. Because the pain neurotag is influenced by any credible evidence of danger in me (a DIM), then the pain neurotag becomes more responsive to all DIMs. Let's take a modulation neurotag such as that which represents the broad concept of *'the low back is vulnerable'*. The more this neurotag is activated, the more responsive it becomes and the more influence it can have on protective action neurotags, most obviously pain, but also on the action neurotag that produces the thought *'my back is damaged'* and makes you say *'my back is damaged'* or *'my back is totally wrecked!'*

The most important implication of bioplasticity is that every neurotag can become more responsive if it is activated enough. This means that every DIM can slowly increase its influence over time – even DIMs you hear, such as *'Bill's got a bad back'* and DIMs you say such as *'it's bone on bone in there'*. This is one reason it is important for people in pain and their well-meaning loved ones to stop saying these things. That every neurotag

can become more responsive if it is activated enough is also reason to find and practice SIMs. The more a SIM neurotag is activated, the more easily it will be activated and the more influential it will become. This principle is at the core of modern pain biology and rehabilitation. It is not easy, but the highest level of scientific evidence tells us that it is doable.

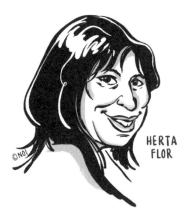

HERTA FLOR

Smudging neurotags

Just a little more hardcore neuroimmune biology – hang in there. Reflect on the exciting discovery that immune cells are critical for healthy synaptic operation. It is the balance between pro-inflammatory and anti-inflammatory cytokines released by the immune cells that modulates the efficiency of a synapse. These cytokines activate receptor sites on pre and post-synaptic membranes. Microglia travel around the central nervous system checking in and monitoring synaptic activity on the hour, every hour, rain, hail or shine. Consider this – these microglia can 'move towards a thought[27]' and in the case of a persistent DIM, such as *'it's bone on bone'*, it is completely feasible that these microglia can 'stake out' the very brain cells that make up the *'it's bone on bone'* neurotag. Wow!

The capacity of microglia to move and create tiny pockets of inflammation at different locations is probably important in causing some pretty profound changes in the stimulus-response profile of specific brain regions. We know these changes occur in people with persistent pain. Perhaps the most important scientist working on this stuff is Prof Herta Flor. Herta is an experimental and clinical psychologist, neuroscientist, brain imager and clinical trialist. Her work has been funded by

---

26 This is a key Target Concept – see Chapter 5, page 128.

27 This luscious phrase would more accurately be 'microglia move towards a thought's neurotag'.

gazillions of euros, pounds and US dollars and is a large part of why the entire pain field has become interested in brain abnormalities as a possible contributor to persistent pain.

A seminal study by Herta and colleagues involved people who were suffering from phantom limb pain years after arm amputation [98]. Herta applied stimuli to either side of their lip and recorded activation in the primary sensory cortex (S1). In order to understand why her study was so important, it is critical to revisit the cortical body matrix theory and the role of S1 and the secondary sensory cortex (S2) in bodily awareness. S1 and S2 are critical for feeling stimuli on our skin (S1) or deeper tissues (S2), but those cells alone are insufficient to 'hold' these sensations.

Let's focus on S1 because we know a great deal about S1 and much less about S2. To reiterate – S1 does not 'hold' the sense of touch. If you have learnt about the sensory homunculus [EP22], you might find this a bit surprising. Experiments have shown that when a tactile stimulus is delivered to the skin, the magnitude of the response in S1 is the same whether or not the person notices they've been touched. That is, whether or not you feel a touch does not depend on activity in S1. The sense of touch actually depends on distributed processing in multiple brain areas [99].

This reality makes total sense when we think about it in terms of neurotags. Remember the principle of single cell insufficiency (page 23). We can be very confident that cells in S1 form part of 'tactile stimulus neurotags'. These 'tactile stimulus neurotags' would be considered modulation neurotags and they would be highly influential over 'touch neurotags'. These touch neurotags would be considered action neurotags because their output is a conscious event. They are highly influenced by tactile stimulus neurotags but, as the experiment mentioned above tells us, tactile stimulation is neither sufficient nor necessary for feeling touch. Experiments have demonstrated the latter – visual stimuli can evoke the sense of touch on areas of skin that are actually numb [100]. The rubber hand illusion also shows that visual stimulus neurotags (modulation neurotags) can also influence sense of touch neurotags (action neurotags) because one *feels* the touch on the rubber hand [101].

Why is this important for understanding Herta's marvellous study? Well, when Herta applied stimuli to both sides of the lip of these amputees, she found that the area of S1 that was activated was different between sides. For the side of the amputation, the lip activated an area of S1[28] that normally

responds to stimulation of the fingers. What is more, they found that the degree to which the lip 'invaded' that of the hand correlated with the amount of phantom limb pain. Since that study, there have been enough studies that show abnormalities of S1 activation in people with chronic pain to warrant a few reviews putting it all into context [74, 102, 103]. The general picture that has emerged is that S1 becomes functionally 'smudged' when pain persists. *This means that outputs become less predictable and less precise.*

Unpredictable. Imprecise. Inflammation.

How does this happen? The most likely explanation is an inflammatory effect at the tripartite synapses in S1. We started this section reminding you of what effect the immune cells can have on the efficiency of the synapse. If the astrocyte, or perhaps the microglia that can transport themselves to different brain areas, turns up its output of pro-inflammatory cytokines, these cytokines escape the local area and have excitatory effects on nearby cells. This means that a targeted input to S1 can evoke a very *un*-targeted response in S1. It's kind of like when someone picks on one member of a gang, the whole gang responds. Because all these S1 cells are part of modulation neurotags that exert influence over a range of action neurotags, one might feel two touches instead of one, or touch in the wrong place, or a large stimulus instead of a small one. Manual therapists may recognise this when a patient says *'you are pushing really hard'* when you are hardly touching them. In this scenario, the detectors might be working perfectly; the transmission mechanisms might be working perfectly; but the perception is very dodgy indeed.

Now remember that brain cells are multitasking cells. This means that the imprecision caused by pro-inflammatory cytokines will affect all the tasks that cell is involved in. For example, when it comes to pain, the pain will spread – not in a classic peripheral nerve or a spinal segmental distribution. The pain might spread in a manner consistent with the sensory homunculus, even in odd anatomically remote sites. If the problem is occurring in S2 cells, the spread will be consistent with S2 – a regional spread (for example, down a whole leg or from the low back to the upper back).

Smudging can be conceptualised in terms of probability gradients. The inflammatory process can make these gradients much flatter, by elevating the probability that surrounding cells will fire in response to a targeted input.

---

28   Of course this is the side of the brain *opposite* to the amputation.

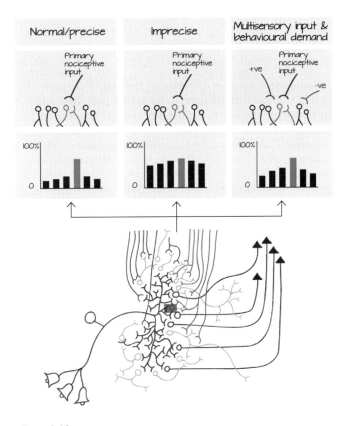

Figure 3.12

As we can see in Figure 3.12, and as we saw in Figure 3.11, in the normal and precise state, the primary nociceptive input is associated with steep activation gradients such that the member (orange) cell is much more likely to fire than its neighbours are.

In the second panel in Figure 3.12, the 'imprecise' state, the member cell and its neighbours are equally likely to fire – the activation gradient is flat. This is probably the result of a local pro-inflammatory state.

The final panel in Figure 3.12 shows how we can reinstate some precision. By adding some specific input, shown by a little +ve and a little -ve sign, the activation gradient is restored somewhat, so that the member cell is more likely to fire than its neighbours are.

Finally, you might see that the last panel is not as precise as the normal situation, but if you keep training it, it gets more and more precise.

Smudging – it's not just an S1 thang

One reason that scientists are attributing smudging to an inflammatory process is that it occurs in other brain areas too. Another highly studied area of the brain when it comes to smudging is the primary motor cortex (M1). Smudging in M1 has direct effects on action neurotags that produce movement. Clinically, this should result in dystonia and reduced fine motor control, both of which are observed in people with persistent pain. In short – the probability gradients become flatter – so that targeted input can result in very un-targeted outputs, just as we see in S1 [103].

There is no reason to suggest that these inflammation-mediated problems are limited to S1 and M1 – it's just that S1 and M1 are relatively easy to assess with current scientific methods. It is reasonable to suggest that similar problems will occur around other brain cells involved in protection neurotags. This will have broad implications, potentially explaining the perceptual problems reported by people with persistent pain, the movement problems, the touch problems and the spatial processing problems. That is, these inflammation-mediated problems might explain all the disruptions we see in the cortical body matrix in people with persistent pain (Chapter 2) [74].

And now for the good news!

Although the impact of smudging can be quite marked and there is a good argument that it generates a range of DIMs, the good news is that normal business can be reinstated reasonably easily by recruiting the brain's inbuilt plasticity mechanisms. Again, it was Herta and her group of willing amputees who kicked off our understanding here – she undertook 'tactile discrimination training' – the patients received stimuli at different locations on their stump with the simple task of identifying the location of each stimulus [104]. In two weeks, S1 activation had become more normal, tactile acuity had improved and phantom limb pain had reduced. Critically, the change in all three variables related really well, strongly suggesting that the location discriminating had produced the changes. There is now a range of techniques that use discrimination training of one type or another to treat persistent pain [105]. Graded Motor Imagery (GMI), devised to treat complex regional pain syndrome (CRPS), is one example [106, 107]. GMI also integrates principles of graded exposure and randomised controlled trials suggest it is helpful for persistent CRPS and phantom limb pain [108] (anecdotally, it is helpful for a range of painful disorders, but clinical trials are still to be undertaken). Along with Tim Beames and Tom Giles, we wrote a book on GMI. *The Graded Motor Imagery Handbook* [109] goes into much more detail on both the rationale and delivery of GMI. Tactile discrimination training is a version of Herta's sensory discrimination training but is now being used for CRPS and back pain [110-112] and others are trialling it in a range of other painful disorders.

Detailed coverage of GMI, tactile discrimination training or other explicit discrimination based approaches is beyond this book, but the general principle takes you halfway there. Any task that requires the participant to discriminate between two similar stimuli or actions, will serve to normalise probability gradients. In theory, you can apply this principle to every situation in which you observe a loss of discriminatory ability. It is often useful to recruit mechanisms that improve precision – most obviously visual feedback or other versions of multisensory feedback. This can have immense explanatory power by using the rapid effects that you impart to reinforce how bioplastic we all are and how important easily modifiable, non-tissue based disruptions can be to someone's pain problem.

The grand finale – a pain mechanisms cheat sheet

A thorough assessment of someone in pain is no trivial undertaking. The up to date health professional will want a full picture of not just the pain, but the impact that pain is having on the person, their wellbeing, their relationships, engagement in work and other meaningful activities, and the person's own goals and expectations moving forward. A critical part of the full assessment, however, is evaluating the likely biological processes that are contributing to someone's pain. We could try to talk you through it, but the deliciously complex cheat sheet (on page 79) summarises it. As is always the case when it comes to biology and to an experience that is as individually unique as any experience can be, the arrows on the cheat sheet are general principles and considerations, not hard fast, non-negotiable rules.[29]

A couple of things from this cheat sheet need a quick explanation. You will see that there are two entries under 'QST'. QST stands for 'quantitative sensory testing' and can only be done properly with rather expensive equipment (like $30,000+) so most clinicians will not have access to it. However, QST is popular at the moment and soon neurologists will not be the only ones with the gear to perform it. German neurologists are particularly fond of QST and they have compiled some impressive databases of what 'normal' results might look like, matched to gender and age [113]. They have also compiled some rough 'signatures' of QST results for particular neuropathic pain diagnoses [114]. Given what we all now know about neurotags and the truly biopsychosocial nature of pain, it's no surprise that these signatures are messy and that no clinician in their right mind would rely on QST results alone to make any sort of diagnosis. In fact, there is sufficient debate about what QST results really mean to wonder whether they will fall off the radar as quickly as they emerged. Time will tell.

The two QST-based metrics that are of most relevance here are wind-up and poor DNIC, or descending noxious inhibitory control. The reason we have singled them out is that they can give some hint as to whether there is impaired or downregulated descending inhibition (anti-nociception) or augmented or upregulated descending facilitation (pro-nociception).

---

29 Note the similarities between the cheat sheet and the pain mechanisms model in Chapter 6 (Figure 6.2)

Some researchers believe that impaired descending inhibition can be tested by comparing the pain evoked by a fixed noxious stimulus, which is called 'the test stimulus' (let's say it is a 44°C thermode), before and after delivering a different noxious stimulus, for example putting one's hand in an ice water bath (known as 'the conditioning stimulus'). If the pain of the test stimulus lessens when it is applied after the conditioning stimulus, this decrease is attributed to descending inhibition. If the pain of the test stimulus is no different between conditions, or is worse after the conditioning stimulus, then descending inhibition is said to be impaired.

The presence of wind-up, or 'temporal summation', is tested by delivering repeated noxious stimuli at less than 1 second intervals [115]. The participant reports the pain evoked by each stimulus. A positive finding of temporal summation is one where the same stimulus evokes more and more intense pain. Temporal summation is clear evidence that there is sensitisation within spinal neurotags concerned with nociception, and some consider this type of response is mediated by descending facilitation. At the time of writing, the jury is still out, so linking temporal summation to upregulated descending facilitation remains a bit speculative.

Back to the very beginning?

Congratulations! You have made your way through what we think are the critical bits of biology to adequately supercharge your Explain Pain endeavours. What! Finished here?! In the spinal cord?! Well, that's the trick, we are really back to the beginning – it might be worth you heading back now to Chapter 2 which focused more on the brain, the concept of neurotags and the truly fearful and wonderful complexity of what goes on inside your skull.

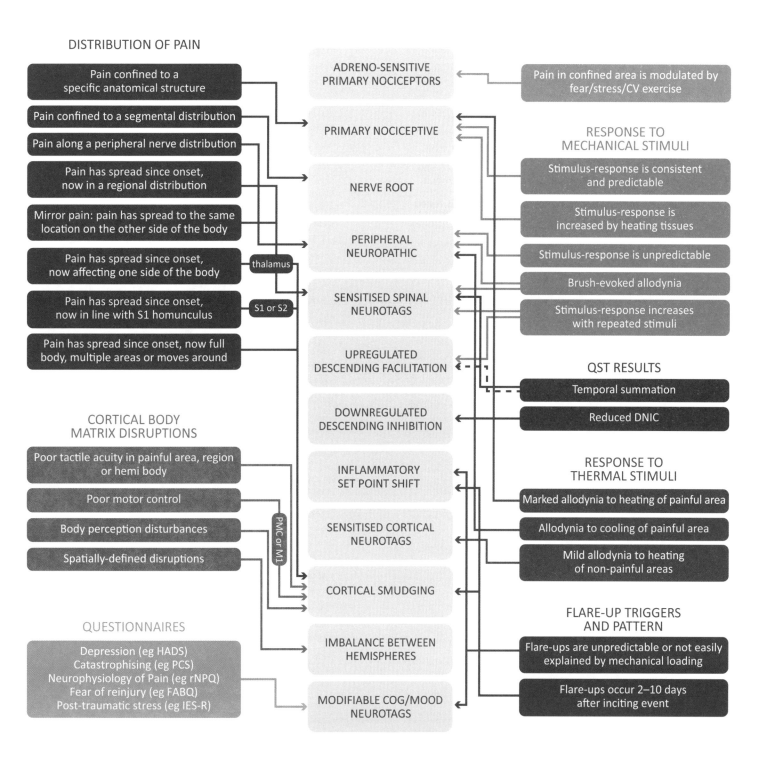

DISTRIBUTION OF PAIN

Pain confined to a specific anatomical structure

Pain confined to a segmental distribution

Pain along a peripheral nerve distribution

Pain has spread since onset, now in a regional distribution

Mirror pain: pain has spread to the same location on the other side of the body

Pain has spread since onset, now affecting one side of the body

Pain has spread since onset, now in line with S1 homunculus

Pain has spread since onset, now full body, multiple areas or moves around

thalamus

S1 or S2

CORTICAL BODY MATRIX DISRUPTIONS

Poor tactile acuity in painful area, region or hemi body

Poor motor control

Body perception disturbances

Spatially-defined disruptions

PMC or M1

QUESTIONNAIRES

Depression (eg HADS)
Catastrophising (eg PCS)
Neurophysiology of Pain (eg rNPQ)
Fear of reinjury (eg FABQ)
Post-traumatic stress (eg IES-R)

ADRENO-SENSITIVE PRIMARY NOCICEPTORS

PRIMARY NOCICEPTIVE

NERVE ROOT

PERIPHERAL NEUROPATHIC

SENSITISED SPINAL NEUROTAGS

UPREGULATED DESCENDING FACILITATION

DOWNREGULATED DESCENDING INHIBITION

INFLAMMATORY SET POINT SHIFT

SENSITISED CORTICAL NEUROTAGS

CORTICAL SMUDGING

IMBALANCE BETWEEN HEMISPHERES

MODIFIABLE COG/MOOD NEUROTAGS

Pain in confined area is modulated by fear/stress/CV exercise

RESPONSE TO MECHANICAL STIMULI

Stimulus-response is consistent and predictable

Stimulus-response is increased by heating tissues

Stimulus-response is unpredictable

Brush-evoked allodynia

Stimulus-response increases with repeated stimuli

QST RESULTS

Temporal summation

Reduced DNIC

RESPONSE TO THERMAL STIMULI

Marked allodynia to heating of painful area

Allodynia to cooling of painful area

Mild allodynia to heating of non-painful areas

FLARE-UP TRIGGERS AND PATTERN

Flare-ups are unpredictable or not easily explained by mechanical loading

Flare-ups occur 2–10 days after inciting event

References

1. Butler DS & Moseley GL (2013) Explain Pain. 2nd Edn. Noigroup Publications: Adelaide.

2. Wall PD & McMahon SB (1986) The relationship of perceived pain to afferent nerve impulses. Trends Neurosci 9: 254-255.

3. Bevan S (1999) Nociceptive peripheral neurons: cellular properties, in Textbook of pain, Wall PD & Melzack R Eds. Churchill Livingstone: Edinburgh.

4. Melzack R, Rose G & McGinty D (1962) Skin sensitivity to thermal stimuli. Exp Neurol 6: 300-314.

5. Meyer RA, Campbell JN & Srinivasa NR (1994) Peripheral neural mechanisms of nociception, in Textbook of Pain, Wall PD & Melzack R Eds. Churchill Livingstone: Edinburgh.

6. Treede RD (2009) The adequate stimulus, in Science of Pain, Basbaum AI & Bushnell MC Eds. Academic: Oxford.

7. Abraira VE & Ginty DD (2013) The sensory neurons of touch. Neuron 79: 618-639.

8. Ruffini A (1894) Di un nuovo organo nervoso terminale e sulla presenza dei corpuscoli Golgi-Mazzoni nel connettivo sottocutaneo dei polpastrelli delle dita dell'uomo. Tipografia della R. Accademia dei Lincei: Roma.

9. Chambers MR, et al. (1972) The structure and function of the slowly adapting type II mechanoreceptor in hairy skin. Q J Exp Physiol Cogn Med Sci 57: 417-445.

10. Melzack R & Wall PD (1965) Pain mechanisms: a new theory. Science 150: 971-979.

11. Merkel F (1875) Tastzellen und Tastkörperchen bei den Hausthieren und beim Menschen. Arch Mikrosk Anat 11: 636-652.

12. Woodbury CJ & Koerber HR (2007) Central and peripheral anatomy of slowly adapting type I low-threshold mechanoreceptors innervating trunk skin of neonatal mice. J Comp Neurol 505: 547-561.

13. Torebjork HE & Ochoa JL (1980) Specific sensations evoked by activity in single identified sensory units in man. Acta Physiol Scand 110: 445-447.

14. Bolton CF, Winkelmann RK & Dyck PJ (1966) A quantitative study of Meissner's corpuscles in man. Neurology 16: 1-9.

15. JÄnig W, Schmidt RF & Zimmermann M (1968) Single unit responses and the total afferent outflow from the cat's foot pad upon mechanical stimulation. Exp Brain Res 6: 100-115.

16. Formby C, et al. (1992) The role of frequency selectivity in measures of auditory and vibrotactile temporal resolution. J Acoust Soc Am 91: 293-305.

17. Thomas PK & Olsson Y (1975) Microscopic anatomy and function of the connective tissue components of peripheral nerve, in Peripheral Neuropathy, Dyck PJ, Thomas PK & Lambert EH Ed. WB Saunders: Philadelphia.

18. Bourane S, et al. (2009) Low-Threshold Mechanoreceptor Subtypes Selectively Express MafA and Are Specified by Ret Signaling. Neuron 64: 857-870.

19. Luo W, et al. (2009) Molecular Identification of Rapidly Adapting Mechanoreceptors and Their Developmental Dependence on Ret Signaling. Neuron 64: 841-856.

20. Li L, et al. (2011) The Functional Organization of Cutaneous Low-Threshold Mechanosensory Neurons. Cell 147: 1615-1627.

21. Millard CL & Woolf CJ (1988) Sensory innervation of the hairs of the rat hindlimb: a light microscopic analysis. J Comp Neurol 277: 183-194.

22. Wu H, et al. (2012) Morphologic diversity of cutaneous sensory afferents revealed by genetically directed sparse labeling. eLife 1: e00181.

23. McGlone F, et al. (2007) Discriminative touch and emotional touch. Can J Exp Psychol 61: 173-83.

24. Seal RP, et al. (2009) Injury-induced mechanical hypersensitivity requires C-low threshold mechanoreceptors. Nature 462: 651-655.

25. Lou S, et al. (2013) Runx1 controls terminal morphology and mechanosensitivity of VGLUT3-expressing C-mechanoreceptors. J Neurosci 33: 870-882.

26. Treede RD, Meyar RA & Campbell JN (1998) Myelinated mechanically insensitive afferents from monkey hairy skin: heat-response properties. J Neurophysiol 80: 1082-1093.

27. Burgess PR & Perl ER (1967) Myelinated afferent fibres responding specifically to noxious stimulation of the skin. J Physiol 190: 541-562.

28. Ploner M, et al. (2002) Cortical representation of first and second pain sensation in humans. Proc Natl Acad Sci USA 99: 12444-12448.

29. Basbaum AI, et al. (2009) Cellular and molecular mechanisms of pain. Cell 139: 267-284.

30. Woolf CJ & Ma Q (2007) Nociceptors – noxious stimulus detectors. Neuron 55: 353-364.

31. Patwardhan AM, et al. (2009) Activation of TRPV1 in the spinal cord by oxidized linoleic acid metabolites contributes to inflammatory hyperalgesia. Proc Natl Acad Sci USA 106: 18820-18824.

32. Hogestatt ED, et al. (2005) Conversion of acetaminophen to the bioactive N-acylphenolamine AM404 via fatty acid amide hydrolase-dependent arachidonic acid conjugation in the nervous system. J Biol Chem 280: 31405-31412.

33. Talavera K, et al. (2009) Nicotine activates the chemosensory cation channel TRPA1. Nat Neurosci 12: 1293-1299.

34. Nagatomo K & Kubo Y (2008) Caffeine activates mouse TRPA1 channels but suppresses human TRPA1 channels. Proc Natl Acad Sci USA 105: 17373-17378.

35. Andersson DA, et al. (2011) TRPA1 mediates spinal antinociception induced by acetaminophen and the cannabinoid Δ^9-tetrahydrocannabiorcol. Nat Commun 2: 551.

36. Kwan KY, et al. (2006) TRPA1 contributes to cold, mechanical, and chemical nociception but is not essential for hair-cell transduction. Neuron 50: 277-289.

37. Ferguson KL, et al. (1997) Tumor necrosis factor activity increases in the early response to trauma. Acad Emerg Med 4: 1035-1040.

38. Keel M, et al. (1996) Different pattern of local and systemic release of proinflammatory and anti-inflammatory mediators in severely injured patients with chest trauma. J Trauma 40: 907-912.

39. Nast-Kolb D, et al. (1997) Indicators of the posttraumatic inflammatory response correlate with organ failure in patients with multiple injuries. J Trauma 42: 446-454.

40. Koller M, et al. (1998) Major injury induces increased production of interleukin-10 in human granulocyte fractions. Langenbecks Arch Surg 383: 460-465.

41. Xing Z, et al. (1998) IL-6 is an antiinflammatory cytokine required for controlling local or systemic acute inflammatory responses. J Clin Invest 101: 311-320.

42. Tilg H, et al. (1994) Interleukin-6 (IL-6) as an anti-inflammatory cytokine: induction of circulating IL-1 receptor antagonist and soluble tumor necrosis factor receptor p55. Blood 83: 113-118.

43. Brøchner AC & Toft P (2009) Pathophysiology of the systemic inflammatory response after major accidental trauma. Scand J Trauma Resusc Emerg Med 17: 1-10.

44. Brederson JD & Honda CN (2015) Primary afferent neurons express functional delta opioid receptors in inflamed skin. Brain Res 1614: 105-111.

45. Lerner UH (2002) Neuropeptidergic regulation of bone resorption and bone formation. J Musculoskelet Neuronal Interact 2: 440-447.

46. Black PH (2002) Stress and the inflammatory response: a review of neurogenic inflammation. Brain Behav Immun 16: 622-653.

47. Kipnis J, et al. (2004) T cell deficiency leads to cognitive dysfunction: implications for therapeutic vaccination for schizophrenia and other psychiatric conditions. Proc Natl Acad Sci USA 101: 8180-8185.

48. Brynskikh A, et al. (2008) Adaptive immunity affects learning behavior in mice. Brain Behav Immun 22: 861-869.

49. Ziv Y, et al. (2006) Immune cells contribute to the maintenance of neurogenesis and spatial learning abilities in adulthood. Nat Neurosci 9: 268-275.

50. Derecki NC, et al. (2010) Regulation of learning and memory by meningeal immunity: a key role for IL-4. J Exp Med 207: 1067-1080.

51. Kipnis J, et al. (2008) Immunity and cognition: what do age-related dementia, HIV-dementia and 'chemo-brain' have in common? Trends Immunol 29: 455-463.

52. Yirmiya R & Goshen T (2011) Immune modulation of learning, memory, neural plasticity and neurogenesis. Brain Behav Immun 25: 181-213.

53. Marchand F, Perretti M & McMahon SB (2005) Role of the immune system in chronic pain. Nat Rev Neurosci 6: 521-532.

54. Uceyler N, et al. (2006) Reduced levels of antiinflammatory cytokines in patients with chronic widespread pain. Arthritis Rheum 54: 2656-2664.

55. Dick BD & Rashiq S (2007) Disruption of attention and working memory traces in individuals with chronic pain. Anesth Analg 104: 1223-1229.

56. Goshen I, et al. (2007) A dual role for interleukin-1 in hippocampal-dependent memory processes. Psychoneuroendocrinology 32: 1106-1115.

57. Yirmiya R, Wincour G & Goshen I (2002) Brain interleukin-1 is involved in spatial memory and passive avoidance conditioning. Neurobiol Learn Mem 78: 379-389.

58. Song C, Phillips AG & Leonard B (2003) Interleukin 1 beta enhances conditioned fear memory in rats: possible involvement of glucocorticoids. Eur J Neurosci 18: 1739-1743.

59. Maguire EA, et al. (2000) Navigation-related structural change in the hippocampi of taxi drivers. Proc Natl Acad Sci USA 97: 4398-4403.

60. Arnold MC, et al. (2002) Using an interleukin-6 challenge to evaluate neuropsychological performance in chronic fatigue syndrome. Psychol Med 32: 1075-1089.

61. Kozora E, et al. (2001) Inflammatory and hormonal measures predict neuropsychological functioning in systemic lupus erythematosus and rheumatoid arthritis patients. J Int Neuropsychol Soc 7: 745-754.

62. Shapira-Lichter I, et al. (2008) Cytokines and cholinergic signals co-modulate surgical stress-induced changes in mood and memory. Brain Behav Immun 22: 388-398.

63. Hebb DO (1949) The Organization of Behavior: A Neuropsychological Theory. Wiley, New York.

64. Schneider H, et al. (1998) A neuromodulatory role of interleukin-1beta in the hippocampus. Proc Natl Acad Sci USA 95: 7778-7783.

65. Balschun D, et al. (2004) Interleukin-6: a cytokine to forget. FASEB J 18: 1788-1790.

66. Kaneko M, et al. (2008) Tumor necrosis factor-alpha mediates one component of competitive, experience-dependent plasticity in developing visual cortex. Neuron 58: 673-680.

67. Tracey KJ (2009) Reflex control of immunity. Nat Rev Immunol 9: 418-428.

68. Wallwork SB, et al. (2016) The blink reflex magnitude is continuously adjusted according to both current and predicted stimulus position with respect to the face. Cortex 81: 168-175.

69. Tracey KJ (2002) The inflammatory reflex. Nature 420: 853-859.

70. Watkins LR, et al. (1995) Blockade of interleukin-1 induced hyperthermia by subdiaphragmatic vagotomy: evidence for vagal mediation of immune-brain communication. Neurosci Lett 183: 27-31.

71. Nicotra L, et al. (2012) Toll-like receptors in chronic pain. Exp Neurol 234: 316-329.

72. Bechara A & Damasio AR (2005) The Somatic Marker Hypothesis: A neural theory of economic decision. Game Econ Behav 52: 336-372.

73. Craig AD (2002) How do you feel? Interoception: the sense of the physiological condition of the body. Nature Rev Neurosci 3: 655-666.

74. Moseley GL, Gallace A & Spence C (2012) Bodily illusions in health and disease: physiological and clincial perspectives and the concept of a cortical 'body matrix'. Neurosci Biobehav Rev 36: 34-46.

75. Moseley GM, et al. (2008) Psychologically induced cooling of a specific body part caused by the illusory ownership of an artificial counterpart. Proc Natl Acad Sci USA 105: 13169-13173.

76. Barnsley N, et al. (2011) The rubber hand illusion increases histamine reactivity in the real arm. Curr Biol 21: R945-946.

77. Madden VJ & Moseley GL (2016) Do clinicians think that pain can be a classically conditioned response to a non-noxious stimulus? Man Ther 22: 165-173.

78. Fitzgerald M (2005) The development of nociceptive circuits. Nat Rev Neurosci 6: 507-520.

79. Andrews K & Fitzgerald M (1994) The cutaneous withdrawal reflex in human neonates: sensitization, receptive fields, and the effects of contralateral stimulation. Pain 56: 95-101.

80. Anand P & Birch R (2002) Restoration of sensory function and lack of long-term chronic pain syndromes after brachial plexus injury in human neonates. Brain 125: 113-122.

81. Reid E, et al. (2015) Spatial summation of pain in humans investigated using transcutaneous electrical stimulation. J Pain 16: 11-18.

82. Stanton TR, et al. (2016) Modulation of pain via expectation of its location. Eur J Pain, 20: 753-766.

83. Chen Y & Devor M (1998) Ectopic mechanosensitivity in injured sensory axons arises from the site of spontaneous electrogenesis. Eur J Pain 2: 165-178.

84. Devor M & Govrin-Lippmann R (1983) Axoplasmic transport block reduces ectopic impulse generation in injured peripheral nerves. Pain 16: 73-85.

85. Han HC, Lee DH & Chung JM (2000) Characteristics of ectopic discharges in a rat neuropathic pain model. Pain 84: 253-261.

86. Korenman EM & Devor M (1981) Ectopic adrenergic sensitivity in damaged peripheral nerve axons in the rat. Exp Neurol 72: 63-81.

87. Pinault D (1995) Backpropagation of action potentials generated at ectopic axonal loci: hypothesis that axon terminals integrate local environmental signals. Brain Res Brain Res Rev 21: 42-92.

88. Serra J, et al. (2014) Hyperexcitable C nociceptors in fibromyalgia. Ann Neurol 75: 196-208.

89. Wall PD & Woolf CJ (1980) What we don't know about pain. Nature 287: 185-186.

90. Woolf CJ (1983) Evidence for a central component of post-injury pain hypersensitivity. Nature 306: 686-688.

91. Moseley GL & Butler DS (2015) Fifteen Years of Explaining Pain: The Past, Present, and Future. J Pain 16: 807-813.

92. Moseley GL & Vlaeyen JW (2015) Beyond nociception: the imprecision hypothesis of chronic pain. Pain 156: 35-38.

93. Drummond PD & Finch PM (2006) Sensory changes in the forehead of patients with complex regional pain syndrome. Pain 123: 83-89.

94. Rommel O, et al. (2001) Quantitative sensory testing, neurophysiological and psychological examination in patients with complex regional pain syndrome and hemisensory deficits. Pain 93: 279-293.

95. Kosek E, Ekholm J & Hansson P (1995) Increased pressure pain sensibility in fibromyalgia patients is located deep to the skin but not restricted to muscle tissue. Pain 63: 335-339.

96. Woolf CJ (2014) What to call the amplification of nociceptive signals in the central nervous system that contribute to widespread pain? Pain 155: 1911-1912.

97. Moseley GL & Butler DS (2015) The Explain Pain Handbook: Protectometer. Noigroup Publications: Adelaide.

98. Flor H, et al. (1995) Phantom-limb pain as a perceptual correlate of cortical reorganization following arm amputation. Nature 375: 482-484.

99. Schubert R, et al. (2006) Now you feel it–now you don't: ERP correlates of somatosensory awareness. Psychophysiology 43: 31-40.

100. Wand BM, et al. (2014) Illusory touch temporarily improves sensation in areas of chronic numbness: a brief communication. Neurorehabil Neural Repair 28: 797-799.

101. Botvinick M & Cohen J (1998) Rubber hands 'feel' touch that eyes see. Nature 391: 756.

102. Moseley GL & Flor H (2012) Targeting cortical representations in the treatment of chronic pain: a review. Neurorehabil Neural Repair 26: 646-652.

103. Wand BM, et al. (2011) Cortical changes in chronic low back pain: current state of the art and implications for clinical practice. Man Ther 16: 15-20.

104. Flor H, et al. (2001) Effect of sensory discrimination training on cortical reorganisation and phantom limb pain. Lancet 357: 1763-1764.

105. Moseley GL (2016) Innovative treatments for back pain. Pain 2016 Dec. doi:10.1097/j.pain.0000000000000772.

106. Moseley GL (2004) Graded motor imagery is effective for long standing complex regional pain syndrome. Pain 108: 192-198.

107. Moseley GL (2006) Graded motor imagery for pathologic pain: a randomized controlled trial. Neurology 67: 2129-2134.

108. Bowering KJ, et al. (2013) The effects of graded motor imagery and its components on chronic pain: a systematic review and meta-analysis. J Pain 14: 3-13.

109. Moseley GL, et al. (2012) The Graded Motor Imagery Handbook. Noigroup Publications: Adelaide.

110. Moseley GL & Wiech K (2009) The effect of tactile discrimination training is enhanced when patients watch the reflected image of their unaffected limb during training. Pain 144: 314-319.

111. Moseley GL, Zalucki NM & Wiech K (2008) Tactile discrimination, but not tactile stimulation alone, reduces chronic limb pain. Pain 137: 600-608.

112. Wand BM, et al. (2013) Acupuncture applied as a sensory discrimination training tool decreases movement-related pain in patients with chronic low back pain more than acupuncture alone: a randomised cross-over experiment. Br J Sports Med 47: 1085-1089.

113. Rolke R, et al. (2006) Quantitative sensory testing in the German Research Network on Neuropathic Pain (DFNS): standardized protocol and reference values. Pain 123: 231-243.

114. Maier C, et al. (2010) Quantitative sensory testing in the German Research Network on Neuropathic Pain (DFNS): somatosensory abnormalities in 1236 patients with different neuropathic pain syndromes. Pain 150: 439-450.

115. Price DD, et al. (1977) Peripheral suppression of first pain and central summation of second pain evoked by noxious heat pulses. Pain 3: 57-68.

116. Traeger AC, et al. (2016) Effect of primary care-based education on reassurance in patients with acute low back pain: Systematic review and meta-analysis. JAMA Intern Med 175: 733-743.

Notes...

4

The evidence base for Explain Pain

Humble (and ignorant) beginnings

To our knowledge, explaining pain biology emerged in the early 2000's as a therapeutic strategy in and of itself. Importantly, it emerged after randomised controlled trials (RCTs) had shown it to be of clinical benefit. While forward thinking clinicians have tried to explain pain for years, as far as *we* know, the first attempt to *evaluate* the effect of sitting someone down and explaining to them the biological mechanisms that underpin pain was undertaken in the late 1990's in a metropolitan rehabilitation practice [1]. Unaware of many of the important aspects of a good clinical trial, the study was underpowered and did not include a follow-up period – two fundamental errors made by a novice researcher. In defence of that work however, the Control group and the Explain Pain group were very similar except for the material that was covered; there were methodological checks that were, we humbly claim, well before their time; the deliverers of both groups thought that they were delivering the active treatment and had very similar expectations of outcome.

That initial study has stood the test of time. It offers clear evidence that a single session of explaining pain with a brief workbook leads to clear improvements in disability, pain-related knowledge, catastrophising, participation in rehabilitation and physical performance for at least two weeks. Those humble beginnings have triggered a range of experiments and clinical trials leading, as effective interventions do, to systematic reviews and meta-analyses.

In this chapter we want to give you a quick tour so as to equip you with what you need to know about the effectiveness and limitations of explaining pain and what might help you in those sometimes frustrating conversations with your patients, their doctors, your parents, your pals, the policy makers and the general public. This is not meant to be an exhaustive account. We can summarise the developments with some oomph by using this quote straight out of *Explain Pain Second Edn* [2]:

'Thanks to those clinical scientists who have not taken our word for it but undertaken their own clinical trials and shown that Explain Pain is not just for Australians – it seems to be equally helpful for Europeans, North and South Americans, Africans, Asians and Arabs.'

That Explain Pain was tested using empirical methods before it was introduced to the wider clinical world as a viable therapeutic approach is of fundamental importance. We both come from a clinical history that is scattered with treatments that change practice first and are empirically evaluated second. When it comes to health and to pain in particular, this is a highly problematic pathway. Just by claiming something works we give it a kind of transient effectiveness. Often a theory is retrofitted to explain why it might work and to this day, we have not heard of a therapy with the tag line 'it works because we claimed it does', even when we realise that is, in fact, the case.

Evidence that explaining pain biology has short term analgesic and behavioural effects

Chapter 2 of *EP Supercharged* urges the reader to think about theories and to consider the hypotheses that are driven by, and drive our theories. We might do well to do the same when it comes to interrogation of explaining pain biology. If then, we consider the hypothesis that 'explaining pain biology reduces protective outputs' we need to ask whether it is a plausible hypothesis and a testable one. We have recently argued the plausibility of such a hypothesis on the basis of the biopsychosocial model and the neurotag theories, and on the clear evidence that modifying one's beliefs about what a stimulus might mean has real time effects on pain [3]. For example, Dr Katja Wiech, a psychology researcher from Oxford, did an intriguing experiment [4] in which she delivered laser stimuli to the foot of 'supposedly normal'[1] healthy volunteers while she recorded their pain ratings and scanned their brains in an fMRI machine. She strategically (and deceitfully)

---

1   Remember – these people are volunteering for pain experiments, which must cast into doubt the assumption that they are in any way 'normal'.

informed participants that one location (randomised between participants) was 'thin-skinned and vulnerable'. Perhaps not surprisingly when a stimulus hit this location, there was more intense pain (and a concomitant shift in brain activation) than when identical stimuli hit any other location. The information the participant received explained the increased protection.

Advising someone they have a 'vulnerable' patch of skin is one thing, but reducing pain by explaining pain biology is a somewhat different thing. Nonetheless, experiments show it is possible, in real time. For example in one of Lorimer's earlier research studies [5], 121 people experiencing chronic back pain participated in either Explain Pain or Back school based education. An independent researcher tested participants' pain thresholds during a straight leg raise, then randomly allocated them to two groups. Each participant was blinded to which treatment was meant to be the active one and they were naive to the study question. The education sessions were about three hours in total and immediately afterwards, the blinded independent assessor came back in to test straight leg raise. Lo and behold, those in the Explain Pain group demonstrated an immediate increase in pain-free straight leg raise but those in the Back school group did not. In fact, those in the Back school group were worse!

Why might this be? Well we think it is not that surprising – the material that was taught in the Back school – spinal physiology, anatomy and ergonomics – is clearly different from the material in *Explain Pain*. Back schools tend to focus on the rationale behind protecting one's back – such as how to lift well, the disc pressures during bending, the precious nature of the spinal cord and its vulnerable location… getting the picture? DIM[2] alert!

Of course, there are many therapies that *seemed* to be effective at first but have ended up, once they have been tested, to be no better than clever shams. This might not necessarily be bad unless the retrofitted theories also claim a non-existent danger. This is one area in which knowing your theories is particularly important. Here are some examples of why: some of the theories are actually catastrophic metaphors – *your disc is slipped and I can put it back in,* or *your spine is out and I will realign it,* or *your rib is stuck and I will get it moving again,* or *your spine is unstable and I will teach you core stability.*

Notice that they all subscribe to an outdated model of pain and they all emphasise (i) that you have a structurally dangerous event happening, and (ii) you need me or my new product or particular approach to fix it. By proving the therapies to be no better than control, the theories are ripped apart, but unfortunately it is too late for the large numbers of clinicians and patients who have bought both the therapy and the theory as a 'package deal'. This pathway is upside down. This is why we are very proud to say that explaining pain biology was tested as a therapeutic approach using empirical methods *before* anyone started claiming it worked and before *Explain Pain,* the book. This is, in our view, a fundamental strength.

Since *Explain Pain* was first published in 2003, research groups around the world have started testing intervention based on the book. To reflect this, and consistent with the scientific literature, from this point on we will use Explain Pain to denote explaining pain biology as a therapeutic strategy. When we refer to the book *Explain Pain,* it will be in italics just like that, or simply, EP.

Clinical trials of Explain Pain

So far, about 20 RCTs have investigated the effects of Explain Pain on pain and disability in people with chronic pain. These trials range in quality, with some scoring quite badly on the usual risk of bias measures and others scoring pretty well. Not surprisingly, the results of the dodgy ones seem more impressive than the results of the methodologically tight ones. Before expanding briefly on the evidence base as it stands, there are two things the reader should remember.

1. No RCT of an intervention that involves interaction between patient and clinician can be blinded. This is not a trivial problem for the pain field because we have no doubt that the beliefs of the clinician can be a DIM or a SIM with substantial clout (see box overleaf).

2. In order to evaluate Explain Pain, there are a few approaches the scientist can take:

    *   She can compare Explain Pain to Explaining Something Else, which would tell her whether the actual material explained is important [eg. 1].

    *   She can compare Explain Pain to an interactive intervention that is thought to have no real effects, for example 'reflecting listening', which would tell her whether there was any effect of Explain Pain beyond that offered by a supportive, caring health care interaction [eg. 6].

---

2   In case you started at this chapter, a DIM is a Danger In Me neurotag and a SIM is a Safety In Me neurotag. See pages 17-18.

- She can compare Explain Pain to another active intervention, for example a GP-driven multimodal management plan, which would tell her how the whole multifactorial package of Explain Pain compared to the whole multifactorial package directed by the GP [eg. 7].

All of these options are appropriate depending on the resources and the most pressing question at hand. However, none of them position Explain Pain as it occurs in the real world – as a range of individually and group-tailored educational strategies that form a preparatory and ongoing component of multimodal, activity-based rehabilitation. Testing Explain Pain as a stand-alone, one off treatment tells us important information, but it lacks a certain real world validity – rarely do we simply just Explain Pain.[3]

- The final option then, is to compare an Explain Pain-based active rehabilitation programme to another kind of rehabilitation, which will allow the scientist to identify which of the two approaches delivers a better return in terms of improvement in pain, disability and quality of life, and which represents the better value for money.

The potentially powerful SIM/DIM role that clinicians beliefs and expectations can play.

Researchers were undertaking a double blind RCT of fentanyl (which should reduce pain), naloxone (which should not) or saline (which should not) after wisdom tooth removal. One group of dentists doing the injections was told that their patient would receive fentanyl or placebo. The other was told they would receive naloxone or placebo. The analgesic effect of the placebo was compared between the two groups. When the dentist thought there was a 50% chance they were injecting fentanyl, the placebo delivered a 3/10 *decrease* in pain; when the dentist thought there was a 0% chance they were injecting fentanyl, the placebo delivered a 2/10 *increase* in pain [8].

The difference?

The clinician's expectations about the chance they were doing something useful!

Back pain is the most common and burdensome of the chronic pains and it is no surprise that more researchers use RCTs to investigate the effects of Explain Pain on people with back pain [1, 5, 7, 9-11] than in any other patient group. RCTs have also tested Explain Pain for lumbar radiculopathy [12], fibromyalgia [13, 14], chronic fatigue syndrome [15] and general chronic pain [16]. There have been four systematic reviews [3, 17-19]. Here's our take on it:

'… the most parsimonious interpretation of the wider body of evidence concerning Explain Pain appears to be that, as a stand alone treatment for a wide range of chronic pain states, Explain Pain improves knowledge of pain biology, improves participation in subsequent biopsychosocially-based rehabilitation, decreases catastrophising and pain and activity-related fear. When combined with other treatments that are also consistent with a biopsychosocial framework, Explain Pain seems to offer clinically important improvements in pain and disability.' [3]

At risk of making this rather beautiful and novel textbook look a bit more conventional, we have included a 'serious data table'. In it we present the systematic reviews and meta-analyses of Explain Pain that have been published up to the moment of writing. We suspect that if you are even interested in this table then you don't need us to hold your hand and walk you through it. Instead, we will round off this chapter by touching on a couple of interesting developments from unpublished work or published studies that are not RCTs.

---

3 The exception here is 'pre-emptive' Explain Pain, which is currently being tested in workplaces and schools in prospective studies. We also like the idea of mass media Explain Pain – we think that mass conceptual change will have the greatest societal impact. However, in a clinical sense, Explain Pain is almost never the only thing we do.

The review	What they did and found
Clarke et al. (2011) [18]	Systematically reviewed three databases from 1996-2010 to investigate evidence for Explain Pain as a management strategy for people with chronic low back pain. They had fairly tight inclusion criteria and a decently high bar when it came to quality of studies to be included. They only found two RCTs that made the grade and both were conducted by Lorimer [5, 20]. Their conclusion was that the evidence base was pretty thin – *'there is low quality evidence that Explain Pain is beneficial for pain, physical-function, psychological-function and social-function'*. They undertook a meta-analysis, but of course there were not much data in it. They concluded that Explain Pain produced clinically small improvements in short-term pain and came short of concluding much else. We reckon their conclusions were really sound, based on the literature at the time. Importantly, this review is the only published so far where none of the authors have a clear potential conflict of interest.
Louw et al. (2011) [17]	Systematically reviewed the evidence for the effectiveness of Explain Pain as a management strategy for people with chronic musculoskeletal pain. This one was not limited to back pain, nor limited to randomised controlled trials. Eight studies were included: 6 RCT's [1, 5, 7, 9, 10, 15], one pseudo-RCT [21] and one comparative study [22]. All studies rated good to excellent quality evidence. No meta-analysis was performed, however narrative synthesis revealed compelling evidence that Explain Pain may be effective in reducing pain ratings, increasing function, decreasing catastrophisation and improving movement in chronic musculoskeletal pain. There are two important caveats here, however. First, the quality of the studies that made it in was a bit lower than the previous one and second, David was one of the authors and three of the four authors had a conflict of interest that might have affected their conclusions.
Moseley & Butler (2015) [3]	Talking about a conflict of interest, this systematic review was undertaken to assess the clinical effects of Explain Pain by the authors of *Explain Pain* – us! We did everything we could to minimise the impact of our conflict, including paying a separate researcher to perform all the searches and analyse and interpret the data. Twelve studies were identified for chronic low back pain [1, 5, 7, 9-11], fibromyalgia [13, 14], lumbar radiculopathy [23], chronic fatigue syndrome [15], whiplash [22] or general chronic pain [16]. The conclusion was that, when combined with other treatments that are also consistent with a biopsychosocial framework, Explain Pain seems to offer clinically important improvements in pain and disability that are maintained at long term follow-up. Obviously you can just read the current chapter for a more comprehensive account of what *we* think about the state of the evidence.
Louw et al. (2016) [19]	A systematic review of RCTs evaluating the effectiveness of Explain Pain for chronic musculoskeletal pain. This review had quite high standards – only accepting RCTs – and they found thirteen that satisfied their a-*priori* criteria [5, 7, 9-16, 24-26]. They concluded that current evidence supports the use of Explain Pain for chronic musculoskeletal disorders. They found that it reduces pain, improves patient knowledge of pain, improves function, positively modifies psychological factors, enhances movement and reduces healthcare utilisation. Again, this review was riddled with serious conflicts of interest on the part of the authors. The conflicts were not declared so it is difficult to know how the authors dealt with them, but the review appeared reasonably solid.

Table 4.1 Serious data table of systematic reviews and meta-analyses of Explaining Pain

Increasing effects over time?

From a curriculum perspective, we think of Explain Pain as targeting key concepts and we identify these Target Concepts for each patient on the basis of a thorough assessment that considers aspects of the learner, the deliverer, the message and the context (see Chapter 5). From a neurotag perspective, we can think of each Target Concept as a neurotag that we are attempting to implant or adapt and then train to make it more influential (see Chapter 2). There are clear principles that we can follow that should achieve this increased influence (and they are hardly rocket science) – promote variability, practice (practice practice!) and foster precision. No matter the theoretical framework in which you consider it, if Explain Pain is successful its effects should increase over time. Whether or not they do is very difficult to evaluate because the participants in studies are, after all, real life humans with busy lives and obligations – to have them wait around in a useless control group is rather problematic. However, early on in our Explain Pain research journey we came across a situation a bit like this one. Here is what we found:

Team Lorimer did an RCT with people who were participating in a four week intensive pain management programme based on CBT principles (and the 'gold standard approach' at the time) [20]. Participants had 'chronic pain' with no exclusions except terminal illness. Let's walk through the graph below (Figure 4.1). There were two groups and about 60 people in each group: one participated in Explain Pain on the afternoon before they started the programme, and they used the *Explain Pain* book [27] as they saw fit to throughout their CBT programme. The other group participated in the usual pre-programme seminar, based on *The Back Book* [28] (a fine book, but without any pain biology education in it), outlining the principles of CBT and the biopsychosocial approach to pain-related disability.[4] We assessed a range of variables but the important ones here are pain and disability. There was no difference in pain or disability between groups at the end of the programme. We were disappointed about this. However, by six months, those in the Explain Pain group were clearly doing far better than those in the other group and at 12 months the difference was even bigger, demonstrating that the Explain Pain group had learnt how to learn and their conceptual changes were durable.

---

4 Mental note: remember that confining the biopsychosocial model to the consideration of pain-related disability rather than pain itself is disappointing and biologically indefensible, but, alas, that was the deal.

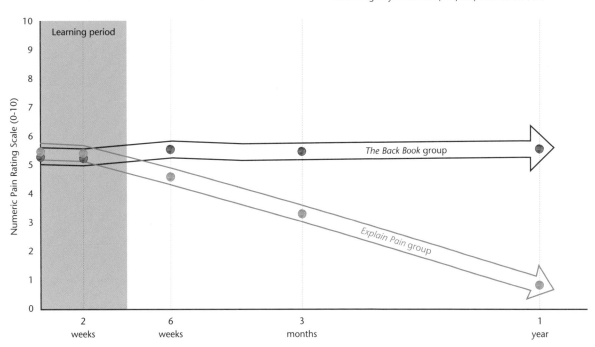

Figure 4.1 Pain scores post pain management programme [20]

We now have audit data that tell a very similar story [29]. Data from about 1000 people who have undertaken an Explain Pain intervention clearly show that improvements in pain knowledge in the first few weeks are associated with important improvements in pain and disability a year later (Figure 4.2).

Dr Hopin Lee, a graduate of the Body in Mind team at Neuroscience Research Australia, analysed these data and discovered an interesting relationship between improved knowledge, catastrophising and long term outcomes [29] (Figure 4.2). In short, he tested whether improved knowledge imparted its effects on pain and disability via a reduction in catastrophising. Hopin showed that at best, the mediating effect of catastrophising was very small. This is really interesting because it confirms what is intuitively sensible to us and we hope also to you – that there are probably multiple mechanisms by which *understanding* one's pain reduces one's pain and disability.[5]

---

5   This work by Hopin followed on the back of his provocative systematic review [30] that showed catastrophising may not be the mediator of change in pain and disability that we all thought it was. Welcome to scientific progress!

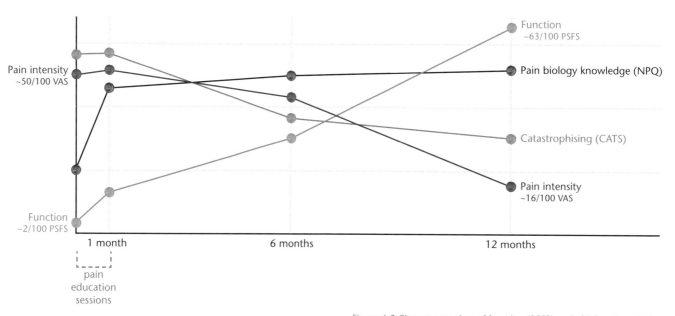

Figure 4.2 Change over time of function (PSFS), pain biology knowledge (NPQ), catastrophising (CATS) and pain intensity (VAS) after an Explain Pain intervention. For exact data we refer you to Hopin's paper [29].

Flare-ups lose their power ...

For people in pain, a key indicator of how they are progressing is the frequency and intensity of their flare-ups. Flare-ups are not a usual outcome variable in clinical studies so we don't have any hard data from RCTs, though clinicians know the importance of dealing with flare-ups. We don't have clear baseline data either – so it is clearly more difficult to detect change. This lack of baseline data is fair enough – people in pain don't want to wait for treatment while we take a couple of months to establish their baseline. However, a few patients have agreed to record their daily pain levels both before and following Explain Pain (Figure 4.3). Flare-ups were both more intense and took longer to resolve before the intervention than they did after the intervention. Remember here though that case reports – even when there are a few cases who seem to do the same thing – do not allow us to attribute the *cause* of the effect to the treatment, and much less to any particular aspect of the treatment.

The other patient group from whom Team Lorimer have collected some decent flare-up data is people participating in treatment for complex regional pain syndrome (CRPS) [31]. In short, each patient was participating in a broad Graded Motor Imagery (GMI) based rehabilitation programme [see 32 for more on GMI]. Data were collected on 204 consecutive patients between 2002 and 2010. In about 2005, a comprehensive 'Explain Pain for CRPS' component was introduced. In about 2007, for reasons beyond our control, that component was cut again such that the next 17 patients did not receive this part of the package. In 2008 it was reintroduced. This presented an opportunity to see whether there was any difference in flare-up data between the periods that included Explain Pain for CRPS and the periods that did not. There was! (Figure 4.4)

When these patients were asked the question *'If you move your affected limb do you think it will make your condition worse?'* they were more likely to say 'no' after Explain CRPS than after Explain Pain.

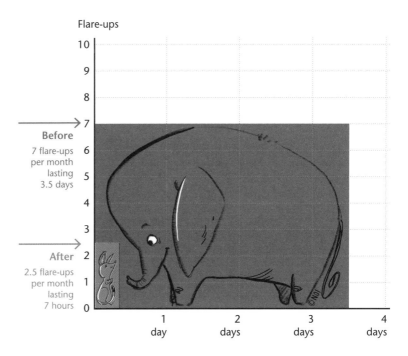

Figure 4.3 Frequency and duration of flare-ups are lower after Explain Pain (bilby) than before (elephant)

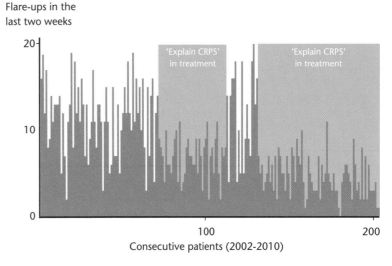

Figure 4.4 Fewer flare-ups after Explain CRPS than after a generic education session [31]

Interpreting and communicating evidence: the basics

It's good and well to know this current Explain Pain evidence stuff, but you need to have some extra skills to make sense of the literature as it continues to move forward. So, we are going to give you some user friendly statistics. Stats are a bit like Vegemite[6] – people either love it or hate it. They generally turn people off – phrases such as 'lies, damn lies and statistics' and 'scientists can prove anything by finding the right statistic' have become common. But stats can hold great power and even be quite exciting.

Statistics are about probability – how likely it is that something is going to happen. Clinically, they can be used to test theories and then provide us with answers to these important questions:

- The probability that a treatment will work – that is, on average, is it likely to have any effect?

- How big is the treatment effect likely to be?

- Is that size effect worth the bother?

Whether or not a treatment works is all about significance

When it comes to research, significance is represented by a 'p value' (eg. p =0.05), which stands for probability. If something is significant, it means that it is at least 95% likely to be true. This magic 95% threshold (or p <0.05) for accepting something to be true is just convention, but most researchers accept it. In fact, if our statistics tell us that something is 94% likely to be true, scientists say it is 'not true' (although they would definitely consider doing another experiment with more participants just to be sure). This 95% rule is a conservative one but it is fabulous for reducing the risk that researchers will say something is true when it is not. Because of the 95% rule, there is a higher risk that researchers will say something is false when really it is true.

So the p value says there is an effect, but how big is it?

Reaching the magic 95% threshold does not mean the result is important, nor big, even if it really excites scientists. You might have heard people try to proclaim that redheads have a higher pain threshold – where did that come from? Well the average temperature at which a hot stimulus becomes painful is significantly lower for redheads than it is for non-redheads. However, the size of the difference is so small it is completely unimportant in the real world. To work out the importance of a significant result, we need to work out the effect size.

Here is an example: explaining pain and a graded increase in activity significantly reduces pain and disability. This means that the statement *'on average explaining pain reduces pain and disability'* is at least 95% likely to be true (the actual statistics suggest it is over 99% likely to be true). However, this statistic tells us nothing about how big the reductions in pain and disability are, nor whether that reduction is likely to be important enough for a patient to spend time going through the programme, nor anything about the risk of Explaining Pain. So we need another statistic to provide this important information.

Effect size and confidence intervals

To have an idea of how well a treatment works on average we can look at the effect size. The effect size tells you how big an effect is. It is calculated by determining the average difference between two measures, eg. pain relief from Treatment 1 versus pain relief from Treatment 2 – and expressing it in terms of differences caused by normal fluctuations and inaccuracies in our assessment tools and methods. Researchers reasonably agree that an effect size (often expressed with the letter d) of 1 is quite a 'large effect'. An effect size of 0.2 would be a small effect. Drug companies become excited if the effect size of a new drug on pain is more than 0.2. If you read a paper that reports a pain treatment with an effect size of 2, then be very sceptical – the study is likely to be a fluke or dodgy. If you read lots of papers that report the same treatment and the same effect size of 2, then invest in the company immediately!

It might work really well on average, but will it work for my patient?

Whenever you see an effect size, you are actually looking at the middle of a range. You need to look for a confidence interval (CI), which will tell you how big the possible range is. A 95% confidence interval means that there is a 95% chance that the true effect size between two measures lies somewhere in this range. The smaller the confidence interval, the better.

To be clear the bigger the effect size and the smaller the confidence interval, the better.

---

6   Insert your own unofficial national dish here. Vegemite is a thick, black, smelly spread made from left over brewer's yeast. As Australians we love it and even if we don't love it, we say we love it.

For example, let's say a study reports an effect size of 0.5 and a 95% CI of 0 to 1. This is a good average effect size, but for any individual, the effect may actually be as small as zero (no effect at all) or as big as 1 (great). This means that the treatment might be very effective, but it might also be a dud. Let's say another study reports an effect size of 0.5 and a 95% CI of 0.4 to 0.6. This means that there is a 95% chance that the true effect size is between 0.4 and 0.6. This is a very effective treatment. Finally, let's say the effect size is 1.5 and the CI is -0.5 to 3.5. This treatment might be outstanding but it might also make you substantially worse.

Consider this: strong scientific evidence shows us that Explain Pain has an effect size on pain and disability of 0.7 (95% CI 0.4 to 1.0). So, we know that it is at least 95% likely that Explain Pain reduces pain and disability (that's 'significance' or the p value), and we now know that it is 95% likely that the true size of the effect is somewhere between 0.4 and 1.0 – a medium to large effect. Therefore, it is 95% likely that Explain Pain will have a medium to large effect on the individual patient. But is that size effect going to be important for them?

Number needed to treat (NNT)

The NNT statistic tells us how good a treatment is at achieving a desired effect and we first decide what the desired effect actually is. For example, we usually say that a 50% reduction in pain or disability six or twelve months after the intervention is important; this effect would be good for someone who has had pain for a long time. We can then work out a NNT for a 50% reduction in pain or disability. To do this, you need to have a comparison, which can be a placebo or no treatment at all. Let's say we use a placebo pill as the comparison. A placebo pill has no medicine in it but still has effects that are caused by a range of other things such as if you believe the pill will work, or if you trust the doctor prescribing it.

The NNT for an experimental pill tells us how many people we would need to treat with the experimental pill for one of them to get better with the experimental pill but not a placebo pill.

An NNT of 1 means a treatment is effective in everyone. In real life, NNT scores are always above 1. For example, the most commonly prescribed drug treatment for neuropathic pain is gabapentin (also known as Lyrica or Neurontin). The NNT for gabapentin is about 6.3. This means that in a group of six sufferers, there will be 1 who will have 50% pain relief from gabapentin but would not have it from a placebo pill and there will be 5 who would have responded similarly to gabapentin and to a placebo. NNTs of over 11 are considered 'clinically useless'. NNTs of under 4 are considered clinically fantastic.

Here's an Explain Pain example: The NNT for a 50% reduction in pain or disability 6 months later, for Explaining Pain instead of usual GP-managed care, is about 4 (95% CI 2 – 6). If you are not used to this concept, an NNT of 4 mightn't sound all that crash hot, but it is actually very good. If a drug company came across a new pain relief drug that provided an NNT of 4 for this outcome, they would be dancing on the rooftops and rubbing their hands with glee! Of course, they would be presuming their drug did no harm....

Number needed to harm (NNH)

Every drug is associated with a risk. The NNH can be quantified in exactly the same way as the NNT can – *how many people are required to find one person who has the negative effect and who would not have it if they were on the placebo.* The bigger the NNH the better. Consider that the NNH for drug, spinal cord stimulator or surgery based approaches range from 25 (which is reasonably good) right down to 2 (which is very bad and not worth the risk). Antidepressants have an NNH of about 13, which is still considered acceptable, but it is common enough to be a warning light for clinical practice.

The NNH for Explaining Pain hasn't been calculated yet because there have not been enough instances in clinical trials of there actually being any harm. That is, the NNH for Explaining Pain is at least a couple of hundred – way bigger than that of any drug. This is a very good thing for Explain Pain.

Number needed to kill (NNK)

Our communities are realising that opioids are not the magic drugs they were claimed to be 20 years ago. In 2016, for the first time, more Americans died from an opioid overdose than from homicide [33]. This has led to a new statistic – Number Needed to Kill (NNK). The NNK for 200 MME[7] per day opioid dose is about 32. That's a worry, there has to be better ways of treating pain.

---

7   MME – Morphine milligram equivalents

Levels of Evidence

There are now many grading systems that tell people how good a treatment is. Most systems report 'Levels of evidence' and they are all quite similar. As a general rule of thumb, you can go with the tables below. Explain Pain fits somewhere in the first row in Table 4.2.

If you are still keen on learning more about how to interpret research on clinical effects, particularly with regards to pain, there is lots to learn! You can start with this paper by Dr Neil O'Connell – it's a cracker [33].

To decide if:	You need:
A treatment is definitely good.	Level 1; Grade 1; Many randomised controlled trials/big 'meta-analysis' level evidence says it is good.
A treatment is probably good.	Level 2 or 2a; Grade 2; A few randomised controlled trials/small meta-analysis level says it is good.
A treatment might be good, but it is too early to tell.	Level 3 or 2b; Grade 3; A single randomised controlled trial says it is good.
We have no idea whether or not a treatment is good, but it is worth doing a clinical trial to find out.	Level 4; Grade 4; Single case studies, expert opinion.
We have no idea whatsoever whether a treatment is good.	A presenter tells you they get excellent results and plays you before and after videos at a conference or course.

Table 4.2 Levels of evidence – good treatments

To decide if:	You need:
A treatment is definitely useless.	Level 1; Grade 1; 'meta-analysis' level evidence says it is useless.
A treatment is probably useless.	Level 2 or 2a; Grade 2; A few randomised controlled trials say it is useless.
A treatment looks quite useless and there is probably no point doing any more research on it.	Level 3 or 2b; Grade 3; A single randomised controlled trial says it is useless.

Table 4.3 Levels of evidence – useless treatments

What can I tell the insurer/referrer/patient?

So as a summary, here is what we currently know about Explaining Pain:

- There is top level evidence that Explain Pain imparts clinically important improvements in pain knowledge, catastrophising and participation in biopsychosocially-based rehabilitation in people with chronic pain.

- There is second-top level evidence that a biopsychosocially-based rehabilitation built around Explain Pain imparts clinically important improvements in pain, disability, work status and quality of life in people with chronic pain.

- The NNT for a 50% reduction in pain or disability at six months after presentation is about 4, which is equal to or better than any other current approach.

- The NNH cannot yet be calculated because no harms have been reported in clinical trials.

- It is quite hard to compare cost-effectiveness between treatments, but Explain Pain based intervention for chronic pain is about as inexpensive a treatment there is and is at least as good as anything else (and probably better). So, it is probably the gold-medallist for cost-effectiveness (but remember, we have a clear conflict of interest here!). We can honestly say however, hand on our heart, that we haven't come across credible data that seems to contradict this claim.

A quick reminder here though, Explain Pain is about bringing the science into practice. It incorporates any evidence based diagnosis-to-treatment approach of primary nociceptor contributions to a pain state. Explain Pain assumes that every patient we see is a human and Explain Pain is equally applicable to every human patient we see.

So, where are we at?

It is worth repeating that Explain Pain refers to a range of educational and conceptual change strategies that aim to alter the way someone understands the biological processes that underpin their pain, allowing them to function differently. Almost twenty years after the first RCT, the evidence is really clear:

1. We can teach people about their pain.

2. We can do that effectively and across cultures and language groups.

3. When we do Explain Pain, people are more likely to take a biopsychosocial approach to their pain, adopt active self-management strategies and, critically, recover.

4. Although effects are impressive, there is no doubt that there is room to improve – our results could definitely be better.

This is where *EP Supercharged* comes in. There is also a very strong argument to say that with very little training or expertise, Explain Pain changes lives. With advanced training, high level expertise and structured, intentional practice, Explain Pain should impart bigger, more durable, and more rapid changes.

Vida longa à revolução![8]

---

8   Long live the revolution!

References

1. Moseley GL, Nicholas MK & Hodges PW (2004) A randomized controlled trial of intensive neurophysiology education in chronic low back pain. Clin J Pain 20: 324-330.

2. Butler DS & Moseley GL (2013) Explain Pain. 2nd Edn. Noigroup Publications: Adelaide.

3. Moseley GL & Butler DS (2015) Fifteen Years of Explaining Pain: The Past, Present, and Future. J Pain 16: 807-813.

4. Wiech K, et al. (2010) Anterior insula integrates information about salience into perceptual decisions about pain. J Neurosci 30: 16324-16331.

5. Moseley GL (2004) Evidence for a direct relationship between cognitive and physical change during an education intervention in people with chronic low back pain. Eur J Pain 8: 39-45.

6. Traeger AC, et al. (2014) Pain education to prevent chronic low back pain: a study protocol for a randomised controlled trial. BMJ Open 4: e005505.

7. Moseley GL (2002) Combined physiotherapy and education is efficacious for chronic low back pain. Aust J Physiother 48: 297-302.

8. Gracely RH, et al. (1985) Clinicians' expectations influence placebo analgesia. Lancet 325: 43.

9. Ryan CG, et al. (2010) Pain biology education and exercise classes compared to pain biology education alone for individuals with chronic low back pain: a pilot randomised controlled trial. Man Ther 15: 382-387.

10. Moseley GL (2003) Joining forces - combining cognition-targeted motor control training with group or individual pain physiology education: a successful treatment for chronic low back pain. J Man Manip Therap 11: 88-94.

11. Pires D, Cruz EB & Caeiro C (2015) Aquatic exercise and pain neurophysiology education versus aquatic exercise alone for patients with chronic low back pain: a randomized controlled trial. Clin Rehabil 29: 538-547.

12. Louw A, et al. (2014) Preoperative pain neuroscience education for lumbar radiculopathy: a multicenter randomized controlled trial with 1-year follow-up. Spine 39: 1449-1457.

13. Van Oosterwijck J, et al. (2013) Pain physiology education improves health status and endogenous pain inhibition in fibromyalgia: a double-blind randomized controlled trial. Clin J Pain 29: 873-882.

14. van Ittersum MW, et al. (2014) Written pain neuroscience education in fibromyalgia: a multicenter randomized controlled trial. Pain Pract 14: 689-700.

15. Meeus M, et al. (2010) Pain Physiology Education Improves Pain Beliefs in Patients With Chronic Fatigue Syndrome Compared With Pacing and Self-Management Education: A Double-Blind Randomized Controlled Trial. Arch Phys Med Rehabil 91: 1153-1159.

16. Gallagher L, McAuley J & Moseley GL (2013) A randomized-controlled trial of using a book of metaphors to reconceptualize pain and decrease catastrophizing in people with chronic pain. Clin J Pain 29: 20-25.

17. Louw A, et al. (2011) The Effect of Neuroscience Education on Pain, Disability, Anxiety, and Stress in Chronic Musculoskeletal Pain. Arch Phys Med Rehabil 92: 2041-2056.

18. Clarke CL, Ryan CG & Martin DJ (2011) Pain neurophysiology education for the management of individuals with chronic low back pain. A systematic review and meta-analysis. Man Ther 16: 544-549.

19. Louw A, et al. (2016) The efficacy of pain neuroscience education on musculoskeletal pain: A systematic review of the literature. Physiother Theory Pract 32: 332-355.

20. Moseley GL (2009) Explaining pain to patients - recent developments. Proceedings of the New Zealand Pain Society Annual Scientific Meeting.

21. Moseley GL (2003) Unravelling the barriers to reconceptualisation of the problem in chronic pain: the actual and perceived ability of patients and health professionals to understand the neurophysiology. J Pain 4: 184-189.

22. Van Oosterwijck J, et al. (2011) Pain neurophysiology education improves cognitions, pain thresholds, and movement performance in people with chronic whiplash: a pilot study. J Rehabil Res Dev 48: 43-58.

23. Louw A, et al. (2015) Preoperative therapeutic neuroscience education for lumbar radiculopathy: a single-case fMRI report. Physiother Theory Pract 31: 496-508.

24. Vibe Fersum K, et al. (2013) Efficacy of classification-based cognitive functional therapy in patients with non-specific chronic low back pain: a randomized controlled trial. Eur J Pain 17: 916-928.

25. Tellez-Garcia M, et al. (2015) Neuroscience education in addition to trigger point dry needling for the management of patients with mechanical chronic low back pain: A preliminary clinical trial. J Bodyw Mov Ther 19: 464-472.

26. Beltran-Alacreu H, et al. (2015) Manual Therapy, Therapeutic Patient Education, and Therapeutic Exercise, an Effective Multimodal Treatment of Nonspecific Chronic Neck Pain: A Randomized Controlled Trial. Am J Phys Med Rehabil 94: 887-897.

27. Butler DS & Moseley GL (2003) Explain Pain. 1st Edn. Noigroup Publications: Adelaide.

28. Roland M (1996) The Back Book. Stationery Office Books: London.

29. Lee H, et al. (2016) Does changing pain-related knowledge reduce pain and improve function through changes in catastrophizing? Pain 157: 922-930.

30. Lee H, et al. (2015) How does pain lead to disability? A systematic review and meta-analysis of mediation studies in people with back and neck pain. Pain 156: 988-997.

31. Moseley GL (2010) Rehabilitation of people with chronic complex regional pain syndrome, in Pain 2010 - An Updated Review: Refresher Course Syllabus, Mogil JS Ed. IASP Press: Seattle.

32. Moseley GL (2004) Graded motor imagery is effective for long standing complex regional pain syndrome. Pain 108: 192-198.

33. Kaplovitch E, et al. (2015) Sex Differences in Dose Escalation and Overdose Death during Chronic Opioid Therapy: A Population-Based Cohort Study. PLoS One 10: e0134550.

34. O'Connell NE, et al. (2015) Interpreting Effectiveness Evidence in Pain: Short Tour of Contemporary Issues. Phys Ther 95: 1087-1094.

Notes...

5

Explaining Pain is all about conceptual change

The Life of Pi

Dave knows something about geometry and pi. At school a long time ago he learnt that π=3.142. His teacher brought in a bicycle, put a chalk mark on the front tyre and then rolled the bike across the room until there were two chalk marks on the floor. The teacher announced that the distance between the marks was something called the 'circumference' and you could always work it out with the formula of twice the radius multiplied by a magical figure called pi. Dave must have been impressed because he can still remember being amazed at the length of a bicycle wheel.[1] This experience is an example of learning a new concept on a blank geometry slate – a complete lack of previous knowledge. The bicycle was an effective metaphor; it was familiar and presented the concept in a novel way. This must have contributed to Dave's now stable, retrievable and reasonably coherent pi neurotag.

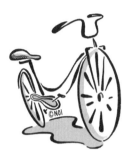

How well you learn a new concept depends on the presence or lack of existing knowledge. If there is no prior knowledge about a concept it is usually much easier to teach, especially if taught well. With little or no existing knowledge there is less reason to reject the idea, even an idea that might be a bit crazy.[2] However, when opposing beliefs are in place it becomes more difficult – this conflicting knowledge can result in resistance to change. While this may be helpful for our survival, it can be a problem when people hold misconceived and inaccurate beliefs.

Conceptual change is a field of education that explores the process of change in our understanding of a phenomenon in the presence of existing knowledge.

We all develop concepts of ourselves and the events occurring in our lives as we try to make sense of our place in the world. Every clinician reading this will know that patients come to the clinical encounter with an extraordinarily wide range of

existing knowledge. When it comes to pain education it is common to find that this knowledge doesn't align with current scientific understanding. We then humbly refer to this inaccurate knowledge as 'misconceptions.' Humility is important – after all we are only writing this in 2017 and we acknowledge that things will change!

Knowledge: the bits of justified information (either accurate or inaccurate) that form a concept

Belief: an attitude towards knowledge

Concept: an overall mental framework

This chapter explores the process of assessing, adapting and replacing inaccurate knowledge neurotags through conceptual change. Conceptual change is both a process and an end result. The number of variables impacting on the process and the educational outcome is massive. Let's dig deeper.

---

1   I must thank my geometry teacher in the Queensland outback for this clear piece of experiential learning and evidence based multimedia!

2   It's pretty easy to convince a child that a fat man in a red suit can fly across the sky, slip down your chimney and deliver you and all the other children in the world presents in one night. Try convincing an adult – previous knowledge may get in the way.

The learner, the deliverer, the message and the context

So many things can influence the outcome of an educational intervention. To make it easier for us all we have categorised these below, adapted from Dole and Sinatra [1], into variables related to the *learner*, the *deliverer*, the *message* and the *context*.

Variable	Definition
Learner	The person engaging in conceptual change
Deliverer	The person facilitating the conceptual change
Message	The information *and* delivery strategies to promote conceptual change
Context	The physical, social and psychological environment in which the conceptual change takes place

Table 5.1 Categories of variables impacting on educational outcomes

These variables are dynamic and interact with each other. Consider motivation – it's a variable relevant to both the learner and deliverer, it can be influenced by the quality of the media used for the message and from time to time societal forces may impact on motivation to change. These four categories of variables form the basis of the Explain Pain (EP) curriculum design discussed in the next chapter. The number and variety of variables reveal the complexity of the conceptual change process for a person with persistent pain. Our job is not easy!

Features of the learner

Lessons from the pain world

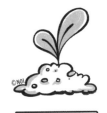

LEARNER

Unlike me prior to my bicycle driven pi revelation, the person in pain, *especially* one who may have constructed a life with chronic pain, will have many existing and varied pain related beliefs. In earlier chapters we discussed how each of these beliefs must be held by brain cells and we can therefore call them neurotags. So as you read this, have nestled in the back of your mind the principles of neurotags – that they are in a constant state of collaboration and competition; they all exert an influence.

A huge number of factors are known to be associated with the development of persistent pain states, although none of them has a large influence on its own. In conceptual change speak, we can think of those variables that are about the person in pain as 'learner variables'. Learner variables are important in determining the outcome of self-management based strategies [2, 3], but they are also important in determining the speed and extent of natural recovery.

We are not reinventing the wheel in this book – so much good research has already been done in this area. The 'flag system' is an example of this (Figure 5.1) [4]. There is much to like about the flag system. There are five flag categories now in use in best practice and they adhere tightly to the biopsychosocial framework we covered in Chapter 2 and on which *Explain Pain* is based. Red flags denote the potential presence of serious tissue-related problems, orange, yellow and blue flags denote the presence of psychological variables associated with poor recovery and black flags denote the presence of social variables associated with poor recovery [3].

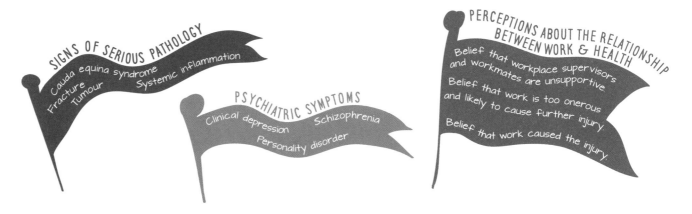

All of the learner variables can be categorised into DIMs (Danger In Me) or SIMs (Safety In Me) and all will be held by neurotags. Make sure you are up with DIMs and SIMs because we discuss them a lot (see Chapter 2, pages 17-18 and [28]). While the flag categories above are very useful, they focus on the negative only – the DIMs if you like. A critical part of EP is to also identify and enhance the SIMs, which are almost like positive versions of these flag categories. In our experience, people don't fit neatly into designated boxes. For example, they may simultaneously feel

SYSTEM OR CONTEXTUAL OBSTACLES
Legislation restricting options for return to work
Conflict with staff over claim
Overly solicitous family & health care providers
Heavy work, few opportunities to modify duties
Lack of qualified health professionals

BELIEFS APPRAISALS AND JUDGEMENTS
Belief that pain equals amount of damage
Belief that pain is an indication of injury
Expectation of poor treatment outcome

EMOTIONAL RESPONSES
Worry, fears, anxiety, catastrophisation.
Distress doesn't meet criteria for diagnosis of mental disorder.

PAIN BEHAVIOUR INCLUDING PAIN COPING STRATEGIES
Avoidance of activity due to expectation of pain and possible re-injury.
Health professional shopping.
Over reliance on passive treatments (massage, hot/cold packs, analgesics).

©NOI

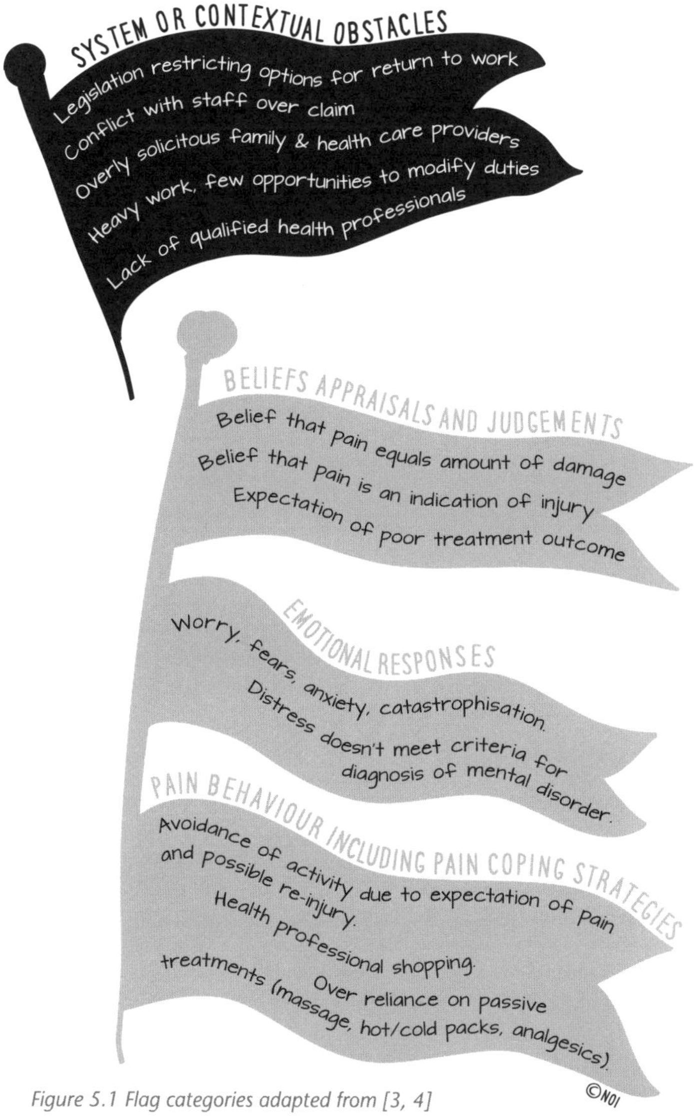

Figure 5.1 Flag categories adapted from [3, 4]

uninspired at work (a black flag and a DIM) but get along well with their workmates (a SIM); they may simultaneously expect that they will return to work in a couple of weeks and expect that they will have a dodgy back forever. Such contrasts fit well with the Protectometer-based model of DIMs and SIMs and also with the principles of neurotags (Chapter 2). Remember, the impact of these contrasting learner variables will depend on their influence, and the principles of neurotags give us clear approaches to adjusting the influence of individual DIMs and SIMs.

Lessons from the education world

Educational research offers its own way of identifying learner-associated variables. After all, the educationalists have been working on this for far longer than we, the health scientists, have. When we dig deeper into this 'Wisdom of the Teachers', the dovetailing with neurotag theory is remarkable. Educationalists are interested in far more than just recognising the presence of a certain concept, they seek to understand its qualities including the *strength*, *coherence* and *commitment* to the concept[3] [1].

The *strength* of a concept is its richness, how strongly it has formed and how 'sticky' it is in the brain. Clearly the stronger the concept the less likely it is to change. Strength occurs on a continuum. Within a population experiencing persistent pain, the strength of a concept will vary within individuals according to biopsychosocial/biomedical orientation, sources of the concept, culture, previous experience, emotional attachment, competing theories and knowledge of physiology among other things. Intuitive beliefs formed directly from experiences (such as pain) can be particularly strong and resistant to change.

Coherence refers to how well the current concept fits together without leaving loose ends. Where ideas lack conceptual coherence, like 'knowledge in pieces' [5] they may be easier to change (look out for the grain metaphors later in this chapter). Incoherent elements of a patient's story that don't fit may provide 'chinks in the armour' where therapists might intervene educationally. Consider Debbie, your inactive patient with chronic pain who says she absolutely can't walk more than 50 metres but tells you that her car broke down last night and she had to walk for 15 minutes to get home. What an opportunity for educational intervention!

There is variation in *commitment* to a concept. Commitment could come from previous experiences, cultural background and social group membership. The learner may not be aware of any other option to his current concept or lose face if he rejects

3   Think of how close this is to the language of the neurotags – the strength and coherence of the belief and the neuronal mass and precision of its neurotag!

the concept. Commitment to a concept will have a large impact on how willing one is to contemplate and consider conceptual change.[4] Some persistent pain sufferers are committed to seeking a passive therapy and a cure rather than playing an active role in their rehabilitation.

Motivation to change is universally recognised as a variable in conceptual change. We like the term 'personal investment' [6]. There are many theories on the place of motivation within conceptual change. Dole and Sinatra [1] propose four key factors that influence motivation that we think are particularly relevant to pain (see Table 5.2).

Features of the deliverer

Health care education is everyone's business. Deliverers include doctors, school teachers, the public, trainers, therapists, journalists, mothers, fathers, you and me. While some deliverers (such as teachers) have had years of formal training, most deliverers, including health care practitioners, have little or no training in *how* to teach. This is remarkable really when you consider that a huge chunk of the work of a health professional is to teach people things such as specific tasks, knowledge, lifestyle skills, behavioural principles. The educationalists are all over this and it is time for the world of health to take a page or two from their books. After all, the capacity for you, the deliverer, to teach is far more likely to impact on someone's health outcome than we ever thought possible.

Leading educationalist Richard Mayer [7] has beautifully summarised the changing role of the deliverer. For many years the most common strategy was *response strengthening* – teaching with reward (strengthening an association with a stimulus) and punishment (weakening an association with a stimulus). Think teachers with canes and rulers and sometimes gentle pats on the head or, as was the case in the class of one primary school student who will remain nameless – Mars bars for everyone who gets an 'A'. For the main part, this has lost traction (yet diabetes rolls on!).

Next in line was *information acquisition,* where the deliverer actively dispensed information and the learner passively received it. Remember rote learning? While this method works in some cases (who fails to reel off 'ellemenopee'?), it often fails to facilitate the deep learning required for true conceptual change.

Knowledge construction is the modern view – it really fits with what we know about pain reconceptualisation. It positions the deliverer as a cognitive guide, presenting information and making sure the learner engages in appropriate cognitive and experiential processing of that information. The learner's role is to make sense of what is being presented. What a sensible idea – an active process for both parties!

Deliverer variables are important but often overlooked. Back in the clinic it's so easy to blame the patient and not ourselves.

Don't be fooled by the brevity of this section on the deliverer – the entire next chapter is dedicated to identifying, exploring and enhancing deliverer variables.

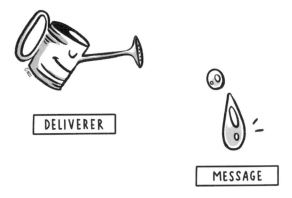

Features of the message

The message is perhaps education at its most basic – what are the concepts that you want the learner to grasp, embed and act on, or in neurotag language, what are the neurotags that you want the learner to develop and use to influence protective behaviours such as pain. It also includes strategies to deliver your educational content.

Message content

The decision of what you want to teach should emerge once you have performed an appropriate assessment of your learner. This assessment should seek specific information and guiding principles such as the learners' current source of information and education targets, all of which will power up your Explain Pain – there is much more on the EP assessment in the next chapter. You'll also need to consider the qualities of your message content. To deliver a persuasive message that brings about conceptual change, it should be comprehensible, plausible, coherent and compelling [1]. We like these terms so much that we have defined them and given some examples in Table 5.3.

---

4   We all know someone who won't eat sashimi or sushi. Can you apply notions of strength, coherence and commitment to their concept and work out why the raw fish is just not on?

Factor	Explanation	Effect on motivation
Conflict	Identification of anomalies between an existing belief and new information creates conflict.	Conflict between existing ideas and new information can motivate adoption of new information.
Personal relevance	Information presented to a learner will have varying degrees of importance, emotional involvement and perceived applicability.	Information that is personally relevant may increase motivation to change. People with pain and those who treat people with pain are likely to have enhanced motivation particularly if personally relevant mutual goals have been established.
Social context	An individual's environment, culture and setting may provide motivational pressure to change.	People in pain may be influenced by their family, their need to work, media, or other people within a pain education group, either towards or away from change.
Intrinsic motivation	Individuals will have a varying innate need to understand their experiences and the world around them.	Individuals with a greater innate curiosity may be more motivated to change and thus enjoy the challenge of considering new concepts.

Table 5.2 Factors that affect motivation to change adapted from [1]

A persuasive message should be:	Definition	How this may relate to EP
Comprehensible	It must be at an appropriate level of understanding and target the kind of misconception (page 113).	Most learners won't be at a level of understanding to comprehend the technical details of nociceptors provided in earlier chapters, but we can make this important information comprehensible by using appropriate metaphor and story.
Plausible	No matter what, the learner must not think 'that's bullshit'.	Information is made more plausible when multiple deliverers speak the same language, present similar stories, back them up with evidence and provide alternative sources of information.
Coherent	All parts of the message must fit together without conflict.	We aim for our curricula to be aligned, meaning that variables related to learner, deliverer, message and context are all attended to.
Compelling	Stories need to use effective multimedia and be relevant, personal, targeted and often emotive.	Make your message novel, a little bit emotional, quirky and at the right time and place, conflict with existing knowledge.

Table 5.3 Features of a persuasive message

Message delivery

There is ample research looking at *how* to best deliver a message.[5] Some clinicians simply give their patients EP to read and then struggle to understand why they don't get it.[6] Perhaps they need to reconsider their delivery. Did you learn maths by just reading your textbook? We know that on average, reading the *right books* [9] leads to an increase in knowledge of pain, a decrease in catastrophising and a change towards a biopsychosocial approach to recovery, BUT, we know that the average effect is small [10]. Copied handouts or library directions alone are not enough!

Multimedia learning

In a world of information bombardment, we want learners to have access to quality multimedia messages that offer the opportunity to accurately convey complex scientific concepts. Multimedia is the presentation of both words (printed or spoken) and pictures (illustrations, photos, animations or videos) [11]. We also include objects, such as pin-boxes (Nugget 14 *Astrocytes, more popular than the Kardashians*) and educational theratube [33] in this definition. This combination of words and pictures promotes construction of coherent mental representations (neurotags) and is known to enhance understanding.

Words and pictures are processed in different ways. We can think of words and pictures as stimuli that can activate verbal neurotags in the case of words, or visual neurotags in the case of pictures. Verbal neurotags can be very influential because they can integrate a large number of neurotags associated with meaning. Visual neurotags can be very influential because they are very precise. By presenting both together, we exploit the benefits of collaboration between already influential neurotags. As such, multimedia is a powerful driver of deep learning and conceptual change because it encourages learners to select and organise relevant information, which in turn avoids overloading working memory with too much extraneous information [11]. We have provided Table 5.4 to summarise the key strategies we have learnt from evidence-based multimedia.

Props

We know that props and pictures are powerful, but it's time to consider whether they're DIMs or SIMs. Anatomical models such as plastic skeletons with red protruding discs and diagnostic images such as x-rays are often used as props to deliver a message. Even frequently used illustrations of a spine that only has bones and discs enhances the concept that the disc can slip. They fail to demonstrate the living, adaptable, force transducing (LAFT) properties of a disc [EP54-55]. Want some first-hand experience? Google 'degeneration', 'arthritis' or 'disc herniation simulator' for some horror DIMs – many of the images you see will be uploaded by well-meaning clinicians, clinical centres or patients themselves. We know that most of these horror images are not related to the likelihood of having pain, but it doesn't seem to stop anyone implying that they do.

Features of the context

Context is the environment in which a thought or an action takes place. The environment consists of physical, psychological, social and cultural domains. You could think of it as the climate perhaps. Contextual variables include the things you see (images on the wall), smell (detergent), hear (crappy elevator music), touch (the moisturiser in the clinic toilet) and taste (maybe the deliverer offers some Toblerone chocolate – see Nugget 60). Context also includes the people you meet, the places you go, the things you think and believe, the things you say and your current biological state. These are the DIM/SIM categories.

A wider view of context also includes societal influences. Is there social security? Are all workers covered by insurance? For how long are workers covered by insurance? How does the media portray pain? Does everybody have equal access to healthcare? What is the quality of the healthcare? Do religious and cultural attitudes impact on health care usage?

Learner variables, deliverer variables, message variables and context variables can all play their part at different times and with different strength during the process of conceptual change. Let's take a look at the process.

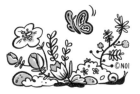

CONTEXT

---

5   We recently tested whether wearing formal attire was perceived as more credible than wearing casual clothing, when the clinician presented the idea of an EP approach to acute back pain management. Rest easy all you casual dressers – there was no difference between groups in treatment credibility [8].

6   We use the term 'get it' in *EP Supercharged* to indicate complete understanding brought on by deep learning.

Multimedia strategies work better when:	Reasoning
• words and pictures are presented together, rather than words alone – narrated words are even more effective	*Words and pictures should be combined for optimal learning. Utilising two cognitive systems, (think here of neurotags) for vision and audition information, increases the influence of the input and its likelihood to embed.* **Keep it together.**
• words and pictures are presented in the same place at the same time (spatially and temporally integrated)	*Avoid materials that require your learner to split attention between multiple sources of information and then mentally integrate them, adding extraneous cognitive load (the total amount of processing that can be supported by both auditory and visual channels at one time).* **If you are drawing on a whiteboard, ask learners to stop writing for a moment and just look and listen.**
• the same information is presented in only one format	*Learning can be impaired when the same information is presented concurrently in multiple forms or is unnecessarily elaborated. If a diagram is intelligible in isolation, it should not be repeated in text.* **If you need to explain an infographic it is not a successful one.**
• cues are added that highlight the key information and its organisation	*Help learners select relevant information by guiding them to essential material. Use colour, highlighting, shading, underline, bolding, italics, size, and spotlight animation. Visually salient information will receive attention.* **Splash out on some colour, but use highlights wisely.**
• extraneous material is excluded, rather than included	*Including information that is not relevant to learning induces extraneous cognitive load, is ineffective for learning and may even hamper it.* **Keep on message.**
• the message is presented in learner-paced segments rather than as a continuous unit	*Too much information will exceed learners' cognitive load. Segmenting slows the pace of presenting to a level that enables learners to carry out essential processing.* **Break up your story.**
• the learner knows the names and characteristics of the main concepts	*Define and draw attention to key words. This reduces cognitive effort and avoids the risk of losing learners while they look up an unfamiliar word.* **Just one unfamiliar word can lose your learner.**
• words are in a conversational style rather than a formal style	*Conversational style activates social cues. Familiarity of words increases their influence because they are already stored in your learner's brain.* **Don't try to sound clever.**
• the learner generates self-explanations during learning	*This encourages learners to think deeply about the material by making inferences and extrapolations. Have them try explaining it to partners, siblings, parents. Start with the cat or dog.* **Get your learner talking.**
• learners draw as they read or listen to educational material	*If your learner tries to represent spatial relationships pictorially (drawings, mind maps) it can help them understand.* **Nothing wrong with scientific doodling.**
• learners receive explanatory feedback.	*Corrective feedback merely provides a measure of right or wrong, whereas explanatory feedback provides the learner with a principle-based explanation of why their answer was right or wrong.* **Explain Pain.**

Table 5.4 Evidence based multimedia strategies adapted from [11]

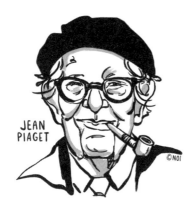

JEAN PIAGET
©NOI

Deep and superficial pathways to conceptual change

Some history

Jean Piaget (1896-1981) was quite a chap. He was never without his pipe and beret, always wore hobnailed walking boots and had a rack full of identical suits [12]. He'd be a real hipster these days. Piaget was a biologist (with papers published on molluscs by the age of 15), a psychologist and an educationalist. He saw no boundaries between biology and psychology and was a real biopsychosocialist before the term was even invented!

While best known for his theories of cognitive development [13], Piaget was also the initiator of the concept of a dual pathway to conceptual change via either assimilation or accommodation of new information [14]. Assimilation means responding by using what you have learnt before. Accommodation means modifying concepts and constructing new neurotags. Later researchers [15-17] further developed this dual pathway concept into deep and superficial learning with Piaget's accommodation linked to deep learning – the deeper the learning, the more effectively the brain accommodates.

Superficial and deep concepts of 'slipped disc'

We can also think of deep and superficial learning in terms of neurotags. Let's think about superficial learning first. Say your learner generates a fresh neurotag that holds the new concept you have been wanting him to learn, for example *'discs can't slip'*. When you ask him *'can discs slip?'* he replies *'no, discs can't slip'*. However, this information does not impact on his behaviour and he do not extrapolate this new

concept. Instead he simply replaces *'slipped'* or *'slipped disc'* with *'herniated'* or *'damaged'* and everything else stays the same – his thoughts, fears, movements and, well, life. He has clearly generated a neurotag that has no influence on other neurotags and no influence on action neurotags that generate movement, pain, thoughts and feelings. This can be considered 'superficial learning'.

Take this other scenario, that of deep learning. Your learner does indeed generate a fresh neurotag that holds the new concept of 'discs can't slip'. When you ask him *'Can discs slip?'* he replies *'No, discs can't slip'*. He then extrapolates that and begins to attempt to bend over. He shift his language from *'I have a slipped disc'* to *'I injured my disc some time ago'*. He looks for other explanations for his pain. In this scenario, the new neurotag is having some influence beyond itself. It is influencing action neurotags that generate movement, pain, thoughts and feelings. This can be considered 'deep learning'.

Using the original work from Piaget and others [eg.18], we have constructed a version of deep and superficial learning that really seems to fit the conceptual change we seek in Explain Pain. This is detailed in Figure 5.2.

The deep pathway is your goal

Optimal conceptual change requires that your learner embraces the material in a deep way. Deep learners want to know the big picture, fill in the gaps in knowledge and enhance the very foundations of their knowledge. This arises from a 'felt need' [19] to engage with the material, that is, an intentional learner driven event. Learners on this pathway may say or think *'I'm in, tell me more'* (Figure 5.2). They reflect on the information, they experiment with behaviour changes related to the information, they extrapolate. Learning on this pathway, though sometimes tough when you are really hurting, is positive, rewarding and can be enjoyable. Most importantly, it is durable and transferable to other situations such as another injury or someone else's problems; however learners may still deviate from the pathway, give up and end at no conceptual change.[7]

Most of us learn superficially – ever crammed in order to pass an exam and then forgotten the content a week later? Health care practitioners will notice patterns in their clients on the superficial pathway such as a reliance on passive treatment and avoidance of attempts to deeply learn – this may show up in

---

7   Think of somebody well into their anti-smoking programme who throws in the towel and goes back to the ciggies, or a slowly improving patient with back pain who is suddenly convinced that a spinal fusion is the answer.

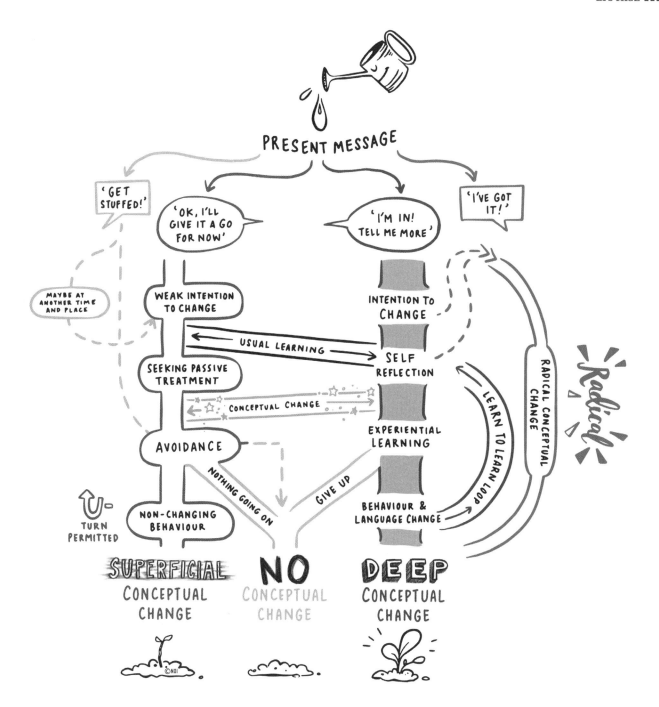

Figure 5.2 Pathways to superficial, deep, radical and no conceptual change

well-known clinical phenomena such as missing appointments, finding other priorities, attending for bursts of therapy before lengthy breaks and a reliance on heuristics ('rules of thumb' such as *'just crack my back in'* or *'my physio knows best'*). It does take great effort, resources and time to deeply process some of the Target Concepts necessary for an optimal Explain Pain outcome and it's not necessarily their fault that learners are on a superficial pathway.

Going deep and encouraging learners from the superficial to the deep pathway is what this book is all about – on the superficial pathway, the deep conceptual change that we seek will never be achieved.

Speed of conceptual change

Conceptual change as proposed by most theorists [20-22] is a gradual process relying on Hebbian mechanisms – where coincident activity in two synaptically coupled neurones results in an increase in the synaptic strength between them [23], crudely referred to as 'rewiring'. This Hebbian thing is often captured with the phrase *'neurones that fire together, wire together'.* The principle that is captured by it still stands, although we now have a more sophisticated understanding of how it works – we talk about it within the wider and more functionally relevant concept of neurotags and the principles that govern the operation of neurotags. We also now know that it is not just neurones that are involved, which is why we prefer the more generic 'brain cells', because it includes both neurones and non-neuronal cells such as astrocytes and microglia.

Integrating the added complexity of the neurotag model with a relatively simple Hebbian synapse-focussed model accommodates instances of rapid, or radical conceptual change (Figure 5.2). Change scientists usually discuss such radical conceptual change from a sociological or behavioural perspective, but seldom touch on the biological substrate. These radical changes are usually seen as positive[8] and most dramatically captured by conversion or revelation type experiences. Both of us have observed patients undergo rapid radical reconceptualisation of pain, even from a single EP session and there is potentially vast value in pursuing a better understanding of how to facilitate this. We also know some clever therapists who are researching and achieving rapid conceptual change using powerful experiential learning, such as deadlifting and headstands for people who thought that these activities were impossible. This rapid and radical change is superimposed on a strong, coherent and guided Explain Pain base, but we also suspect that the more we learn about this, the better.

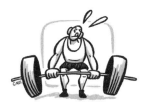

Existing knowledge frameworks and misconceptions

The patient's existing knowledge framework is an important learner related variable. But if you, the deliverer, are not aware of the importance of this variable or are unable to deal with it, then it becomes a deliverer related variable – yours! So this is one you definitely don't want to miss, because it's a big one.

Why don't they 'get it'?

Every one of us who has tried to formally educate, tell a story or joke will have had the experience of feeling we are talking to a blank wall – that our story is bouncing off the would-be recipients, their eyes glazing over.[9] No one, deliverer nor intended recipient, likes a story that falls flat, especially when it's your best joke. We admit that we have previously thought *'why don't they get my pain story, they must be really thick'* – not only patients but a few colleagues too! Let's explore the very nature of misconceptions about pain.

---

8 Though these days negative radical reconceptualisation away from societal norms seems frequent. At the time of writing, the term 'radicalisation' refers to complete endorsement of extraordinary beliefs and attitudes that are perceived by all but a tiny minority of the world as wholly negative. This radicalisation is a profound example of deep learning and can be considered in terms of learner, deliverer, message and context variables and also in terms of collaboration of neurotags and their collective influence. Critically, there are clear examples of both gradual radicalisation and rapid radicalisation.

---

9 Even when it looks like they 'get it', we might have missed the mark – check out Dimos in Painful Yarns [PY97-104]!

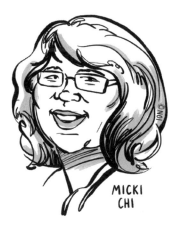

MICKI CHI

Introducing *kinds* of misconceptions

We draw heavily from the theoretical framework of conceptual change developed and researched by cognitive learning scientist Michelene (Micki) Chi [24, 25]. Other conceptual change frameworks exist [26], and they have much in common, but we think Micki Chi's work fits well with our notions of neurotags, changeable brains, conceptual change in pain and what we've seen in the clinic for years. Broadly, we believe that we can identify five kinds of misconceptions, usually overlapping, in our patients. For clinical utility we have linked some of these misconceptions to the metaphor of grains of sand (Table 5.5). Educational interventions should be more effective if they take into account the kinds of misconception that the learner may have.

Kinds of misconceptions	
Missing bits	*Gaps in the overall coherency of the knowledge*
Single grain misconception	*Simple, non-sticky, 'grain of sand' misconceptions*
Sandcastle misconception	*'Flawed mental model' – single grains now sticking or clumping to each other*
Sandstone misconception	*Grains in the sandcastle stuck tightly to each other*
Lack of neurotag for emergent patterns	*No framework for information to stick to*

Table 5.5 Five kinds of misconceptions

Missing bits – filling in the gaps

The simplest category presents when the misconception is based on 'missing bits'. Educational interventions here can be relatively smooth sailing, avoiding the conflict, emotion and hard work that is sometimes required to facilitate conceptual change. Here information 'fills in the gaps' and we can think of this category as 'knowledge enrichment' [27]. Learners who are already active knowledge seekers and searching for the increased control that quality information allows may respond dramatically when you just fill in a few gaps for them – we call them 'gap info responders'. All health care professionals would be aware of this form of education. We, the deliverers, usually feel quite pleased with ourselves as gap filling education can be instantly rewarding and pleasant. At this point the learner's knowledge could be considered incomplete or in the form of 'knowledge in pieces' [5]. Gap-filling education should provide a stronger and more coherent mental frameworks for ongoing future knowledge absorption. From a neurotag perspective, we can think of facilitating the generation of neurotags that are more likely to collaborate with existing neurotags, rather than compete with them.

Gap filling still requires considerable educational and interactional skill. You will need to find the gaps and there is no algorithm or educational recipe even at this level. Gap filling often involves more than the provision of verbal information (gap filling in real time) – it may include suggestions of websites, books, YouTube clips and any other relevant multimedia. It often involves affirmation or even negating existing conceptions.

Examples of gap filling in real time
- Affirming that what the learner says is correct (if it is)
- Comparing different tissue healing rates – disc tissue heals slower than muscle
- Providing various nuggets to fill in the gaps (Chapter 8)
- Giving reasons why a review or treatment from another professional is necessary (or unnecessary)
- Linking symptoms to common pain mechanisms (Figure 6.2, page 126)

Facilitating conceptual change in the next four categories is more difficult than simply filling in missing bits and may engender some conflict. But don't panic…

Unhelpful knowledge and beliefs at the 'single grain level'

We use grains of sand as metaphor here – a 'grain of knowledge' is a single concept or a small cluster of concepts. Remember that concepts must be held by neurotags and that neurotags obey the same broad principles (page 21) regardless of what their outputs are – cognitions, movement, autonomic responses etc.

A learner's pain knowledge may be held in grains that are not deeply anchored, sticky[10], related to each other or elaborated into a more mature concept. Misconceptions at the single grain size are very common[11] and are likely features of superficial learning (see box below). They can be identified during routine evaluations or responses to questions such as *'what do you think is going on in your body?'* Many common DIMs are misconceptions that exist at the single grain level, such as the conceptual metaphors – *'I've done a disc',* and *'I need to push through the pain barrier'.*

> **Examples of common single grain misconceptions**
>
> *It's just old age*
>
> *My back is out*
>
> *Open wounds heal well in sea water*
>
> *Pain is weakness leaving the body*
>
> *I have a dodgy back*
>
> *My physio knows my body better than anyone*
>
> *I've got a disease – Scheuermann's Disease*

Take *'my knee – it's just old age'* as a frequently heard misconception held at single grain level (old age is not a pathology!). This conceptual metaphor may exist as a single isolated grain of information without links to any other grains of information. Everyone knows that exercise is good for them, but the misconception may create a belief that *'exercise is no longer for me'.* Such a grain could develop further and become 'stickier' in the brain – your patient's neighbour might have had a total knee replacement and relentless TV advertising for

arthritic supplements (now that your patient sits all day) may have added more grains making the original misconception even stickier. Now the misconceptions have strengthened to a sandcastle level of *'I am finished and ready for the scrapheap'.*

Single grain misconceptions should be easy to manage. Because they are not deeply elaborated they can be refuted, often 'head on' or explicitly, perhaps with something like *'age has nothing to do with it – we know age does not link to pain and if it was an age problem, both knees would hurt the same'.* It is basically acknowledging what the learner says, offering the alternative (the truth as we know it), inevitably creating a bit of conflict, but helping your patient weigh all the information. This hopefully leads him to a helpful revision of his previous knowledge. With some banter back and forth, a good physical examination of the knee and introduction of some better metaphors, perhaps something like *'sure, your knees are oldies but goodies'* and *'we all have a few kisses of time',* the original, unhelpful metaphor *'my knee – it's just old age'* can be revised.

Yet a belief that there is a singular blame for one's pain can be powerful. For learners in pain and particularly for those who have lost money, happiness and jobs and have encountered denial of their pain state, there may seem to be a one directional blame for their problem such as *'it's all the supervisor's fault'.* This is hard to refute and can't be easily denied and challenged. Even though this may seem like a really strong singular grain, this misconception might now be held at 'sandcastle' level.

Misconceptions at sandcastle level

With ongoing pain and troubles, unhelpful knowledge and beliefs may be held as well elaborated and increasingly coherent misconceptions[12]. Although there may be many underlying misconceptions, they might be summarised for the person in pain as a single statement, such as *'I am broken'.* We refer to this category or misconception as being held at 'sandcastle' level. From the perspective of neurotags, we can consider that many concept neurotags (or grains) are collaborating – remembering the principles that govern neurotags include mass, precision, and bioplasticity. When many concept neurotags collaborate, both mass (the number of brain cells involved) and precision (the relative probability of member and non-member brain cells firing) increase. These two principles mean that this sandcastle

---

10 We like the term 'sticky' to suggest a more influential neurotag. We picked the term up from Mark Jensen, Professor of Everything at the University of Washington, Seattle and genuine nice guy.

11 Still think you can catch a cold from cold weather? Still think you shouldn't swim for 30 minutes after eating? Still think your leg hairs grow back thicker when you shave them? Still think Australia is really 'down-under'?

12 Make sure you are okay with 'coherent misconceptions', that is, coherent to the holder.

level misconception will be highly influential. The more influential, the more it can engage pain and other outputs, such as behaviours, then the more difficult it is to change.

Misconceptions at the sandcastle level present more conceptual change challenges than missing bits or single grain misconceptions. Some possible contributing grains to the common belief at sandcastle level that *'I am in pain therefore I am damaged'* for an individual experiencing chronic pain are shown in Figure 5.3.

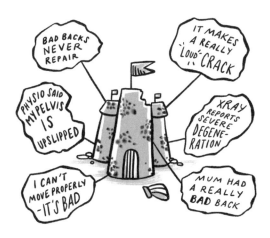

*Figure 5.3 Grains which may construct a '**I have pain therefore I am damaged**' sandcastle*

Many common 'sandcastle' concepts held by individuals experiencing chronic pain have been identified and included in what became known as 'yellow flags' – psychosocial factors known to predict pain chronicity (Figure 5.1). Some common misconceptions at a sandcastle level are listed below.

Common misconceptions likely held at sandcastle level

It's not safe for me to move that way, it's sure to do damage'

'It's all work's fault'

'My pain will be worse today, it's Wednesday'

'With all the technology around they should be able to fix it'

'If only they could just reach in and pull it out'

'If I bend over, one of those discs could slip out'

'My pain is different to the one I read about in Explain Pain'

Misconceptions held at a sandcastle level are so well established that any new knowledge is often assimilated without updating the erroneous misconception. The individual now has more grains of knowledge, but the misconception remains.

> *We strongly believe that when attempts at pain education interventions fail in the clinic, or as p art of research, it is possible that clinicians and researchers are just throwing more grains of sand at the learner without addressing their level of misconception.*

We do not have a questionnaire (yet) to identify whether a learner holds single grain, sandcastle or sandstone misconceptions. However, we trust you're clever enough with clinical reasoning judgements to distinguish between them. Therapists collecting E-flags (page 133) or DIMs may suddenly think, *'hang on, all these single grain misconceptions have formed a sandcastle. And increasingly they are no longer open for change'*.

There are a number of ways of managing unhelpful sandcastles; including presenting an alternative sandcastle and dealing with one grain at a time.

Presenting an alternative sandcastle

'Holistic confrontation' [24] is usually about utilising multimedia depictions to compare and contrast the entire misconceived mental model with a more accurate alternative. This provides alternative knowledge at the same level as a person's misconception. During an Explain Pain intervention this may involve asking the learner to express her pain experience with words, pictures and diagrams and then to contrast this with material showing the correct visual representation. Visually encoded data are very precise and reasonably high mass, making them highly influential. If they collaborate with other neurotags, they can 'lend' their high precision to those neurotags. Examples of multimedia that may present an alternative sandcastle include the conceptual change pathway map (Figure 5.2), drawings of sandcastles with labelled grains (Figure 5.3) and contrasting normal and perturbed output systems using media in [EPH28].

Visual representation: friend or foe?

We might ask in relation to someone's painful body part *'do you have a picture in your mind of what this looks like?'* Daniel – a rower with thoracic pain putting his Olympic three-peat at risk – answered *'absolutely – my first rib gets stuck'*. He then pulled out a drawing, done for him by an internationally renowned 'stuck rib specialist', that clearly showed one rib jammed against the sternum, straining a muscle and squashing a lung. It was biologically daft but artistically quite clever. In contrast, Tori – a hairdresser with cervical pain, headaches and exactly the same diagnosis, answered *'no idea – I was just told it was getting stuck'*. Daniel had a clear visual representation of his problem, based on the advice of a 'guru'; Tori had no visual representation of her problem. The structural misconception was probably more influential for Daniel than it was for Tori. She responded very well to Lorimer saying *'that's nonsense really'* – for her it was a single grain misconception. Daniel needed the drawing deconstructed (holistic confrontation) and a great deal of work besides – his structural misconception had become a well elaborated sandcastle. Or, the structural misconception neurotag had become very influential over protective output neurotags.

Waves of knowledge wear away sandcastles – grain-by-grain

If we continue the seaside metaphor, then waves of knowledge may erode and demolish sandcastles. In contrast to the single-grain misconception where more explicit education is possible, a sandcastle misconception requires a bit more finesse and work. We suggest identifying the key grains in the sandcastle, affirming and enhancing the correct concepts (SIMs) and removing the unhelpful ones (DIMs). This is where the sandcastle metaphor helps – the imagery of waves of knowledge slowly altering the mental sandcastle until it is completely revised. Sandcastles erode at different rates. Sometimes one wave flattens it. In this case, there may be a core assumption – a key grain (major DIM) with lots of edges that interlock with other grains holding the sandcastle up, but which can be liberated with knowledge.

So with this advice, you wouldn't say to someone who complains that Wednesdays hurt, *'what do you mean it hurts on Wednesday, it's just a day, just imagine it's Tuesday or Thursday'*. Rather you would identify the grains that make up the *'I hurt on Wednesday'* sandcastle. It might be a supervisor, hump day, the injury occurred on a Wednesday or other family demands occur on a Wednesday.

These two methods, 'presenting the alternative sandcastle' and 'grain-by-grain', can be used together. Deciding which method to start with will depend on your learner's situation and your delivery skills. For example, you may not confront the woman who has a strong, almost impenetrable belief that her back is damaged with 'pain doesn't equal damage' – she may require an implicit grain by grain method, at least initially. However, another client may benefit from you planting conceptual change seeds such as 'pain doesn't equal damage' or 'pain has become over protective'.

Sandstone – firmly fixed mental models

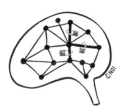 Therapists know rejection well. Remind yourself of the two possible paths ('get stuffed' and 'give up') that lead to 'no conceptual change' (Figure 5.2). A learner's knowledge framework may be so coherent to them that it's extremely difficult to change. Repeated experiences with biomedically based clinicians may also cement sandstone concepts. There may be clear religious (*'It's God's will for me to suffer'*), cultural [29], cognitive disability and language barriers to conceptual change. In some situations, we have no right or moral authority nor sufficient skill to alter the concept. But keeping our goal of an NNE of 1[13] alive, we can have a go by adapting our approach. Broadly, educational therapy can be carried out within the confines of the patient's concept, but without directly challenging it.

Examples that might infer a sandstone misconception

'It's God's will'

'I must suffer'

'The glass is broken'

'It's a massive disc herniation – four specialists have told me and I can see it on the MRI. You can't help that.'

Misconceptions might be so strong that they exist at a sandstone level. But even sandstone can be chiselled and will crumble. For best management of a sandstone concept, a biopsychosocially-aware clinician will recognise the need to upskill his or her knowledge where needed, to understand the role of religion, culture and long-term biomedical exposure. Many learners may not have been given the educational opportunity of another viewpoint. Even if a concept is coherent for that person, it can

---

13 NNE equals number needed to educate, see Chapter 6, page 123.

still be used as a discussion prop. For example, a good way to extract DIMs from a religious person may be to ask 'why would your God want you to have a sore knee?'[14]

Lack of neurotags for emergent patterns

In fields such as science education, people are known to have difficulty adopting new concepts that involve *emergent properties* if they have very little experience with them. This is important for learning about pain because pain itself can be thought of as emergent. So, what does that really mean?

Emergent patterns occur, often surprisingly, when a collection of agents interact with each other in complex ways. Examples of agents might be water molecules, brain cells, insects, humans, or cars. The patterns or phenomena that *emerge* from their collective activity could be a snowflake from water molecules, a thought from brain cells, a swarm of insects, a crowd at a water fountain during a music festival in summer, a traffic jam or weather. Pain can be considered an emergent process arising from the collective activity of cells, especially, but not limited to those in the brain. Don't forget, agents also include other people and places. This suggests that to understand pain and other phenomena with emergent qualities such as love and anger, a person requires neurotags for emergent concepts *and* neurotags for linear concepts to allow ideal absorption and management of incoming data.

One person clapping is pretty boring, but when ten, a hundred, or ten thousand people *applaud,* the emergent rhythms and patterns, lulls and surges in the sound can be as interesting as the performance itself. A few neurones firing may not mean much, but when millions fire in a complex dynamic pattern, thoughts and movement and perhaps pain emerge. An ant on the west side of the anthill probably doesn't know what his ant mate on the north side is doing, but the overall anthill construction works and that, my friend, is truly astonishing.

Emergent and Linear Patterns

A great way to understand emergent patterns is to contrast them with linear patterns (contrasting is a great way to learn). Of any observable phenomenon or pattern, it could be said that some are more linear, while others are more emergent, with examples at either end of this continuum being strong examples of either. Consciousness could be considered to be

toward the emergent end of the spectrum and moon phases toward the linear end.

Linear patterns usually have a dominant initiating event and the sequential nature means that something has to happen and perhaps be completed before the next step can occur. You eat, then swallow, then digest, then poo. The ventricles of the heart contract and blood flows along pre-determined pathways (vessels) in a defined and ordered direction. People tend to understand these patterns with linear features. Many people are less able however, to understand and use more emergent patterns.

Emergent patterns can be directly contrasted with linear patterns by the interactions between the parts, objects or 'agents' that make up the pattern. Consider the difference between a mother duck leading her ducklings across a road (a more linear pattern) and an emergent swarm of locusts[15] (Table 5.6).

In the example below (Table 5.6), swap a locust for a brain cell and you have a reasonable analogy for how the brain probably works. Can you distinguish between emergent and linear patterns? Test yourself with Figure 5.4 (answers at the end of the chapter).

Mother duck leading ducklings	Locust swarm
The mother duck is the clear leader and pattern controller.	There is no clear leader; all the locusts interact with one another.
There is a collective and shared goal of crossing the road.	Each locust is doing its own thing with the pattern of the swarm emerging as a result of the millions of interactions.
The ducklings follow the mother duck in an order, one after the other.	All of the locusts are simultaneously interacting with many others all of the time.
The pattern will start when the mother duck decides to move to another location and stop when the destination is reached.	There is no defined start or end point of the swarm – it literally emerges from nowhere and then can spontaneously dissipate.

Table 5.6 Contrasting patterns that are more linear and emergent adapted from [25]

---

14 We're really chuffed that the Bible supports Explain Pain, for example Proverb 12:18 *'The words of the reckless pierce like swords, but the tongue of the wise brings healing'.*

15 Google 'starling murmuration' for some incredible emergent bird behaviour.

EPS PAGE **118**

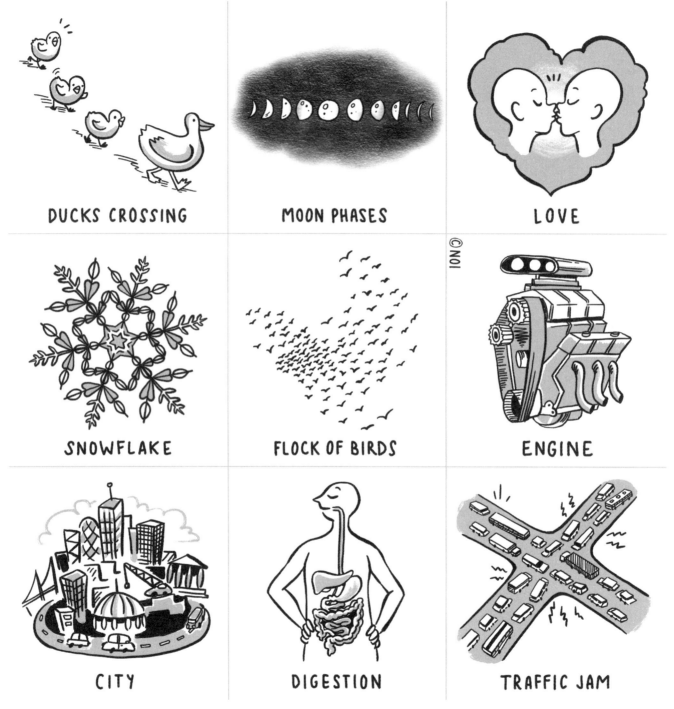

Figure 5.4 Which processes are more linear or emergent?

Problems with lack of neurotags for emergent patterns

As we suggest above, in order to deeply understand pain, you probably need to have accessible neurotags for understanding emergent patterns. It's likely that we will have a well developed, perhaps over-developed framework for understanding linear patterns – they are easier to understand and most educational strategies are linear. Most of the childrens stories we grew up with are linear, for example *Little Red Riding Hood*.

Research tells us that most people's framework for understanding emergent patterns is likely to be a little dormant [25, 30]. Problems arise when people try to understand emergent patterns by applying well-rehearsed and deeply embedded linear frameworks. This is well known in the teaching of science [25, 31, 32]. Such students have problems when they are taught about processes that are emergent (diffusion, electricity, natural selection and evolution), but don't have such difficulties when they are taught about processes that are linear. Micki Chi observed this and had a eureka moment – perhaps these students just don't have a framework into which they can build emergent phenomena. So she taught them about emergence. Great!

Reflect on these clinical experiences:

- If someone seeks and blames a single 'cause' for a problem, this is a dead giveaway that they have a linear explanation for their pain. For example, *'I have done a disc'*, or *'that surgeon did a bad job'*, as an explanation for a three year old spinal problem is classic, single 'leader' linear thinking.

- Clinicians may reflect on how easy it usually is to educate about tissue healing (a more linear process) and then how the learner's eyes glaze over when the discussion turns to pain or emotions (a more emergent process). This switch from neurotags for understanding linear patterns to neurotags for understanding emergent patterns can be hard for many and likely impossible for some when their neurotags for understanding emergent patterns are under-developed or even completely absent.

- Sometimes learners can't 'see the wood for the trees'. They may have a plethora of knowledge but it is in pieces. They can't draw it together, make it coherent and then extrapolate it, perhaps due to the lack of an emergent neurotag.[16]

- Maybe it is obvious in passing comments – *'Yes I know I have hurt a disc, but work is tough, the kids are driving me up the wall and my car has broken down – lucky my wife's such a gem!'*. This suggests an emergent appreciation of experience.

Can emergence be taught?

Yes it can [25]! We think for really good quality *Explain Pain*, the learner's neurotag for understanding emergent phenomenon needs to be activated. We've included a short emergent neurotag module in Chapter 9 (Novella 12 *Traffic jams, cakes, snowflakes and pain*).

Maybe we also need to ask – does the deliverer have a framework that allows her to engage emergent phenomena? It's time to take a good hard look in the mirror. Look at your own capacity to grasp modern pain science and emergent patterns. What do you see? Do you find it easier to make sense of linear phenomena? Do you find yourself thinking that your patients are biopsychosocial beings but *your* pain, well that is 'physical'? One of the most challenging parts of really joining the Explain Pain Revolution is recognising where your own barriers are. If you find emergent thinking difficult, do not despair – you can learn. And you can learn the same way your patients will! By getting your hands dirty, so to speak – Novella 12 is for you too.

Helping others construct neurotags for understanding emergent patterns could make a real and positive difference to how they understand their pain experience. How helpful might a quick explanation of traffic jams or locust swarms be for a person reporting that his or her entire body and life is falling apart as a result of chronic pain following a minor injury? How much more powerful could an explanation of pain be for a person who is convinced that surgery and *'cutting the painful bit out'* is going to fix the problem if it is accompanied by a discussion about the complex interaction of self and environment and the emergence of pain? Here's a thought; if you have a patient who is a keen baker, how might a story about baking a cake be relevant to his understanding of pain? Or if she enjoys a wine, how making pain is like making a fine wine. Many such stories describe emergence.

---

16 When Dave marks assignments where the question requires some understanding of emergence, such as *'describe pain as a brain output rather than an input'* some students are all over the place with piecemeal answers and lists. Others pull it together and extrapolate and infer. Maybe the latter have more emergent neurotags?

Answers to linear and emergent patterns (Figure 5.4)
LINEAR – Ducks crossing, Moon phases, Engine, Digestion
EMERGENT – Love, Snowflake, Flock of birds, City, Traffic jam

References

1. Dole JA & Sinatra GM (1998) Reconceptualising change in the cognitive construction of knowledge. Educ Psychol 33: 109-128.

2. Pinheiro MB, et al. (2015) Symptoms of Depression and Risk of New Episodes of Low Back Pain: A Systematic Review and Meta-Analysis. Arthritis Care Res 67: 1591-1603.

3. Nicholas MK, et al. (2011) Early Identification and Management of Psychological Risk Factors ("Yellow Flags") in Patients With Low Back Pain: A Reappraisal. Phys Ther 91: 737-753.

4. Kendall N, Linton S & Main C (1997) Guide to Assessing Psycho-social Yellow Flags in Acute Low Back Pain: Risk Factors for Long-Term Disability and Work Loss. ACC: Wellington.

5. diSessa AA (2013) A bird's-eye view of the "pieces" vs. "coherence" controversy (from the "pieces" side of the fence) in International Handbook of Research on Conceptual Change. Vosniadou S. Ed. Routledge: New York.

6. Ambrose SA, et al. (2010) How Learning Works: 7 Research-Based Principles for Smart Teaching. Jossey-Bass: California.

7. Mayer RE (2012) Cognitive Learning, in Encyclopedia of the Sciences of Learning, Seel NM. Ed. Springer US: New York.

8. Traeger AC, et al. (2016) What you wear does not affect the credibility of your treatment: A blinded randomized controlled study. Patient Educ Couns 10: 104-111.

9. Moseley GL (2008) Painful Yarns: Metaphors and stories to help understand the biology of pain. Dancing Giraffe Press: Canberra.

10. Gallagher L, McAuley J & Moseley GL (2013) A randomized-controlled trial of using a book of metaphors to reconceptualize pain and decrease catastrophizing in people with chronic pain. Clin J Pain 29: 20-25.

11. Mayer RE (2014) The Cambridge Handbook of Multimedia Learning. 2nd Edn. Cambridge University Press: Cambridge.

12. Bliss J (2010) Recollections of Jean Piaget. The Psychologist 23: 444-446.

13. Piaget J (1936) La naissance de l'intelligence [The Origins of Intelligence in Children]. Delachaux et Niestlé: Switzerland.

14. Piaget J (1970) The science of education and the psychology of the child. Grossman: New York.

15. Marton F & Saljo R (1976) On qualitative differences in learning: 1- outcome and process. Brit J Educ Psychol 46: 4-11.

16. Entwistle N & Ramsden P (1979) Understanding Student Learning. Croom Helm: London.

17. Biggs, J. (1979) Individual differences in study processes and the Quality of Learning Outcomes. J High Educ 8: 381-394.

18. Gregoire M (2003) Is It a Challenge or a Threat? A Dual-Process Model of Teachers' Cognition and Appraisal Processes During Conceptual Change. Educ Psychol Rev 15: 147-179.

19. Biggs J (2011) Teaching For Quality Learning At University. 4th Edn. McGraw-Hill Education: London.

20. diSessa AA & Sherin BL (1998) What changes in conceptual change? International Journal of Science Education 20: 1151-1191.

21. Smith JP, diSessa AA & Roschelle J (1993) Misconceptions reconceived: a constructivist analysis of knowledge in transition. J Learn Sci 3: 115-164.

22. Siegler RS (1996) Emerging Minds. Oxford University Press: New York.

23. Hebb DO (1949) The Organization of Behavior. Wiley: New York.

24. Chi MTH (2013) Two kinds and four sub-types of misconceived knowledge, ways to change it, and the learning outcomes in International Handbook of Research on Conceptual Change Vosniadou S. Ed. Routledge: New York.

25. Chi MTH, et al. (2012) Misconceived causal explanations for emergent processes. Cognitive Sci 36: 1-61.

26. Vosniadou S. Ed. (2013) International Handbook of Research on Conceptual Change. Routledge: New York.

27. Carey S (1991) Knowledge acquisition: enrichment or conceptual change? in The Epigenesis of Mind: Essays on biology and cognition, Carey S & Gelman R. Eds. Lawrence Erlaum Associates: New Jersey.

28. Moseley GL Butler DS (2015) The Explain Pain Handbook: Protectometer. Noigroup Publications: Adelaide.

29. Morris D (1991) The Culture of Pain. University of California Press: Berkeley.

30. Slotta JD & Chi MTH (2006) Helping Students Understand Challenging Topics in Science Through Ontology Training. Cogn Instr 24: 261-289.

31. Chi MTH (1992) Conceptual change within and across ontological categories: examples from learning and discovery in science, in Cognitive Models of Science: Minnesota studies in the philosophies of science, Giere R. Ed. University of Minnesota Press: Minneapolis.

32. Chi MTH (2005) Commonsense Conceptions of Emergent Processes: Why Some Misconceptions Are Robust. J Learn Sci 14: 161-199.

33. Neuro Orthopaedic Institute NOI (2015) Nerves, knowledge and theratube - with David Butler, viewed 21 March 2017, <https://www.youtube.com/watch?v=gdKldyXgkgs>.

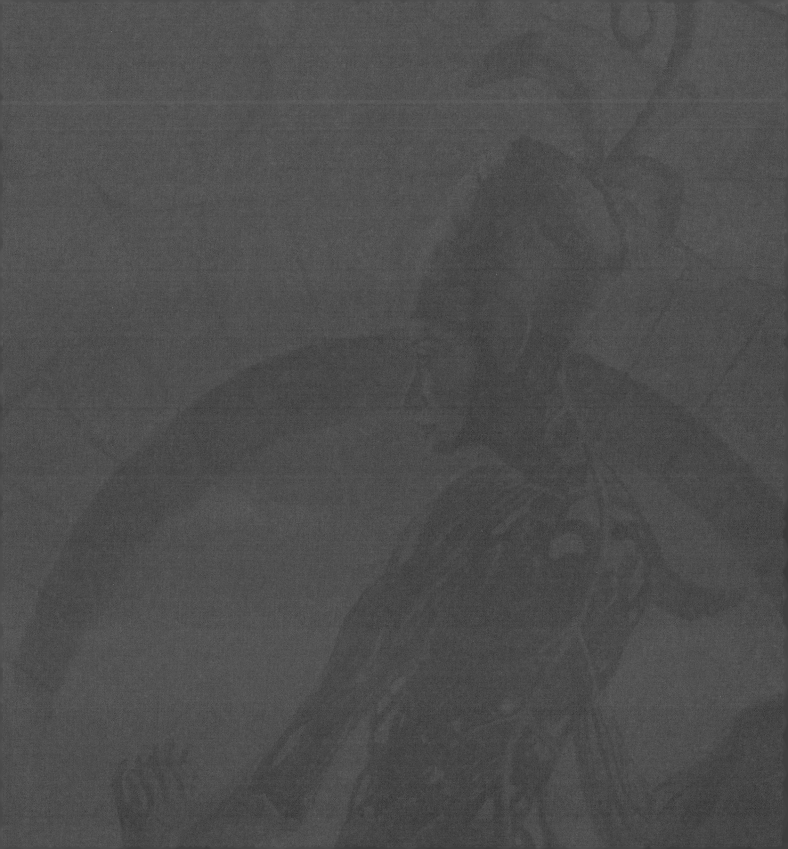

6

Deliverer competencies, assessment and curriculum

Education for everyone

Our target is effective, up to date, behaviour-changing and pain-reducing education for all. We are not alone with this goal. In 2015 the World Education Forum created a global challenge to *'ensure inclusive and equitable quality education and promote lifelong learning opportunities for all'* by 2030 [1]. Such a goal would mean that every person educated (or 'treated') with Explain Pain would have a defined successful learning outcome. That is, they would undergo knowledge enrichment and/or conceptual change that eased their pain in some way. In epidemiological terms, the number needed to treat (NNT) will be 1. We offer a new consideration, that the number needed to *educate* (NNE) should also be 1 (in other words everyone benefits from Explain Pain). This is the goal of the Explain Pain Revolution. Such a goal requires attention to all the variables that may impact on the outcomes of an educational intervention.

> **Education** – we use this term broadly. We like the following adapted definition: education is the wise, hopeful, skilled and respectful facilitation of learning undertaken in the belief that all should have the chance to share in life [2]. Conceptual change is a part of education.

In Chapter 5 we categorised variables that could impact on conceptual change into features related to **the learner, the deliverer, the message** and **the context**. In this chapter we explore the often forgotten features of the deliverer and suggest desirable deliverer competencies in order to facilitate effective conceptual change for a learner. We also introduce an Explain Pain assessment, all leading to the development of an Explain Pain curriculum.

'Curriculum!' you might gasp! As clinicians we have probably never thought about developing curricula for our patients, yet if you are teaching anything you would have to have a curriculum, though it may lurk unconsciously in your brain. Despite not being a healthcare tradition (yet), our view is that curricula are fundamental to education and health and our goal of an NNE of 1.

A curriculum is the linking framework between the learner, the deliverer, the message and the context. It's all about the educational materials, methods, measurements and planned experiences that a learner undergoes in order to achieve conceptual change. A developed curriculum should provide answers to questions that a competent deliverer should have, such as *'what do they know now?'* and *'what do they need to know?'* and *'how and when and where will I deliver the information?'*. Curricula are fun and trendy. When we meet clinicians who tell us they are educating using EP or researchers investigating EP, we will often ask: *'tell me something about your curriculum.'* We frequently receive blank looks, but feel that if we can induce some reflection, then it is a worthwhile question.

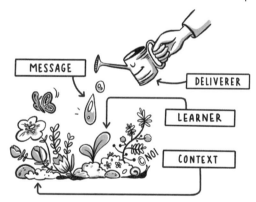

Key deliverer competencies

Physiotherapists require certain competencies before they touch a patient; so do doctors before they prescribe a drug; psychologists before they treat; and electricians before they rewire your house. Indeed, teachers need certain competencies before they are let loose on our kids. All professionals require intervention-related competencies. For anyone delivering education, and this includes health professionals, educational skills are necessary competencies. Competencies are critical to optimal curriculum development and we suggest 11 key Explain Pain competencies.

1. Perform a comprehensive initial assessment

We assume that a comprehensive, valid and up-to-date assessment, as is appropriate to the deliverer's profession and within a biopsychosocial framework, has been carried out prior to the educational intervention. Hopefully, the deliverer's profession endorses a current view of pain sciences,[1] such as the Interprofessional Pain Curriculum from the International Association for the Study of Pain (IASP) [3]. In particular, all professionals require an awareness of 'red flags' and a responsibility to refer for further medical or psychological assessments where they are indicated. The medical profession excels at identifying the sometimes nasty but rare issues that require medical attention. The assessment should be at a depth that allows identification of education targets, informs the best way to educate an individual or group, and ultimately provides the information to make an effective curriculum.

2. Have the biopsychosocial framework deep in your guts – understand, endorse and spread the Grand Poobah Pain Theory

You might have to quickly turn back to Chapter 2 and reaffirm your ties with the biopsychosocial model and the Grand Poobah Pain Theory. Until you really have these ideas deep inside your belly, you will be half-hearted and half-arsed in helping others understand why their pain is not quite as simple as they might have thought, why it doesn't respond predictably, why it is worse some days than others and why it hasn't gone away even though the injury should have healed.

All of the potential contributors outlined in the biopsychosocial diagram have biological substrates and consequences. We are of the school of thought that our biology subserves all we think, feel and do, and that there are no supernatural or non-biological mechanisms by which we detect, process and store information. This is particularly clear when it comes to the 'psycho' bits – sophisticated brain imaging studies clearly show patterns of brain activity associated with a range of psychological variables.[2]

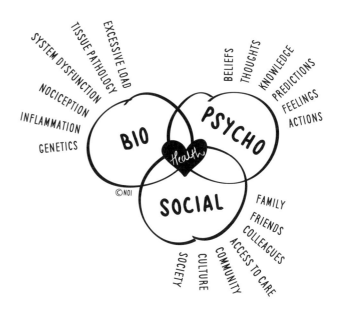

Figure 6.1 The biopsychosocial framework and a reminder: 'Pain involves the intricate variable interaction of biological factors (genetic, biochemical, etc.), psychological factors (mood, personality, behaviour etc.) and social factors (cultural, familial, socioeconomic, medical etc).'

One thing that comes up time and time again however, is that no two people have exactly the same results – we all have slightly different ways of producing the same types of feelings, thoughts or perceptions. Remember – thoughts are biological events, always real and constructed by neuroimmune networks that we call *neurotags*.

Now that you have just reviewed Chapter 2 and are in love again with the biopsychosocial model (Figure 6.1), remember the cortical body matrix theory in Chapter 3, because this takes the implications of the biopsychosocial model to new heights. In short, it reminds us that we are truly so interconnected, a combination of machine, garden and biology as the metaphorical cover of the book suggests, that we can't really think, feel or experience something without having additional bodily effects.

---

1   If not, get out there, make noise and push your profession to catch up.

2   Although clear patterns of brain related activity with psychological variables have been shown, keep your radar up, there is a great deal of fluff around – check out this paper [4] for some sobering news that up to 40,000 functional brain imaging studies may be fundamentally flawed.

The 'social' part of biopsychosocial is often neglected or understated – some of you will be cognisant of it, but many don't give it much thought. Some of the problems that patients describe may well be problems in society as a whole. Social constructs such as culture, gender [5], class and socioeconomic status impact on pain. Smoking, drug abuse and pain misconceptions are also examples of societal problems that can have an influence on a person's body and may benefit from a societal 'treatment'.

These days it's trendy to proclaim *'I am biopsychosocial'*. Lip service rules! But it's no use just having or proclaiming a biopsychosocial framework – you need to implement it as well. This can be tough. Even when clinicians recognise the importance of using a biopsychosocial framework, when it comes time to treat they often revert back to a biomedical approach [6-8]. This is a common retreat with many possible reasons: time constraints, patient expectations, the 'too-hard basket', too tired, seeing the last patient on a Friday afternoon.

More worryingly, perhaps some don't truly *believe* psychosocial factors are important, or at least not *as* important as biomedical factors. Superficial rather than deep learning looms for their patients. One thing is for sure, Explain Pain requires the best of a biopsychosocial mental framework for both the deliverer and learner. There's great healthy narrative in each of the three linked domains.

Don't get us wrong, there are some really good bits in current biomedical thinking so long as they can be integrated into the bigger biopsychosocial framework. Some readers may not be alive today if an aggressive biomedical search for a lesion was not carried out. However, as George Engel made clear half a century ago (Chapter 2), a purely biomedical approach is at best suboptimal – none of those readers for whom the aggressive biomedical search was life-saving would have been less saved if the biomedical search was integrated within a biopsychosocial model (and there may be less post-intervention problems). Just so you remember what it is we are ranting about here, contrast the two frameworks below (Table 6.1).

A more biomedical perspective	A more biopsychosocial perspective
Involves a search for a single cause.	Recognises multiple causes from biological, psychological and sociological domains.
A focus on the disease process.	A focus on disease and the responses to disease (illness).
Strongly focuses on anatomical and biomechanical principles.	Strongly acknowledges interactions between brain and body.
More disease focused.	More health focused.
Patient management often passive – 'what can medicine do for you?'	Patient management more active, including self-management - 'what can you do for yourself?'
Curative monotherapies attempted (such as surgery, injection, manipulation).	Therapies more rehabilitative/interdisciplinary.
The dominant response is to cut it out, turn it off or replace it.	The dominant response is train it.
Higher perceived harmfulness of physical activity, yet an emphasis on physical activity.	Lower perceived harmfulness of physical activity.
Research aimed more at cellular, molecular and genetic levels, some engagement with neuroscience.	Research aimed more at psychosocial contributions with increasing engagement with neuroscience.
May fail to recognise preventative medicine.	Includes psychosocial contributing factors as precursors to injury/disease.

Table 6.1 Contrasts between biomedical and biopsychosocial mental frameworks

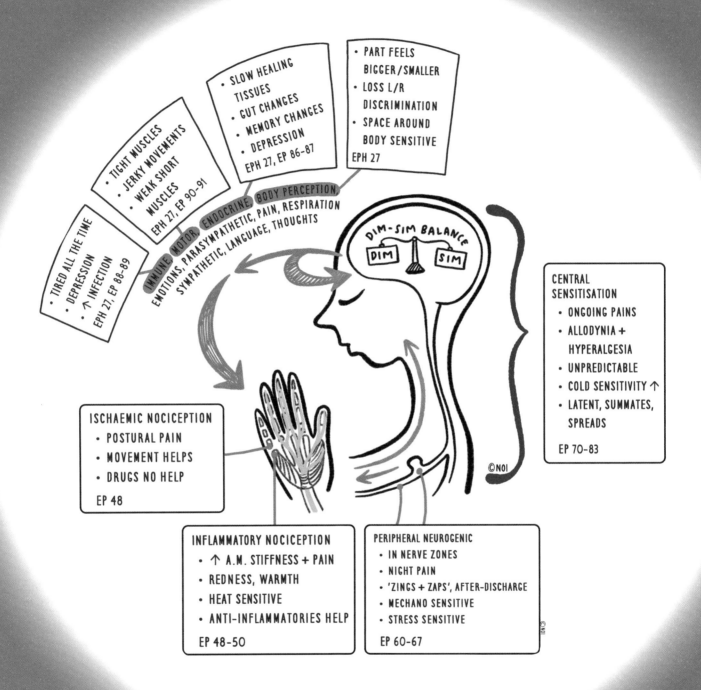

Figure 6.2 Pain mechanisms model with examples of clinical findings, adapted from [12]

3. Be biologically literate – really know your stuff!

There is a new goldmine available for humanity – a biological knowledge store, ever increasing in size and powered up by a neuroimmune revolution! The bare minimum knowledge level for a clinician who ever sees anyone in pain is that presented in *Explain Pain* [9]. We are often asked *'where is the best place to find all this info'* and *'how do I make sense of it?'*. We recommend the pain mechanisms framework [10-12] as a way to source, categorise and make sense of all this info (Figure 6.2). Note how this aligns with the cheat sheet in the end of Chapter 3 (page 79). These categories include mechanisms or processes that are more related to input (such as inflammatory processes associated with an acute ankle sprain), more related to processing in the central nervous system and some more related to perturbed homeostatic systems. The term 'more related' is important as overlap always occurs and bidirectional feedback between mechanisms also occurs. Note that the model is circular with no start and finish. Clinical patterns can be broadly allocated into mechanisms [13, 14]. This is important in education because it is the clinical pattern that often needs explaining and if it can be linked to known biological processes then the story grows richer and closer to the truth.

But you can dig deeper and deeper. If you're up for a challenge and have strong arms, try books such as *'Wall & Melzack's Textbook of Pain'* [15] and *'Science of Pain'* [16] where you can identify a pain mechanisms framework. If you do delve into these books you will begin to see which authors 'get' the Grand Poobah Pain Theory and which are stuck in old, linear models; you will see the true biopsychosocialists and the quasi-biopsychosocialists; you will see how much EP and *EP Supercharged* simplifies the biology to make it digestible.

The final point when it comes to biological literacy is to remain aware that knowledge is changing rapidly. Remember the grand old man Piaget, from Chapter 5. He wasn't into pain but he said, *'scientific knowledge is in perpetual evolution, it finds itself changing from one day to the next'*. Maintaining an up-to-date, accurate message is an essential deliverer competency.[3]

4. Know the difference between declarative and functional knowledge

Critically relevant here for your curriculum design is the distinction and relationship between *declarative knowledge* and *functional knowledge* [17]. Declarative knowledge[4] is knowledge about things that you can state – facts such as *pi = 3.142*, and *there is no such thing as a pain receptor*. Functional knowledge[5] is knowledge that informs action. This is 'know how' knowledge, such as how to use pi to calculate the volume of your home brew kit or if you know there are no pain receptors it should stimulate a wider search for contributions to pain. There is overlap between declarative and functional knowledge. When you have finished your home brew kit calculations, pi still sits in your brain in the pi neurotag waiting to be called upon at a future date. Metaphors are usually functional knowledge – *'motion is lotion'* is a good example. Think of the declarative knowledge around the health benefits of motion that might allow you to use that metaphor with confidence.

This declarative/functional knowledge relationship is important because it is functional knowledge that underpins conceptual and behaviour changes. Functional knowledge encourages experiential learning that can lead to a positive cycle of ongoing learning. It is functional knowledge that we try to measure. If you peek ahead at the table of objectives for an Explain Pain intervention (Table 6.5), notice that the objectives begin with verbs that demand functional knowledge – verbs such as *have, apply, explore, function* and *extrapolate*. If we were just aiming to provide learners with declarative knowledge our objectives might start with *list, tell* or *repeat*.

But this doesn't mean you as a deliverer are off the hook – you need a deep reservoir of declarative knowledge (recall Figure 1.1) from which to draw and create your own therapeutic stories and not just rely on ours.

5. Be aware of kinds of misconceptions

Various levels or kinds of misconception were discussed in detail in Chapter 5, so this is a reminder. They may range from simple 'missing bits', increasingly flawed mental frameworks, to unchangeable paradigms and missing frameworks to engage emergence. We ask that you, the deliverer consider the kind of misconception that the learner has and adapt your educational strategies accordingly.

---

3 To help keep up to date, you could join the IASP, your national pain society, and find more readings at www.noijam.com and www.bodyinmind.org.

4 You may read about declarative knowledge as content, propositional or public knowledge; it's out there in libraries and the internet. Most of the exams you would have done relate to how well you can regurgitate the knowledge back.

5 Also known as procedural knowledge.

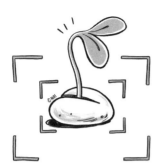

6. Know common Target Concepts

'Pain involves distributed brain activity' and *'We are bioplastic'* are examples of Target Concepts. These are broad concepts based on banks of declarative knowledge. If the learner adopts and internalises a Target Concept then functional knowledge should follow. So from the Target Concept *'Pain involves distributed brain activity'*, the functional knowledge may be *'well, that's good, many things can influence my pain, perhaps I need to explore how I can modify these things!'*

Note that Target Concepts align with the Grand Poobah Pain Theory, the topics covered in *Explain Pain* [9], *Painful Yarns* [21], and they are used/adapted in the curricula in Chapter 10. This is actually no accident! There will be other Target Concepts for different situations and individual deliverers may frame them differently.

In our experience, some Target Concepts are universal. Here are 10 of the most common Target Concepts (Table 6.2). In Chapter 10, we have listed multiple ways of expressing these concepts.

Target Concept	Explanation
1. Pain is normal, personal and always real.	All pain experiences are normal and are an excellent, though unpleasant response to what your brain judges to be a threatening situation. All pain is real.
2. There are danger sensors, not pain sensors.	The danger alarm system is just that – there are no pain sensors, pain pathways or pain endings.
3. Pain and tissue damage rarely relate.	Pain is an unreliable indicator of the presence or extent of tissue damage – either can exist without the other.
4. Pain depends on the balance of danger and safety.	You will have pain when your brain concludes that there is more credible evidence of danger than safety related to your body and thus infers the need to protect.
5. Pain involves distributed brain activity.	There is no single 'pain centre' in the brain. Pain is a conscious experience that necessarily involves many brain areas across time.
6. Pain relies on context.	Pain can be influenced by the things you see, hear, smell, taste and touch, things you say, things you think and believe, things you do, places you go, people in your life and things happening in your body.
7. Pain is one of many protective outputs.	When threatened the body is capable of activating multiple protective systems including immune, endocrine, motor, autonomic, respiratory, cognitive, emotional and pain. Any or all of these systems can become overprotective.
8. We are bioplastic.	While all protective systems can become turned up and edgy, the notion of bioplasticity suggests that they can change back, through the lifespan. It is biologically implausible to suggest that pain can't change.
9. Learning about pain can help the individual and society.	Learning about pain is therapy. When you understand why you hurt, you hurt less. If you have a pain problem, you are not alone – millions of others do too. But there are many researchers and clinicians working to find ways to help.
10. Active treatment strategies promote recovery.	Once you understand pain, you can begin to make plans, explore different ways to move, improve your fitness, eat better, sleep better, demolish DIMs, find SIMs and gradually do more.

Table 6.2 Common Target Concepts

7. Ponder whether you possess an emergent framework

Anthills, flocks of birds, love, cities, traffic jams and pain are phenomena with emergent qualities. They are the result of individual agents (ants, birds, brain cells, cars, molecules etc.) interacting simultaneously and collectively [18]. In contrast, mitosis, phases of the moon and to some degree tissue healing and digestion are more linear phenomena (Figure 5.4).

In the section on 'deliverer variables' in Chapter 5, we suggested deliverers need to possess an emergent framework to fully embrace the current understanding of pain. There is no test (yet) to check whether a person has linear or emergent frameworks or is more or less emergent or linear – so we ask you to 'ponder it'.

Both linear and emergent frameworks are useful and necessary – we need to be aware of both frameworks and know when to apply them. It would be of little use being emergent when thinking about linear phenomena. Our view though, based on educational research [19], is that we are more likely to be missing emergent frameworks and incorrectly apply simpler linear frameworks to complex (emergent) phenomena – after all, this is how formal education is often structured.

Deliverers who understand emergence are likely to be better at treating people with chronic pain. We have no hard data to support this view, so why do we think this? Because really understanding the biopsychosocial framework requires acknowledgment that multiple, simultaneous and diverse agents contribute to an output such as pain.

We contend that deliverers with a healthy emergent framework and with a depth of knowledge to apply it to the correct phenomenon will naturally use the biopsychosocial framework, be comfortable using the Protectometer [20] and understand that a singular blame for chronic pain is indefensible. In Novella 12 *Traffic jams, cakes, snowflakes and pain*, we have suggested a module to give learners access to an emergent framework. Deliverers may want to have a look as well.

8. Develop your Explain Pain library

A library is a collection of something. An Explain Pain library refers to a categorised collection of educational pain stories. There is no doubt in our minds that pain sciences can be packaged into appropriate, highly adaptable and reasoned therapeutic narratives, metaphors, similes and analogies that can be integrated into a clinically reasoned biopsychosocial approach.

Deliverers require a working collection of these stories, the knowledge of when to use them, the ability to continually develop them and multimedia strategies to deliver them. The bigger the library the better. We have provided our library of Nuggets and Novellas (Table 6.3) as a starting point in Chapters 8 and 9, but we really hope that you will develop your own as well.

Category	Description	Examples
Nuggets	Short, perhaps around a minute or less. Explicit learning, targeting 'singular grains of misconception'. Often emergency analgesia.	*24. Pain strips for you* *63. Motion is lotion*
Novellas	Longer stories, around 1-5 minutes. Explicit and implicit learning, requires significant multimedia. Targets 'multiple-grains' or 'sandcastles'.	*15. Smudged maps and what to do about them* *2. The drug cabinet in the brain*

Table 6.3 Nuggets and Novellas as part of an Explain Pain library

9. Be a reasoner – no place for recipe treatments

We don't have a one size fits all recipe for Explain Pain. How boring that would be! We advocate clinical reasoning. Clinical reasoning can be defined as: *'thinking through the various aspects of patient care to arrive at a reasonable decision regarding the prevention, diagnosis, or treatment of a clinical problem in a specific patient'* [22].

This process is necessarily emergent across repeated clinical encounters – we avoid reliance on linear processes such as algorithms, questionnaires, pre-set modules and simplistic models that feed off individual researchers' pet theses. We prefer face to face interviews.

It is quite a call, but we think that reasoners are more likely to have access to and appropriately use emergent frameworks in their thinking than non-reasoners. We also think that use of an emergent framework is more likely to capture the 'whole of life' influences on an individual's health state via broad Target Concept identification. Your other choice, which we really hope you don't make, is to sink into recipe-based practice – the 'if you see this, do that' model. We strongly advocate that you think, don't sink. Sinking stinks.

10. Cultivate educational skills

If you are this far into *EP Supercharged*, you are now something of a budding educationalist and you will become more so as you read this book. While some people are 'naturals' at education, we can *all* have our Explain Pain outcomes enhanced with some educational science. We recommend three textbooks for those who want to go deeper into the world of education [17, 23, 24]. Here are some tips around *self-explanation* – a fundamental Explain Pain skill.

Self-explanation is explaining a concept to yourself or others [25, 26]. This has been shown to deepen learning, enhance problem solving and it helps turn declarative knowledge into functional knowledge. When self-explaining, learners elaborate on the knowledge they have been given by linking it to their own prior knowledge, making inferences, providing examples and extrapolating from their own life experiences. Asking *'what did you make of last session'* is an example of encouraging self-explanation. You could ask your learner to first tell themselves what is going on and then to explain it to someone else. One of our patients tried to first explain her pain to her dog! Learners can use images, flow charts, art, words, gesticulation and whatever else they need to self-explain. Within self-explanation strategies,

you might encourage learners to *elaborate* with their own examples to help foster a deep understanding of the associated concept and *compare* their examples with peers and experts.

We encourage learners to provide several examples rather than one. This enables deeper elaboration and contrasting. Examples prompted by self-explanation are usually functional knowledge – *'I noticed my pain was not there when I was laughing, but also when I was doing those stretches, so I have a lot to go on now'*.

Now, because you too are a learner, go and do some self-explanation! We are always explaining stuff to each other, our family, our pets, blank walls...

11. Live Explain Pain as a cognitive lifestyle

In a broad sense, Explain Pain is a way of thinking about pain, a 'cognitive lifestyle' if you like. In a more targeted sense, Explain Pain is not a singular and isolated therapy [27], but a range of conceptual change strategies based on current knowledge of the pain sciences. Explain Pain always links, merges and utilises experiential elements of other evidence based approaches which could include Graded Motor Imagery (GMI), graded exercise and activity, Pilates, yoga, Tai chi, hypnosis and psychological techniques, pharmacology and surgery among others. Education has a place in every intervention. But be aware that mixed messages can be trouble [27]. An Explain Pain intervention carried out at the same time as a competing biomedical treatment is not conducive to deep learning.

The integration of Explain Pain with psychological therapies is particularly relevant here. We are not aware of any clinical trials (except the ones we are currently running) that compare combinations of Explain Pain and other therapies. However, we are wholly supportive of strategies such as Motivational Interviewing [28], Cognitive Behavioural Therapy [29], Acceptance and Commitment Therapy [30], hypnosis [31], health coaching [32] and behavioural approaches [33].

One exciting example is the potential of integrating hypnotic suggestions prior to an Explain Pain intervention and using hypnotic language during education. Bona fide world leader in pain related hypnosis research and practice Professor Mark Jensen reckons the best Explain Pain-ers do it hypnotically anyway and adding specific hypnotic strategies should enhance the 'stickiness' of the message.

Combining two effective treatments should be useful *as long as both subscribe to the biopsychosocial model and the Grand Poobah Pain Theory* [27].

The Explain Pain assessment: Eight Great Questions

In order to power up your curriculum and optimise your Explain Pain intervention, there are some systematic steps you can take – steps that are based around the answers to some key questions.

1. Does the learner really want to know about pain and science?

The notion of learning a bit of science can really frighten some people. The person in front of you may have had a negative experience at school, failed biology or chemistry or couldn't handle the frog dissections. Perhaps they have always seen themselves as 'arty types' and avoided science altogether. Saying that you will 'provide *information*' may be better than 'provide *education*' as the term 'education' is often linked to unfortunate school days, propaganda or may even come across as condescending. You could say something like, *'We want to help you understand the situation as best as possible because you're going to have to make some decisions based on some new information.'*

Not everyone wants to learn about pain either. There will be people who *'just want it fixed'* and say *'I don't want to know about that stuff'*. Remind yourself of the 'get stuffed' pathway in Figure 5.2. In this situation, it will be essential for you to communicate the Target Concept that *'learning about pain can help the individual and society'*. You will need all your deliverer skills to keep the learner on board and inspired. When learners realise science can be translated into stories such as those in *Painful Yarns* [21] or the Nuggets and Novellas described in Chapters 8 and 9, that learning about science and pain can be fun and exciting, their curiosity may awaken. They may like to know that scientific discoveries make great stories.

2. How does the learner like to learn?

'How do you usually like to learn stuff?' This is a reasonable question for an educator to ask. Or *'think of something you learned in the past – what was it that made it memorable?'* This may open up an important discussion to find the best educational delivery methods and facilitate trust. It is also a polite way to seek information about literacy. Consider that 15% of the global adult population are illiterate [34] and 1 in 10 people are dyslexic [35]. Your patient could be offered a number of ways of participating in conceptual change, some of which may include movies, video clips, group discussion, one on one discussion, images, drawing and texts of varying complexity.

3. Does the learner have an impaired ability to learn?

Some disease and traumatic states affect access to learning via impairments in hearing, vision, cognition, movement, language and communication. Additionally, we are increasingly aware that pain is often associated with other perturbed brain outputs such as alterations in endocrine, motor and immune function, each of which can affect learning and memory. Vagueness, memory retention problems or enhanced sensitivity in a group environment may relate to the same biological processes that are underpinning someone's pain [36]. Persistent pain states are associated with mental inflexibility [37]. You are highly likely to find some learning difficulties in people with persistent pain states.

Memory changes and consequently learning, are possible side effects of many medications including antidepressants, tranquillisers, statins, chemotherapy ('chemo brain' is well known), benzodiazepines, long term opioids, oxycodone, gabapentin and pregabalin, incontinence drugs and some cold and flu medications. There is not much clear research on this but it seems that most long term medications may influence memory and learning.

4. Does the learner have access to digital media and know how to use it?

Access to computers, tablets, smartphones and the internet can permit a wide range of multimedia approaches that are likely to improve learning [38]. Not everybody is that lucky though. A digital divide exists between developed and developing countries in terms of access to the internet [39]; older people are less likely to be comfortable with computers and tablets and the software required to use them; some people have skill limitations or indeed simply don't like using the internet or electronic devices. It is critical to determine someone's access to, and preference for electronic materials and have non-digital materials available for those who need them. Have your coloured pencils at the ready!

5. Where does the learner currently seek health knowledge?

A person's source of health knowledge will be diverse – we learn much from our parents, our friends, formal and informal training, our experiences and, more and more, from Professor Google (the accuracy of which is rather unpredictable!). When your health is affected by something, your sources of health knowledge will probably expand to include your health providers, your friends in health fields and, more and more, anecdote and rumour from well-meaning acquaintances who 'knew someone with that problem'.

Make a point of finding out where someone is sourcing information on their situation. You will need to make a respectful judgement on the quality and source of the information and you may need to provide some learners with a framework for evaluating the quality themselves. If conceptual change is required, you may be up against some formidable opponents! If a person's information sources are more diverse rather than singular you may find conceptual change easier to orchestrate. But overall, it is likely that previous information received is not what we might consider modern Explain Pain, otherwise they would not be seeking help.

6. What is the learner's current pain literacy?

Health literacy is the degree to which individuals have the capacity to obtain, process and understand basic health information and services needed to make appropriate health decisions [40]. Pain literacy could be defined similarly – the degree to which individuals have the capacity to obtain, process and understand pain-related health information.

It's difficult to judge someone's level of pain literacy, at least in the first session. As a starter, we are aware that around 60% of Australians have a less than optimal health literacy [41]. Most people also have a misconstrued understanding of pain that considers it to be a purely tissue-based phenomenon – that pain is detected by pain receptors and pain signals are transmitted to the brain where they are registered [42]. Very few people will present for care with a modern understanding of pain such as that presented in The Grand Poobah Pain Theory outlined in Chapter 2, which is why conceptual change knowledge, skills and science are so important.

Clinicians can make a judgement about pain literacy levels during an assessment, from questions like *'tell me what you*

know about the problem', *'do you have a theory about what is causing your pain?'*, *'what do you know about your diagnosis?'* or *'how do you think I can help?'*. It is our overwhelming experience that, with careful and respectful questioning, most people have a theory even if they are reluctant to share it for fear of being made to feel silly. We have also found that the first answer is often along the lines of *'I don't know what's causing it – you're supposed to be the expert'*, to which we might respond with *'Thanks! But why see me and not another kind of expert?'* or *'Thanks! I am also very interested in what* you *think is going on because this is a really helpful indicator of how your brain will be processing all kinds of information from and about your body'*.

7. What kind of misconception does the learner hold?

Although we haven't yet constructed a test that will identify the 'kind of misconception', we suggest that the deliverer can make a reasoned judgement on the kinds of misconception that a learner may have (Chapter 5). Remember that the kinds of misconceptions include missing bits, single grain, sandcastle and sandstone misconceptions and interpreting emergent processes using linear frameworks. Adapting your Explain Pain intervention according to the kinds of misconception held by the learner will be a key element in the actual content and delivery of the intervention.

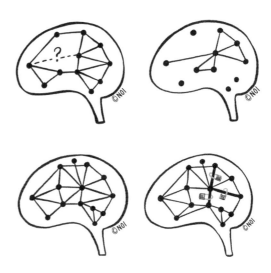

Figure 6.3 Misconceptions include missing bits, single grain, sandcastle and sandstone misconceptions

8. What are the relevant Target Concepts for the learner?

We've helped you here by providing a list (Table 6.2) of common Target Concepts – feel free to use them and add your own. The points below will help you further refine your selection.

Predetermined Target Concepts

Group settings lend themselves to predetermined Target Concepts, especially if the group setting is likely to be repeated. Chapter 10 provides an example of group curricula using these predetermined Target Concepts.

E-flags to help select appropriate Target Concepts

We have used the E-flag (education flags) approach for many years now [14]. An E-flag is a piece of information picked up in an assessment and for which you want to provide an explanation. We identify these in our notes and put a small flag with an E on it as a reminder to come back and address. There are some examples below and while each flag could be addressed individually, note how some may relate to the same Target Concept – for example, the first three relate to *'pain is one of many protective outputs'*.

- *'My gut really aches too!'*
- *'I seem to get sick really quickly.'*
- *'I'm just really wound up and stressed all the time.'*
- *'Some days I can vacuum the house no problems and other days I can't even finish one room.'*
- *'I think it's getting worse, sometimes I feel it in my good leg!'*
- *'My pain is strange, it goes from the outside of my leg to the top of my foot!'*
- *'My back hurts when I duck my head to get into the car!'*

DIM SIM analysis as a deeper way to uncover appropriate Target Concepts

We have taken the E-flag concept further in recent years with the release of the *Protectometer* [20] and the allied concepts of DIM (Danger In Me) and SIM (Safety in Me) as discussed earlier. The E-flags mentioned above are DIMs and while we believe that *'every DIM deserves a story'*, the *Protectometer* also picks up the SIMs which help identify and solidify which Target Concepts are truly specific to your patient.

Measuring pain education outcomes

It's not easy to measure what someone knows. Educationalists have grappled with this for years and still do. In healthcare, we often rely on *possible* correlates of knowledge change, such as returning to work, mood status and altered behaviour and these can be all influenced by many variables. Perhaps the bluntest of all measurements is whether or not that patient comes back for the next appointment.[6] Let's assume she does – although there are challenges in assessing conceptual change, we can offer you some guidance on how best to measure. In short, we should implement both *formative* assessment – continual checking and rechecking of progress along the way and *summative* assessment – stopping and assessing the whole lot at the end of the process and further down the track.

Formative assessment

Formative assessment occurs during the educational process. It relies on learner feedback and it will nearly always be qualitative. There is a bit of 'picking up on the vibe' here and it relates to the critical skill of observing – really observing and hearing what the person in front of you says and does and how they say and do it[7]. This could be new words and phrases used, it could also be the right amount of nodding (definitely not too much), but also how comfortable they are in their chair, whether their arms are crossed, shoulders lifted or they seem relaxed and at ease.

More detailed formative assessment could include the depth of your patients' questions, their ability to repeat information back to you, the quality of preformed questions before follow-up sessions and responses to quizzing and questioning. Of course, how well you do this will also depend on whether you, the deliverer, have truly taken on board the biopsychosocial approach and the Grand Poobah Pain Theory.

You may have hit the mark when the learner starts extrapolating the information to other circumstances such as a previous injury or another person's pain state, or perhaps they say *'why wasn't I given this treatment earlier?'* or *'this is a great place for learning'*.

If your learner is really on the deep learning pathway, they should act differently. This could be picked up in changes in any of the homeostatic systems [EP Section 4] and most obviously in movement, emotional and cognitive wellbeing.

---

6   They may well have taken it on but wouldn't it be great if they'd ring you and tell you?

7   Review Chapter 2 page 9.

Summative assessment

Any educational objective, by definition, should be linked to some form of assessment. This may be qualitative – we think it is always worthwhile asking patients if they think each of the educational objectives have been met. On a more formal note, questionnaires could be used, though most don't identify an individual's unique beliefs and existing knowledge. There are many questionnaires out there being used to assess pain, behaviour and function but not many on what people actually know about the biology of their pain. The obvious exception is the Neurophysiology of Pain Questionnaire (NPQ) [43] – a Rasch analysis showed the 11-item revised version to be a good way to assess knowledge in a way that allows us to measure change and to position people on a scale of 'pain biology knowledge is very weak' to 'pain biology knowledge is very strong' [44]. We think the NPQ is worth using before and after every Explain Pain programme.

Construction of an EP curriculum

What's your curriculum?

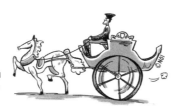

The original Latin meaning for the word curriculum is a *course* – the kind one runs around (the Latin verb *currere* means *to run*). If you're a fan of Jane Austen you may have read about the *curricle* – a light, two-horsed carriage used in the late 18th century. The original meaning of the word can be seen in the term *curriculum vitae*, which is quite literally the *course of one's life.*

The idea of curricula (or 'curriculums' for our American friends) is fundamental in education, although it may be new in health. However, if you are educating in any capacity, then you will have a curriculum of sorts, even if you have never thought much about the term. We could (very humbly and quietly) sit next to you while you educate a patient or take a group and extract your educational framework, which we could call a curriculum.

This section will guide you through the construction of an EP curriculum. This involves more than just figuring out what you want someone to learn, updating your PowerPoints and checking if the data projector still works. Let's start at the very concept of curriculum.

Four broad and overlapping concepts of curriculum exist [45]:

1. **A body of knowledge** to be transmitted – *this is the stuff you want someone to know*
2. **A product** held together with clear objectives – *so you can measure and repeat it*
3. **A process** – a living, adaptable, problem solving relationship between deliverer and learner – *it actually takes two or more to conceptually tango*
4. **A practice** – as an extension of the process into life and activities of daily living – *don't think it all stops when the treatment time is up – make it a way of life.*

Curriculum as body of knowledge, product, process and practice

The **body of knowledge** in a curriculum is more than just a list of the contents to be transferred. The body of knowledge needs to be defined in terms of the target problems and expected outcomes, philosophy, opposing views, and the vision of the teaching group.

The perspective of curriculum as a **product** emphasises the need for aims, objectives and measurement of the product. It invites critical testing. *Product* also highlights the need to consider all elements that may contribute to an outcome. There is no harm in asking *'Is my educational product saleable, worthwhile, testable, repeatable?'* and *'How should I market it?'* It should be part of the procedures manual for groups.

When curriculum is conceptualised as a **process**, it proposes a dynamic and reciprocal interaction of deliverer, learner, message and environment – transforming it into a living thing, a journey with continual formative assessment and levels of understanding. It is an implementation of product and body of knowledge. It also suggests that there may be no end, that your patient/learner achieves deep learning and that you, the deliverer, also improve for the next learning encounter.

Curriculum as **practice** is an extension of the curriculum as process concept. This is living the curriculum with new practical wisdom. It suggests informed, committed and reflective action during education, and particularly post education. It suggests a focus beyond the individual's current treatment to the use of this wisdom for future life, analysis of past circumstances, knowledge to translate or relate to others – or even in helping to deal with societal problems in the broader sense. This is an important part of Explain Pain education if we have a goal of an NNE of 1.

A good quality Explain Pain curriculum will also have a *hidden curriculum* (unexpected impacts). These are those unintended (but hoped for) developments in the personal values, beliefs and problem solving skills of the learner.

Constructive alignment for deep learning – keeping it all together

The notion of constructive alignment is widely used in modern curriculum design [17] and we see it as fundamental to an Explain Pain curriculum. It simply means all the 'bits' must align and fit together, especially a curriculum based on the four concepts just listed and one which links learner, deliverer, message and context. Have a quick peek if you want, at one of the detailed curricula in Chapter 10. They are quite complex documents and all parts must link together to achieve deep learning outcomes. If it is out of balance, for example, by missing a key aspect of any of the variables, it is likely that learning will be limited to superficial conceptual change. Basically we want to create the best possible situation so our learners won't escape deep learning.

Well stated objectives are the glue that hold a curriculum together. They are what your patient or group does and are therefore the foundations for learning. Objectives help you define the Target Concepts for educational intervention. An objective will also have some level of attainment in it, which is why any good objective will begin with a verb – something the learner has to enact, such as: *understand, apply, discuss* and *function*. The verbs leading the objective can range from not too taxing (*describe, list, be aware, carry out simple procedure*) to more taxing (*compare, analyse, integrate, explore, apply, reflect*). In this way, they align with content, delivery, assessment and outcomes [17]. Earlier in this chapter we linked these verbs to the notion of functional knowledge.

If you're an avid reader and into this stuff, you might want to further explore the Structure of Learning Outcomes (SOLO) taxonomy [46]. We use the SOLO concept all the time to develop our curricula and to mark exam papers. The SOLO taxonomy places learning outcomes in a hierarchy, usually four levels of cognitive complexity. The simplest level is uni-structural (identify, memorise) progressing to multi-structural (describe, list). The higher levels of understanding are more qualitative, from relational (compare, relate, analyse) to extended abstract (theorise, extrapolate, reflect). Note how the progressive complexity of the verbs dictate the level.

The process of curriculum development

The information extracted from a health professional's assessment, along with information from the Explain Pain assessment and the Eight Great Questions, should provide most of the information to construct a curriculum. Here are some suggested steps to complete your curriculum.

1. Extract essential demographic and practical data

Our suggestions are below in Table 6.4.

Key questions	Examples of details sought
Who are the stakeholders in the outcome?	Other than the patient, stakeholders could be family, friends, referrers, payers, employers and anyone who requires a report.
Features of the deliverer(s)	Skills, knowledge, background, philosophy, vision, competencies, 'fit' with other deliverers.
Features of the learner(s)	Number of participants, age, gender, injuries, diagnoses, unique needs, health and pain literacy, language/communication challenges, potential outliers in a group.
Features of the context	
• Time available	Time, number of sessions, period of time, follow up.
• Place	Space, design, media available, parking and access.
• Cost	Equipment and facility hire, material costs.
• Other issues	There are sure to be some.

Table 6.4 Essential demographic and practical data for a curriculum

2. State your aims and objectives

Here is the glue for constructive alignment. If you are educating now, and you all will be to some degree, then you would already have some basic aims and objectives, but you probably don't realise it. It's just a matter of identifying, extracting and articulating them. We do know that people find aims and objectives a bit confusing, even a touch boring sometimes but the more you create and use them, the easier and more refined it will be and the more you will realise their power.

To make it clearer, think about it in this way:[8]

- Aims are what the *deliverer* intends to do and they ideally will be statements prefaced by – *I will*:

- Objectives describe what you hope your *learner* does and what he or she will gain or graduate with. The answers will be prefaced by – *The learner will*:

We have provided some generic examples of aims and objectives that might be appropriate for a range of Explain Pain situations in Table 6.5. Note the use of the verbs to suggest enactment, level of enactment and possible assessment. Between three and seven aims and objectives are usually quite workable. Each aim will give rise to one or more objectives which should be numbered so that you can link them to the Target Concepts of the curriculum, ensuring constructive alignment – you should have a sense of all of this coming together now! If you note that there are objectives with no Target Concepts or Target Concepts with no linked objectives, then you are missing something and you could be constructively misaligned.[9] Aims and objectives development also provides an unrivalled opportunity for a shared process between deliverer and learner.

Some educationalists focus on objectives, and while these do frame the curriculum, we suggest that a statement of what you intend to do, that is – the aims, will help define the objectives.

AIMS The deliverer will:	OBJECTIVES At the end of the sessions the learner will:
Provide current knowledge about pain and other protective mechanisms in a healthy group-learning environment.	*1. Have* up to date, functional knowledge of pain and other protective mechanisms, as it relates to them.
Deliver information to allow participants to generate realistic prognoses.	*2. Apply* bioplasticity knowledge to set short and long term goals with the expectation of improved outcomes.
Provide a framework that integrates Explain Pain with graded exposure and cognitive behavioural therapies.	*3. Explore,* use and develop personalised practical applications of Explain Pain knowledge.
Use multimedia, storytelling and metaphor to explain and transform the pain and stress experiences of the learner(s).	*4. Function* better with reduced pain and stress, and use healthy linguistic expression.
Make learnt skills applicable to 'whole of life'.	*5. Extrapolate* the material and the group skills for future personal pain states of self and others.

Table 6.5 Generic aims and objectives for an Explain Pain curriculum

We know what you're thinking. *'Do I really need to do this before every patient?'* The answer is yes, but read on…

As we've said before, if you are educating you are already using a curriculum. We're just giving you some sharper tools to write it down and use it better. If you are taking a group, we think that a curriculum is essential. Once you've created one it's easy to copy, change, and adapt. If you are treating one-on-one there's rarely enough time to fill in a full curriculum for each patient. Our suggestion is that you at least have Target Concepts listed in your plan and have methods of assessing if they have been achieved.

Maybe every now and then, construct a full curriculum for a patient. Don't do Explain Pain research without one.

---

8   If you have a medical research background or training, these ideas of aims and objectives will probably be a bit different to how you have thought of them before. For instance, you might have learnt that aims are what you will achieve and objectives are what you will do to achieve the aims. *EP Supercharged* is all about conceptual change and is deeply grounded in conceptual change theory and literature. That's why we are talking about aims and objectives in the way we are here.

9   Nothing worse!

3. Define your Target Concepts

We have already provided a list of common Target Concepts that we've used over the years (Table 6.2). You can select from our list if you want, or make up your own. You can see how we've adapted some Target Concepts for curricula in Chapter 10. The important thing is to answer the question *'What Target Concepts need to be addressed to meet the objectives that the deliverer(s) and learner(s) have raised?'*

4. Populate the columns

The columns in the curriculum table below are divided up into the message, the learner, the context and the deliverer. That should be nice and familiar for you. The message is further divided into 6 columns, not that it's more important than the others, but curriculum does have a focus on the message.

There are many ways to create a curriculum, not necessarily one 'right' way. Completing this document is by no means a linear process. It doesn't necessarily flow from left to right or top to bottom. It will come about as an emergent construction of thoughts and considerations relating to the message, the learner, the deliverer and the context and the linkage of these variables to the aims and objectives to make it all align. We hope that this 'template' provides sufficient scaffolding for you to become confident constructing your own curricula.

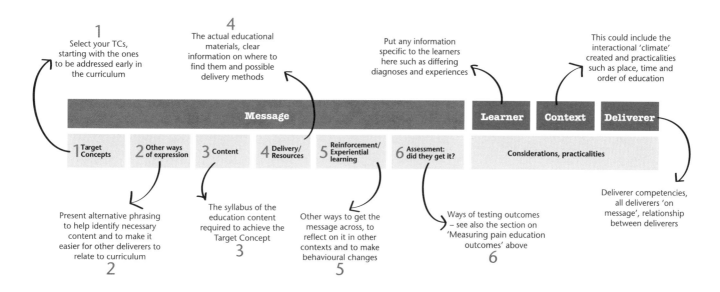

Figure 6.4 The columns in a generic curriculum document for a group. Multiple examples of material for each column are given in Chapter 10.

Recording what you have done

We suspect that many deliverers are just writing *'explained pain'* in their patients' notes along with details of other interventions. In the light of evidence, this is a bit lazy as it downgrades the place and power of education and it won't help someone else trying to read your notes. If you are seeing a few patients then you may well have forgotten what you said.

For groups with defined curricula you can easily tick off what you have done following a group session. It's a bit harder one on one because the intervention will change during and between sessions.

As a minimum, your educational objectives should be recorded, as well as the Target Concepts. Further details could include the resources used, any linked experiential activity and a tick if you and the patient believe he or she has adequately conceptualised the Target Concept.

If you are using NOI resources, the Protectometer book and App allow collection and management of DIMs and SIMs.

It's really cool to be curriculo-centric!

There are lots of advantages including:

- You can be sure that you are doing the best possible EP intervention
- Workmates will marvel at your organisation
- You will identify the strengths and weaknesses of your EP intervention
- Teachers will want to be your friend
- After you do it once it becomes much easier
- It supports and helps develop your clinical reasoning practice
- You will be invited to join the committee of your local club
- You can reflect and see why things sometimes don't work out for the best
- The word curriculum slides off your tongue without making spit go everywhere – it has a lovely dry sound.

References

1. UNESCO (2015) Education 2030: Towards inclusive and equitable quality education and lifelong learning for all. World Education Forum: Incheon Declaration.

2. Smith MK (2015) What is education? A definition and discussion. Viewed 25th January 2017: http://infed.org/mobi/what-is-education-a-definition-and-discussion/.

3. International Association for the Study of Pain (2012) IASP Interprofessional Pain Curriculum Outline. Viewed 25th January 2017: http://www.iasp-pain.org/Education/CurriculumDetail.aspx?ItemNumber=2057.

4. Eklund A, Nichols TE & Knutsson H (2016) Cluster failure: Why fMRI inferences for spatial extent have inflated false-positive rates. Proc Natl Acad Sci 113: 7900-7905.

5. Racine M, et al. (2012) A systematic literature review of 10 years of research on sex/gender and pain perception – Part 2: Do biopsychosocial factors alter pain sensitivity differently in women and men? Pain 153: 619-635.

6. Bishop A & Foster NE (2005) Do physical therapists in the United Kingdom recognize psychosocial factors in patients with acute low back pain? Spine 30: 1316-1322.

7. Bishop A, et al. (2008) How does the self-reported clinical management of patients with low back pain relate to the attitudes and beliefs of health care practitioners? A survey of UK general practitioners and physiotherapists. Pain 135: 187-195.

8. Valjakka AL, et al. (2013) The association between physicians' attitudes to psychosocial aspects of low back pain and reported clinical behaviour: A complex issue. Scand J Pain 4: 25-30.

9. Butler DS & Moseley GL (2013) Explain Pain. 2nd Edn. Noigroup Publications: Adelaide.

10. Siddall PJ & Duggan AW (2004) Towards a mechanisms-based approach to pain medicine. Anesth Analg 99: 455-456.

11. Woolf CJ, et al. (1998) Towards a mechanism-based classification of pain. Pain 77: 227-229.

12. Gifford LS (1998) Pain, the tissues and the nervous system. Physiotherapy 84: 27-33.

13. Smart KM, et al. (2010) Clinical indicators of 'nociceptive', 'peripheral neuropathic' and 'central' mechanisms of musculoskeletal pain. A Delphi survey of expert clinicians. Man Ther 15: 80-87.

14. Butler DS (2000) The Sensitive Nervous System. Noigroup Publications: Adelaide.

15. McMahon SB, et al. (2013) Wall & Melzack's Textbook of Pain. 6th Edn. Elsevier: Philadelphia.

16. Basbaum AI & Bushnell MC (2009) Science of Pain. Elsevier: Oxford.

17. Biggs J & Tang C (2011) Teaching For Quality Learning At University. 4th Edn. McGraw-Hill Education: London.

18. Johnson S (2012) Emergence: The Connected Lives of Ants, Brains, Cities, and Software. Scribner: New York.

19. Chi MTH, et al. (2011) Misconceived causal explanations for emergent processes. Cognitive Sci 36: 1-61.

20. Moseley GL & Butler DS (2015) The Explain Pain Handbook: Protectometer. Noigroup Publications: Adelaide.

21. Moseley GL (2008) Painful Yarns: Metaphors and stories to help understand the biology of pain. Dancing Giraffe Press: Canberra.

22. Hawkins DR, Elder L & Paul R (2010) The Thinker's Guide to Clinical Reasoning. Foundation for Critical Thinking: California.

23. Mayer RE & Alexander PA (2016) Handbook of Research on Learning and Instruction. 2nd Edn. Routledge: New York.

24. Vosniadou S (2013) International Handbook of Research on Conceptual Change. Routledge: New York.

25. Chi MTH, Bassok M & Lewis MW (1989) Self-Explanations: How Students Study and Use Examples in Learning to Solve Problems. Cognitive Sci 13: 145-182.

26. Fonseca B & Chi MTH (2011) The self-explanation effect: A constructive learning activity, in The handbook of research on learning and instruction, Mayer RE & Alexander PA Eds. Routledge: New York.

27. Moseley GL & Butler DS (2015) Fifteen Years of Explaining Pain: The Past, Present, and Future. J Pain 16: 807-13.

28. Miller W & Rollnick S (2002) Motivational interviewing: Preparing people to change. 2nd Edn. Guildford Press: New York.

29. Keefe FJ, Dunsmore J & Burnett R (1992) Behavioral and cognitive-behavioral approaches to chronic pain: recent advances and future directions. J Consult Clin Psychol 60: 528-536.

30. McCracken LM & Vowles KE (2014) Acceptance and commitment therapy and mindfulness for chronic pain: model, process, and progress. Am Psychol 69: 178-187.

31. Jensen MP & Patterson DR (2014) Hypnotic approaches for chronic pain management: clinical implications of recent research findings. Am Psychol 69: 167-177.

32. Gale J (2012) Health Coaching Guide for Health Practitioners: Using the HCA Model of Health Change. Health Change Associates: Sydney.

33. Main CJ, et al. (2015) Fordyce's Behavioral Methods for Chronic Pain and Illness: Republished with Invited Commentaries. Wolters Kluwer Health: Philadelphia.

34. UNESCO (2015) Fact Sheet 32 - Adult and Youth Literacy. Viewed 25th January 2017: http://www.uis.unesco.org/literacy/Documents/fs32-2015-literacy.pdf.

35. Dyslexia International (2014) Dyslexia International Report: better training, better teaching. Viewed 25th January 2017: http://www.dyslexia-international.org/wp-content/uploads/2016/04/DI-Duke-Report-final-4-29-14.pdf.

36. Berryman C, et al. (2013) Evidence for working memory deficits in chronic pain: a systematic review and meta-analysis. Pain 154: 1181-1196.

37. Berryman C, et al. (2014) Do people with chronic pain have impaired executive function? A meta-analytical review. Clin Psychol Rev 34: 563-579.

38. Clark RC & Mayer RE (2011) e-Learning and the Science of Instruction: Proven Guidelines for Consumers and Designers of Multimedia Learning. 3rd Edn. Wiley: California.

39. International Telecommunication Union (2015) ICT Facts & Figures - The World in 2015. Viewed 25th January 2017: http://www.itu.int/en/ITU-D/Statistics/Documents/facts/ICTFactsFigures2015.pdf.

40. US Department of Health and Human Services (2010) Healthy People 2010: Understanding and Improving Health. US Government Printing Office: Washington.

41. Australian Commission on Safety and Quality in Health Care (2014) Health literacy: Taking action to improve safety and quality. Sydney.

42. Lee H, et al. (2016) Does changing pain-related knowledge reduce pain and improve function through changes in catastrophizing? Pain 157: 922-930.

43. Moseley GL (2003) Unravelling the barriers to reconceptualisation of the problem in chronic pain: the actual and perceived ability of patients and health professionals to understand the neurophysiology. J Pain 4: 184-189.

44. Catley MJ, O'Connell NE & Moseley GL (2013) How Good Is the Neurophysiology of Pain Questionnaire? A Rasch Analysis of Psychometric Properties. J Pain 14: 818-827.

45. Smith MK (2000) Curriculum theory and practice. Viewed 25th January 2017: http://infed.org/mobi/curriculum-theory-and-practice/.

46. Biggs JB & Collis KF (1982) Evaluating the quality of learning: The SOLO taxonomy. Academic Press: New York.

Notes...

7

The malleable magic of metaphor

*Metaphors are not to be trifled with. A single metaphor
can give birth to love.*
Milan Kundera, The Unbearable Lightness of Being

My back is stuffed

Our goal for *EP Supercharged* is to help you and your patients navigate a deep learning pathway to pain literacy. So far we have covered neurotags, theories, some hard core biology, concepts, planning curricula and more. Before we proceed to the science and art of therapeutic storytelling, let's take a closer look at language, in particular the role of metaphor in the interactions between health professional and patient; between deliverer and learner. How we move, learn, sweat, repair, plan, hurt, heal, talk – how we live our lives – is influenced by how we think metaphorically.

We're definitely not linguists and this chapter is by no means a comprehensive analysis of metaphor and health – rather our goal is to explore the concept of metaphor and pain, recognise the ubiquitous nature of metaphor in clinical encounters, and highlight the transformative power of metaphor. In this book we draw heavily on the seminal work of Lakoff and Johnson [1, 2] who proposed the neural theory of metaphor. We find great overlap with their work on the neural basis of metaphorical thought and our understanding of the principles that govern the operation and influence of neurotags.

If we were linguists, at this point we might stop and point out that *my back is stuffed* is a metaphor, *it's like bone on bone* is a simile, *I'm into McKenzie* is a metonym, and *how's your waterworks?* is a euphemism. Linguists go much deeper into this of course and it's very easy to mix up these categories especially when using more complex language.

Table 7.1 presents four commonly used linguistic structures. If you find yourself in a bar fight with a linguist you might want to remember them, but as far as *EP Supercharged* is concerned we will broadly refer to all four as metaphorical or figurative language. Importantly, all four examples have a conceptual nature: they are more than words, they are thoughts and language based on reasoning and conceptualisation and they will be held in our brains in neurotags.

Metaphorical language is our focus here, although we acknowledge and encourage a wider view including metaphorical non-verbal expressions such as art and dance. The non-verbal elements of interaction such as silence, pauses and gesticulation may at times be more expressive than words alone. Reflect on a time you experienced an acute injury – descriptive language other than swearing probably eluded you. Words perhaps only emerged when everything calmed down and even then your descriptions were probably in the past tense and relied on homeostatic responses other than pain – *that was a real shock to the system, it took my breath away*. Altered language and particularly loss of language are common features of post-traumatic stress states. They are also common in chronic pain states, with sufferers sometimes resorting to art and music to express what they are experiencing. We ask you to consider not just what is said, but what is not said and how it is not said. In health, where we seek to promote liberated expression, *silence is not always golden*.

Linguistic structure	Definition	Examples
Metaphor	Directly equates something from one domain with something from another domain.	*Petrol prices are sky-rocketing* *My pain is a real killer*
Simile	Directly compares something from one domain with something from another domain.	*My knee is like a rusty hinge* *The pain is as sharp as a razor blade*
Metonym	Stands for another term within the same domain. Often used as a shortcut.	*Hoover the floor* *I use Maitland* *Healthy workplace* *Give you a hand*
Euphemism	Replaces words and terms considered harsh, offensive or impolite. Often used to prevent embarrassment and maintain respect.	*Passed away* *Sleep together* *Passing wind* *Willy and lady-bits*

Table 7.1 Common linguistic structures used in the language of pain

Metaphors We Live By

The use of metaphor in pain can be conveniently explored via the themes in *Metaphors We Live By* [1]. Consider this view – metaphors allow two or more people to converse on a deep level and discuss something unfamiliar to *one* person in language that *both* people understand. Dave doesn't really understand computers, but he is quite the expert on how a bucket works – so explaining one aspect of how a computer **stores information like a bucket**, and how that **storage can become full** will help him understand that he might need to **empty the bucket out a bit** (delete files) to make room for some more information. Dave's computer **leaks information** too, but he is trying to **plug** that! This is known as the conceptual theory of metaphor, essentially how metaphor structures our conceptual systems.

Three key elements that emerge from Lakoff and Johnson's [1] influential work are:

1. The notions of primary and secondary metaphors.

2. The ubiquitous, unavoidable and unconscious nature of metaphor.

3. How metaphors emerge from our bodily experiences in the world and ultimately shape us.

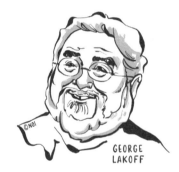

GEORGE LAKOFF

Primary and secondary metaphors

A primary metaphor provides the foundation from which other metaphors are conceptualised by linking two domains. Secondary metaphors are thoughts and language that arise from this linkage. LOVE IS A JOURNEY[1] [1] is a primary metaphor from which numerous secondary metaphors can arise – *it's been a bumpy road, highway to heaven* and *time to part ways*. The target domain of a metaphor is the idea or notion that a metaphor seeks to explain, in this instance, love. The source domain of a metaphor is the concept from which the primary metaphor is constructed, ie. journey (Table 7.2).

---

1   We write the primary metaphor in upper case, following the convention of Lakoff and Johnson.

Target Domain	Source Domain	Primary metaphor	Secondary metaphors
What you want to explain	Concepts used to explain the target		
Love	Journey/travel/pathway	LOVE IS A JOURNEY	*It's been a bumpy road* *Look how far we've come* *We're at the end of the line*
Theories	Building/architecture	THEORIES ARE BUILDINGS	*Your theory needs more support* *You need to construct a better argument* *What's your theory framework?*
Brain	Machine/computer	YOUR MIND IS A MACHINE	*Rusty cogs in my head* *Steam coming out my ears* *The workings of the mind*

Table 7.2 Examples of target and source domains of primary metaphors

Primary metaphors in health and pain

A common, powerful and persistent primary metaphor is MEDICINE IS WAR [3]. Following on from this primary metaphor, medical investigations and surgical and pharmacological interventions are *weapons of war* [4]. The term *fight* and *battle* are used a lot. Often, treatment *targets the source* of the disease and approaches range from *scattergun approaches* to *looking for the silver bullet*. When people receive an unfortunate diagnosis of cancer they may say *I will fight this to the end*. No doubt some fight and spirit is helpful but you are fighting your own cells – conceptualising them as *invaders*. Perhaps it would also help to get to know them?

A primary and linked metaphor that we repeatedly challenge in this book is PAIN IS ENEMY. This suggests that pain has found its way into language almost exclusively through powerful and evocative metaphors of weaponry and things that can damage the body [5]. Metaphors arising from PAIN IS ENEMY including *fight pain, shooting* or *stabbing pain* and *attack of pain* are probably not helpful. Such metaphors suggest an external blame rather than an internal understanding – fighting and killing are stressful things! Repeatedly using these metaphors will strengthen their neurotags which are most likely DIMs.

A primary metaphor that is more in line with current pain biology is PAIN IS A PROTECTOR. The secondary metaphors or linguistic expressions that arises from this primary metaphor include *you can be sore but safe* and *pain is a gift* (Table 7.3). This raises an important issue – while we may offer alternatives to a learner's metaphorical thoughts and language, it may be a better and longer term strategy, perhaps a societal strategy, to try to alter the PAIN IS ENEMY primary metaphor. This will be a difficult task. Take for example the metaphor *painkillers* – this is so embedded in our language that it will be difficult to change.

The primary metaphor of PAIN IS ENEMY is hinted at in the International Association for the Study of Pain's (IASP) definition of pain as '*an unpleasant sensory and emotional experience associated with actual or potential tissue damage, or described in terms of such damage*' [6]. It has been noted that this definition is somewhat negative and restricted to metaphors of damage [7]. If pain can only be negative, then pain will only be used for negative purposes and have negative effects. Perhaps future definitions will integrate the glorious, protective, life-enhancing properties of pain.

Target domain What you want to explain	Source domain Concepts used to explain the target	Primary metaphor	Secondary metaphors
Medicine	War	MEDICINE IS WAR	*War on cancer* *I can't fight the insurance company anymore* *The clinical battlefront* *Attack the source of the problem*
Pain	Enemy/conflict	PAIN IS ENEMY	*Burning, stabbing, shooting* *Attack of back pain* *Pain is killing me* *Painkillers target the pain*
	Protection	PAIN IS A PROTECTOR	*Sore but safe* *Hurt doesn't equal harm* *Know pain, know gain* *Pain stops you in your tracks*

Table 7.3 Examples of medicine and pain primary and secondary metaphors

Metaphors are everywhere

The second element in Lakoff and Johnson's work is that metaphors are so pervasive in all aspects of our lives that we are rarely aware of them. How many metaphors can you recognise in this description provided by one of our clients who was experiencing chronic pain in his back and right leg.

The pain can be a real killer. It goes around and down the inside of the driver muscle to my old knee which I stuffed up years ago. Sometimes it goes into my right ball. That drives me crazy. I get pins and needles in the bloody right foot too. I can't put my finger on why it's happening, but I am ready for the scrapheap! The treatment so far has been bullshit.

What a great way to communicate! Reflect on the enormous amount of medical information that has been expressed by a non-medical person through this short statement – everything from anatomical, diagnostic, psychological and prognostic information and even a blunt view of the health system. It has also facilitated discussion of more intimate issues such as testicle pain and the statement has opened negotiations *Well, let's go back a step and put it all on the table.* By the way, we counted around twenty-eight metaphors! (No arguments here, see end of chapter.)

If you really think about it, we *have* to use metaphors to communicate our pain experiences. Our concept of pain is not complete without metaphor. Just as love is not love without metaphors of journey, madness, magic and union [1], pain is not pain without metaphors of invasion – *burning inside*; bodily damage – *tearing, ripping*; objects – *a vice on my head*; the future – *back pain is forever*; disembodiment – *I hate my leg* and orientation – *it goes down my leg.*

Reflect for a moment on the place of metaphor in health education. The *heart as a pump, gate control theory,* the *brain as a computer*, the *lock and key principle* of drug action – they are all metaphors, but it is likely we've not been aware that we have been taught via metaphor. We forget that *core stability, pelvic floor, nerve root, pins and needles, arch of the foot, trigger points* and *double blind study* are all metaphorical language. Pain questionnaires inevitably seek information using metaphorical descriptors – *Is your pain burning or stabbing?* We also see metaphors entrenched in radiology reports – *degenerated, desiccated* or *prolapsed disc*. Metaphors – they're everywhere!

Metaphors shape us

Another central theme in *Metaphors We Live By* and one that follows on from the ubiquitous nature of metaphor, is that metaphors help make us who we are.[2] Our life stories, full of metaphor, mould us. Reflect on how you know or knew your grandparents from their stories. Notions of embodiment are much loved and argued about by philosophers who, in our readings, can only agree that embodiment is a difficult concept. Lay people take embodiment easily into metaphor though – *she is the embodiment of all our dreams* and on a somewhat more aggressive line, boxing champion Joe Frazier's strategy was to *kill the body and the head will die!* [9].

We take a simple view of embodiment here along the lines of how the state of the body and perceptions of that state shape the mind. What might be the difference if a person holds the primary metaphor that LIFE IS A STRUGGLE compared to another who holds the primary metaphor LIFE IS A DANCE. How would they react in times of difficulty and in times of joy? We suggest that repeated use of a metaphor such as *I am riddled with arthritis* puts self-imposed limits on a person's life. And it is not just the physicality that is embodied. Metaphor has allowed a linguistic form and thus a linguistic physicality for non-physical things – *what you said made me g low* and *when I heard the diagnosis, I felt my life was ripped away*. The importance here is that pain states not linked to physical change can be expressed. As Denis Donoghue says in his lovely book on metaphor, '*it ensures that nothing goes without a name'* [10].

On a more specific note, metaphors will influence how we think about other aspects of life too – those who hold a BODY IS A MACHINE primary metaphor may only seek mechanical fixes and regard any other option as absolute nonsense and a sleight on their character. A yoga lover, with a primary metaphorical

concept of BODY IS A GARDEN, is likely to behave and act very differently from that; he might be reluctant to consider any mechanical explanations for his pain. Tricky isn't it?

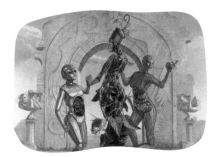

DIMs, SIMs and the inviting metaphorical fuzziness

The conceptual view of metaphor links nicely to the Danger in Me (DIMs) and Safety in Me (SIMs) neurotags that we introduced in *The Explain Pain Handbook: Protectometer* [11] and discussed earlier in *EP Supercharged* (pages 17-18). We proposed seven categories of DIMs and SIMs and in each category there are potent and evocative metaphors (Table 7.4).

An Explain Pain intervention will seek to acknowledge but also highlight and challenge some of the DIM metaphors. If a woman associates the movement of her knee with breaking and grinding glass fragments, how willing might she be to embark on a program of movement and activity? In fact, based on this visceral and evocative (but ultimately inaccurate) metaphor, she would be quite right *not* to move.

If appropriate, you might offer a SIM metaphor, which may evoke multisensory imagery, to replace a DIM. Rather than *my disc is like a doughnut with jam oozing out,* your transformative response could be *your LAFT[3] is more like a tyre that you can inflate with exercise, time and understanding.*

Metaphor provides a '*fuzziness and openness'* that invites a way into the patient's world through understanding and story [4]. Simply telling a patient that he is wrong is not likely to get you (or them!) very far, but carefully listening for his metaphors and offering back a combination of literal explanations and transformative metaphors can be a respectful way to begin to challenge unhelpful conceptualisations.

---

2   Would Usain Bolt run as fast if his name was Usain Plod? [8]

3   LAFT is a Living Adaptable Force Transducer. We think it is a much better name for the disc [EP54-55]

Metaphorical DIM	DIM SIM Category	Metaphorical SIM
Each time I move it *feels and sounds like broken glass*	Things I hear, see, smell, touch and taste	'The Three Graces' in Botticelli's 'Primavera' are so *uplifting*
I keep doing the same thing over and over like *I'm stuck in a rut*	Things I do	I'm moving and *exploring* my surroundings again, just *like a chameleon*
The disc will *slip* if I bend over	Things I think and believe	I have enough info to make *new flight plans*
It's got me this time	Things I say	I'm *bouncing* back
Work is a *cold, dark* place	Places I go	Going to work gives *structure to my life*
He makes my *skin crawl*	People I meet	My friends have really *carried me through this*, but now it's time to *stand on my own two feet*
Everything inside me is just *falling apart*	Things happening in my body	When I exercise, it feels like everything *runs like a well-oiled machine* *Motion is lotion!*

Table 7.4 Examples of metaphors related to the DIM SIM categories

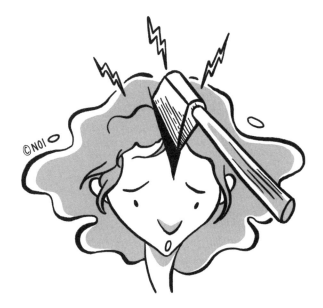

SPLITTING HEADACHE

*Figure 7.1 **Splitting headache** may be an example of a DIM which is an invasive metaphor*

Classification of metaphors in the clinic

Clinical encounters are a metaphorical fountain! Metaphors gush from the patient and the clinician and from all over the clinical environment. We have collected hundreds of health and pain associated metaphors from patients, from discussions with course participants, and from an informal survey of over 200 practising physiotherapists enrolled in a postgraduate pain management course.

We've put together a classification of pain-related metaphors based on the work of Lakoff and Johnson [1] and Kövecses [12] but have also added some classifications to include metaphors linked to pain and clinical encounters. These categories are somewhat artificial, particularly because some metaphors will fit into a number of categories, but the suggested categorisation will help deliverers contemplate the role of metaphor in their intervention (Table 7.5).

Classification	Examples of DIMs and SIMs
Structural Metaphors Provide a rich knowledge structure to understand a target domain These are often anatomical	*My knee is like a rusty hinge* (DIM) *Those extra bits of bone that I can see on my x-ray mean my back is a stable platform* (SIM)
Orientational Metaphors Relate to space, direction and movement These help objectify a problem	*The pain goes down and around my leg* (DIM) *I'm at the peak of health* (SIM)
Invasive Metaphors Suggest physical and/or psychological invasion	*Like a knife in there, Splitting headache* (DIM) *I am getting to the guts of the problem* (SIM) (Invasive SIMs are difficult to find)
Disembodiment Metaphors Imply separation of body and self	*My arm doesn't feel like mine* (DIM) *I'm loving my leg again* (SIM) (more embodiment)
Ontological Metaphors Objectify things that are not actually objects such as feelings or thoughts Can be further grouped into: • Journey Metaphors • Container Metaphors	*Walking on eggshells* (DIM) *It's all coming together* (SIM) • **Journey** *I'm in quicksand* (DIM) *Light at the end of the tunnel* (SIM) • **Container** *I'm full up to here with all these appointments* (DIM) *I think my meditation releases some pressure* (SIM)
Diagnostic Metaphors Label an injury or disease	*Whiplash, Frozen shoulder* (diagnostic metaphors are nearly always DIMs unless explained)
Prognostic Metaphors Suggest the future course of the condition	*I'm totally stuffed* (DIM) *You're cruising along nicely* (SIM)

Table 7.5 A pain related metaphor classification with examples of DIMs and SIMs

Structural metaphors

In structural metaphors, the source domain provides a relatively rich knowledge structure for the Target Concept. Structural metaphors are common in the health domain and are so deeply embedded within our language that we can forget they are metaphors at all. They often emerge from an anatomical base such as *my pelvis is twisted*, can be quite descriptive, and to some extent may offer self-diagnosis – *I've slipped a disc*. For many, the metaphor may be the limit of their knowledge about the problem. Until it is identified as metaphorical, deconstructed and reconceptualised, it may also limit their ability to learn more about their problem.

All metaphors, but particularly structural, health-related metaphors, can be geographically and culturally specific – *I was as sick as a dog* is quite Australian (meaning really ill) and *my dogs are barking* is very American for sore feet, while *I am all stoved up* (meaning really stiff) seems to be only heard in the southern states of the USA. *It's munted* belongs to New Zealand where it means the body part is not working as well as it could or one is drug and alcohol afflicted. A welder once said to one of us *my knee has been arcing up* – I should have asked him what kind of welder he was using!

Structural metaphors as an invitation

Metaphors are open ended and we see them as an invitation for deeper analysis. Questions may arise from these descriptions, such as *so what do you mean when you say the knee is going to buckle?* and *are there certain movements that make your shoulder catch?* or *can tell me more about this feeling of a pinched nerve?* They also enhance clinical interaction. You have clearly been listening and engaged if, at your patient's next visit you can ask *is the knee still arcing up?* or *do your muscles feel less knotted now?*

Use the invitation to seek the source of the metaphor. You might ask *where did you get the idea that your pelvis is twisted* or *why do you think your disc has slipped?* Such metaphors will ideally be challenged in an Explain Pain intervention and the challenge may be more powerful and directed if you know the origin of the metaphor.

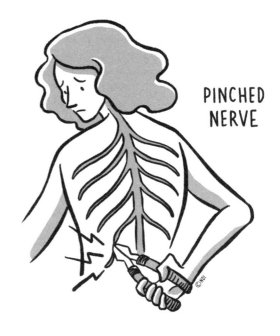

PINCHED NERVE

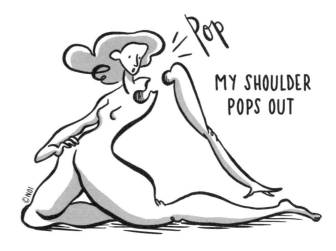

POP

MY SHOULDER POPS OUT

*Figure 7.2 **Pinched nerve** and **my shoulder pops out** are examples of structural metaphors*

Structural metaphors offer potential to convert DIMs to SIMs

Note that the structural metaphors we've been discussing so far are all DIMs. We hope that you can look at them eagerly as they all invite a creative transfer to SIMs via alternative language and metaphor. Take *my knee is like a rusty hinge* – a transformative response may be, *Okay. Knees are more complex than hinges though, they also rotate and glide, they love movement – even some compression – knees are self-lubricating too. I can help you work out some strategies to encourage your natural joint oils to flow*.

In this case the word *joint* has replaced *hinge*, the knee has been elevated from a mere bendy thing to a more complex, living structure and you've provided hope along with self-management advice.

Some metaphors invite careful responses

If your patient comes out with a structural metaphor such as *my muscle is knotted,* it may be best not to say *let's stretch it* but instead *let's work out how we can relax it*. Why? Because stretching a knot will only tighten it of course. *Let's slip it back in* is not appropriate for *I've got a slipped disc*. This would be maintaining the DIM as it infers that a disc is a slippable object. Better to say something like *There is nothing slippery about a disc. Discs are Living Adaptable Force Transducers (LAFTs) that are firmly connected to the bones in your back and supported by really powerful ligaments. Diffs[4] slip, soap slips, discs definitely don't slip.*

More examples of structural metaphors
– note how they are all DIMs

- *The muscles are knotted*
- *My back is out*
- *A catch in my shoulder*
- *Pinched nerve*
- *My elbow creaks like an old door*
- *My knee buckles*
- *The pain came in waves*
- *I've got a glass back*
- *My hand is all pins and needles*

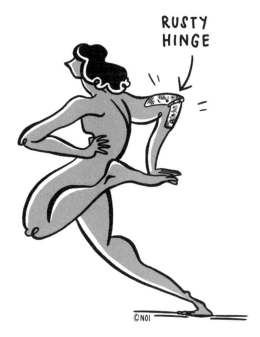

Figure 7.3 *My elbow is a rusty hinge* invites transformative SIM language

---

4 For those of you who are not *petrolheads* or *gearheads*, a diff is a differential – an essential part of a car that drives the wheels and allows them to rotate at different speeds so you can turn corners.

Orientational metaphors

Health professionals will hear (and use) orientational metaphors with every patient. Take **the pain goes up to my head** – 'goes **up to**' makes this an orientational metaphor. These are well embedded in our language and until terms like **up, down, front** and **back** are viewed up close and personally, we often don't think of them as metaphorical. Reflect on **the pain goes down my leg**. You rarely hear someone say **the pain goes up my leg**. These metaphors are common and can often be categorised as DIMs or SIMs (Table 7.6).

Diagnosing and grounding the problem

Learners ground their pain states by adding orientational descriptors. This gives meaning, substance and language to objectify their symptoms. Along with aiding communication, orientational metaphors should help you, the deliverer, understand some of what is going on in your patients' minds, in particular how language may be helping them to **get a grip** on their problem.

Orientational metaphors can be extremely helpful in diagnosis. **Down and around** and **into** or **it goes from here to here** may provide information about a known neural zone such as a dermatome. This can be illustrated, explained and dethreatened (Nugget 24 *Pain strips for you*). Equally, **pressure deep in my chest going up to my jaw** should raise suspicions of heart ischaemia.

Perhaps the suggested changeability of symptoms that might be captured by metaphors such as **it runs down** and **it travels around**, hint at processes more related to upregulation of the central nervous system. Perhaps **stuck in**, **wedged** and **out** hint at more tissue-based pathophysiology, or at least a tissue-based explanation. What an open and currently untouched potential area for research!

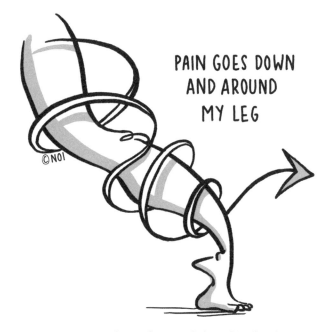

PAIN GOES DOWN AND AROUND MY LEG

©NOI

Figure 7.4 Orientational metaphors may help to objectify pain

DIMs	SIMs
Laid me low	Looking ahead and moving forward
Down in the dumps	Everything is in front of me
Pain goes right through my body	Things are looking up
My body has let me down	The bruising has come out to the surface and everything is healing inside
Something is wedged in there	Reaching new heights
My life is upside down	I'm feeling grounded
Fell ill	Bounced back quickly
Teetering on the edge	Clawed my way back from the precipice
Listing to the left	I'm straight as an arrow and as flexible as well cooked spaghetti
Pain is peaking	My pain levels are way down
Pain is deep inside	I'm back on the straight and narrow
Back to square one	The worst is behind me now

Table 7.6 Examples of orientational metaphors – DIMs and SIMs

Transformations – from down to up and DIM to SIM

The notion of **up** in orientational metaphors is usually linked with positive conceptualisations – **on top of it all today; upbeat.** Whereas **down** is usually more negative – **fell ill; down in the dumps.** This pattern has always been strong in health with primary metaphors of HEALTH AND LIFE ARE UP and SICKNESS AND DEATH ARE DOWN [1]. An awareness of these primary orientational metaphors offers opportunity for DIM to SIM transformations and also enhancement of the language of SIMs. By including **up, front** and **forward** in metaphorical language offered back to learners we promote the positive, ie. we promote SIMs.

Other positive metaphorical language might include words like **goal, reach** and **balanced.** Avoid negative metaphorical language for example **under, out, imbalance** and **behind** because they promote the negative and thus promote DIMs. Just when it's looking all neat and tidy, like everything else in this book, things are more complicated than they seem – it's usually a good thing to be **under control,** and you don't want pain to **ramp up** – see how this breaks the 'rules'? Metaphors are clearly malleable.

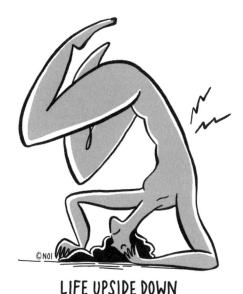

LIFE UPSIDE DOWN

Figure 7.5 **Life turned upside down** can be transformed to **upright and on track again**

Invasive metaphors

Invasive metaphors imply that a person has conceptualised an invasion from an external agent, or an invasion in some way from within his or her body. At their most overt, invasive metaphors range from direct descriptions such as *it feels as though there is a knife in me* to milder descriptions such as *I'm a bit worn out*.

Some invasive metaphors may have been passed on by health professionals or picked up from websites – *my neck is out* or *it's bone on bone*. Radiology reports often include invasive language like *degenerative, compressing, invading, occupying, protruding* or *sequestrated*[5] when describing disc changes. Note also how many of these metaphorical labels are verbs, implying that this is happening right now as they read it or hear it. Scary stuff! These words and the phrases they are in suggest an invasion from within – something inside has gone wrong (or is actually going wrong), with notions of the unknown, unseen and often unexplained.

There are also common metaphorical external invasions as well – *it's like ants crawling on me* or *my head is in a vice*. The adjectives *squashed* and *burning* suggest external physical invasion from various agents. On reflection, *ingrown toenail* is not a pleasant term. Neither is *splitting headache* – a rather visceral metaphor that may evoke an unpleasant feeling deep in your guts. Other invasive metaphors may suggest more psychological invasion – *the insurance guy is getting under my skin* or *my employer is playing mind games with me*.

Consider the likely neuro-immunological consequences

Think for a moment about all these metaphors from the perspective of the cortical body matrix theory and the notion that all metaphors are held by modulation or action neurotags. Invasive metaphors, perhaps more than other conceptual metaphors, clearly have the potential to influence protective neurotags and therefore feelings (such as pain and stiffness), immune and motor responses (remember the Roman ruins in Chapter 2 pages 30-31). Invasive metaphors can contribute to the stories that become part of us – both metaphorically and literally.

Take repeated use of the simile *it's like there is a knife in my back*. If the neurotag that holds this simile becomes very influential, one might have a protective response to visual or other cues of knives, sharp objects, or even kitchens. This is clearly speculative but it is not at all outrageous speculation. A strongly held metaphor (ie. an influential metaphor neurotag) of, for example *a fire inside me* may become sufficiently influential to shift thermal heat pain threshold; or might be sufficiently influential to bring a radio news item of bushfires into consciousness; it might be sufficiently influential to cause one to lose interest in cooking marshmallows on an open fire.

Again, these are all speculative examples, but insofar as our theories allow us to generate predictions, these predictions are certainly plausible, if not easily testable. What is more, the field already knows that neuroimmunological changes that can be brought around by threatening inputs can persevere for months or years beyond the removal of threat [13, 14].

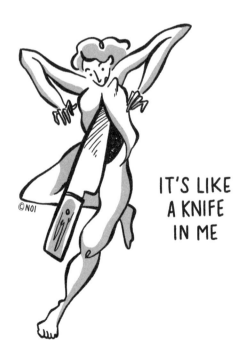

Figure 7.6 Powerful invasive metaphorical language

---

5   *Sequestrated* may send the reader straight to Google where they will learn that 'sequestrate' means to *take possession of someone's property until they pay something*, but also read about disc fragments breaking free and moving into the spinal canal and compressing nerve roots.

More examples of invasive metaphorical language

- *It feels like there's a screw left rubbing after the surgery*
- *There is someone inside in my head with a hammer*
- *Feels like a fire in there*
- *Something is eating me from the inside*
- *They told me the vertebrae were unstable in there*
- *Disc derangement*
- *This whole process is grating on my nerves*
- *What he said went straight to my heart*
- *It's flared up again*
- *Joints are eroding*
- *Down-slipped pelvis*

Invasive language calls for care and creative interpretation

Avoid offering new invasive metaphors

Invasive metaphors include some of the most potent and evocative language patients can use to express their pain and situation – they are nearly always DIMs. Health professionals may like to consider why this patient is choosing to use this particular metaphor. Possible answers include everything from simply having no other language or understanding, to an urgent need to deeply express how distressing their problem is. Clearly you need to put some thought and care into this before proceeding. Our first consideration is not to introduce invasive metaphors to your learner. Perhaps we can all collectively acknowledge that clinicians, with the very best of intentions, have been responsible for giving birth to some of the horrible invasive metaphors that have become social standards today – *slipped discs, backs out, pelvic upslips, bone on bone* and so on.

Acknowledge the patient's invasive metaphor

Invasive metaphors, indeed all metaphorical language, invite careful clarification such as *what do you think it might take to relieve the stabbing/pressure/tearing/knife inside feeling?* Here you are acknowledging and using your learner's invasive metaphor, without introducing any further invasive elements. Acknowledging learners' metaphors demonstrates that you are listening carefully, and given the fuzzy nature of metaphors, engaging with them is often just a small step away from modifying them and eventually converting them to SIM metaphors.

Reframe an invasive metaphor

One educational technique would be to reframe the invasive metaphor. A response to *it feels like a knife in me* could be *it's not a knife, though its a bit stiff and inflamed where you're pointing and the tissues inside would love some special movements*. A response to *it's burning inside when I move* would be to suggest water-associated imagery or hydrotherapy.

Further reframing of a notion such as *my joints are eroding* could be *your joints are showing the natural and healthy signs of use – the hallmarks of experience representing everything you have done, and everywhere you have gone in life*. Rather than tell a learner that it's desirable to *tear adhesions* or *break up scar tissue* (which you can't do anyway), try reframing their concept by suggesting that appropriate *movement will encourage healthy, elastic, strong and flexible healing*.

Reframing. Watzlawick et al. [15] describe reframing as *'changing the conceptual and/or emotional setting or viewpoint in relation to which a situation is experienced and to place it in another frame which fits the 'facts' of the same concrete situation equally well or even better, and thereby changing its entire meaning.'*

Provide an explanation to encourage change

A still more powerful educational intervention in the presence of invasive metaphors is to provide information to help your learner understand why holding invasive metaphorical thoughts and language, including CAMPs (Cognition Associated Molecular Patterns page 60), can keep danger surveillance systems on alert. This may help give your patient reason to seek and experience new language and thoughts and to open up pathways to find more SIMs, including safer language.
(Novella 5 *Protection has a long memory*)

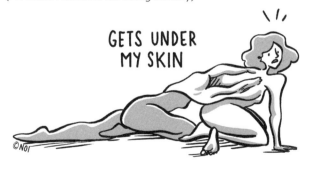

Figure 7.7 There are psychological elements to invasive metaphors

Disembodiment metaphors

Disembodiment refers to the feeling of no longer owning one's body, or not having agency over it. Use of disembodiment metaphors suggest that a person perceives that his or her body or body part no longer belongs to them, is different or unlikeable. Language that suggests disembodiment may range from overt statements such as *I can't find my feet* or *I've got a wooden arm,* to more subtle statements such as *the back's a real problem*. When people use *the, this, that* or *it* rather than *my* to describe a body part, it hints that they may have some kind of disconnect with that part of their body.

We also identified metaphors and statements such as *no one knows my body as well as my physiotherapist* and *I get my neck put back in once a month*. These suggest that the person's body has been left to someone else and is no longer his/her responsibility. The metaphor *I've got Mum's knees* is clearly incorrect and also defers responsibility of your own body. You might respond *no you haven't – you have your own knees*.

Disembodiment metaphors hint at loss of precision of neurotags

Take care when making judgements on the potential meaning of language that suggests disembodiment. Peripheral phenomena such as nerve injury or tissue swelling can make a limb feel odd and unfamiliar. Disembodiment metaphors in these cases can be important diagnostic cues when taken into account with other signs and symptoms. Of course, disembodied language may have always been a part of a person's vernacular – they may have always unconsciously said *the leg* or *it's killing me* and yet still be quite in touch with their body. Careful questioning will tell you if this is the case.

Sometimes however, disembodiment metaphors may form part of an overall pattern that suggests nervous system upregulation, including alterations in the precision of bodily neurotags. Disembodiment metaphors may be linked to physical findings such as impaired two-point discrimination and altered left/right discrimination. In this case it makes sense to adapt or change disembodiment metaphors. Describe the problem biologically – explain that avoiding, not loving and rejecting the body part can cause problems, and then give them something to do about it. This may include language shifts but also imagery strategies such as Graded Motor Imagery [16] and sensory retraining. For further suggestions see Nugget 51 *I ache in the places where I used to play*.

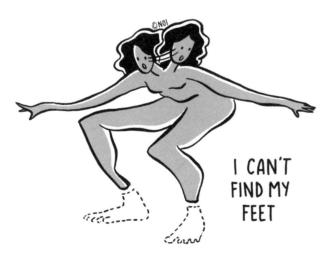

Figure 7.8 Language hinting at disembodied lower limbs

> **More examples of metaphors suggesting disembodiment**
> - *The leg has gone out with the fairies*
> - *It's like a block of wood*
> - *I just block that part of my body out*
> - *I can't find my feet sometimes*
> - *Trade me in on a new one*
> - *It feels swollen*
> - *I hate it, just cut the leg off*
> - *My legs feel foreign*
> - *The back is a problem*
> - *The right leg is my bad leg*

Are you contributing to the solution or the problem?

Health professionals may inadvertently be providing disembodiment metaphors. Asking *how's the back today?* rather than *how are you today?* Or failing to acknowledge the potential danger of people with a stroke naming their neglected part *Suzy* or *George* may encourage disembodiment. Some patients' language emerges from perceptions of blame, such as *look what they have done to it* and *this back is out of bounds to all health professionals*. Leaving these statements unchallenged may further strengthen a disembodied state.

Disembodiment metaphors often include the concept of *out* for instance – *my back is out* or *I am out of alignment* or *put me back in*. It suggests a body part has periodically gone somewhere else. This highlights a lack of knowledge and the presence of misconceptions about anatomy and physiology. *Slipped disc* would also fit under this category. This language and the knowledge that goes with it is danger enhancing (DIMs).

More DIM to SIM opportunities

Anger, disrespect, hate and disgust frequently emerge in language that hints at disembodiment, suggesting a negative emotional connection between someone and his body or body part. It could be as simple as *trade me in on a new one* or *it's that shitty knee again*. Encourage your patient to become aware of the negative emotions he may have towards his body through thoughts and language. Where possible try to offer more SIM-enhancing language – *that knee has been a great part of life's journey* may be an appropriate response.

Quick real-time fixes are available. Downgrade the DIM power of *bad arm* or *injured side* to *left or right arm, or side*. Challenge *wooden leg* with *it's not wood – wood burns, decays and disintegrates – your leg lives and regenerates*. And *get rid of the nickname – it's your arm* (Nugget 65 *It's not out, it's never out*). This reminds us of one intriguing survey response of *my leg needs mediation* – what an invitation for education! You might ask *who is fighting whom?*

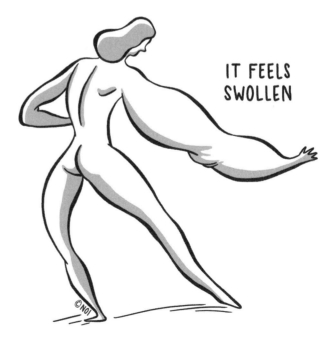

IT FEELS SWOLLEN

*Figure 7.9 The limb may **feel swollen** but rarely is*

Ontological metaphors

A friend once described his partner's grief at a funeral by saying *she broke up like a biscuit*. This is an ontological metaphor – the language gives structure and objectifies something that is not an object. In this case emotion was objectified by linking it to a crumbling biscuit. An ontological metaphor objectifies abstract concepts such as life, mind, love and pain – giving them an existence you can grab onto, hold and personify. Winston Churchill used an ontological metaphor to describe his depression that became so well endorsed it has even been adopted by a major research institute – *The Black Dog* Institute in Sydney, Australia.

Pain, especially chronic pain, is difficult to articulate and many have said it has no voice – which is perhaps why some of the most powerful descriptors of pain have come from art, poetry and prose [17, 18]. We see the moon, smell the coffee, we hear Bob Marley wail and we stroke sensual silk. While the redness, swelling, deformation and bandages associated with an acute pain experience give it a voice and engender understanding, chronic pain rarely has these obvious signs. *I am falling apart at the seams* links to clothing, or *I feel fragile today* associates with crockery and glassware. Everyone likes to talk about the weather and perhaps it is no surprise that the sky and climate features in ontological metaphors like *it comes out of the blue* and *I am under the weather*. We all use these metaphors to objectify things so we can talk, quantify and act accordingly.

A call for grounding, anchoring and reality

Altered nervous system functioning associated with upregulation and sensitisation may lead to repeated use of ontological metaphors. The patient's use of ontological metaphor is an implicit call for deeper understanding of what is really happening in her body. Therapeutic story is required here to objectify the pain experience, grounding it so someone can imagine, construct and believe what is going on and share it publicly. By doing this, we give words to things that currently have no words.[6]

Holding onto words makes sense

Patients often desperately cling to the words provided by health professionals – even throwaway lines like *just a minor disc bulge*. Radiology reports can be a rich source of ontological metaphor – seemingly innocuous words for a clinician such as *degeneration* might be the only tangible thing for a patient to grasp onto.

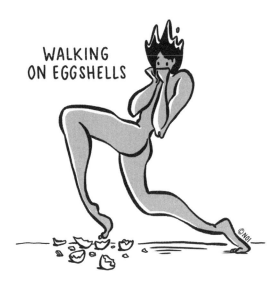

Figure 7.10 Metaphor to describe a delicate situation in life

Remember, there will always be *something* reported in a radiology report! Perhaps patients are seeking to anchor their experience – to objectify it and to make a clear operational diagnosis for themselves. It is no wonder they hang onto the past when there may have been an object – a break, a bandage, a clear MRI finding, an infection. You can't blame them.

Consider when a patient says *I have damaged my leg* despite the injury occurring over two years ago – which is plenty of time for healing! Think of how common it is for people with persistent pain to conclude they have *a bad back* whereas what they might mean is that they have bad back pain. One response might be to ask *'how do you know your back is bad?'*, to which the response may be *'because I have back pain'* and there is the trigger for helping the patient identify their circular argument. You might have heard *I wish we could open a little door to my back, have a peek inside and see what is really going on,* also a call for objectification.

> **More examples of ontological metaphors**
> - *I have paid the price for doing this*
> - *My back sucks*
> - *His back pain defeated him*
> - *It hurts like hell*
> - *My pain is at 12/10*
> - *It's a prick of a thing*
> - *Back pain is a real killer*

---

6   Wittgenstein famously said, *'whereof one cannot speak, thereof one must be silent'* [19] – the silence of your patient might be an indication that they just don't have the words or metaphors to express their experience.

The journey and the container in ontological metaphor

Journey lends itself well as a source domain, giving rise to primary metaphors such as LIFE IS A JOURNEY [1, 12]. Secondary metaphors are born such as *I'm at a crossroads in life* and *it's been a rocky road*. Journey metaphors are particularly apt and common in health with WELLNESS IS A JOURNEY as a primary metaphor. The pain experience and the disease or injury that may be associated with it can be given structure, objectification, a sense of time, a start and a finish. *It's been a highway to hell but I am on the road to recovery* are examples. Equally, journey metaphors can be more positive – *it's been smooth sailing* or *I'm travelling like Speedy Gonzales* even *going OK,* or more negative – *I feel like I am in quicksand* or *end of the road,* or simply *stuck*. Some ontological metaphors emerge from the primary metaphor of BODY IS A CONTAINER [1] – *I'm up to my eyeballs with the pain* or *I can't hold it in anymore*. Journey and container metaphors can be either DIMs or SIMs (Table 7.7).

Journey DIMs	Journey SIMs
It's a downward spiral	Onward and upward
Can't get off the merry-go-round	I'm at a crossroads
It's been a rough ride	Onward Christian soldiers
End of my rope	Smooth sailing
It's an uphill battle	Got new flight plans
I'm swimming against the tide	I am all over it now
Sinking in quicksand	It's all fallen apart, let's rebuild
I'm up shit creek (sometimes without a paddle)	One small step at a time
I'm in struggle street	I'm cruising
I'm at my wits' end	Back on the road again
Container DIMs	**Container SIMs**
Can't hold it all in	Let out a little bit at a time
I have had a gutful	I'm full of hope
Full up to the eyeballs	Let's refill you with some good stuff
I can't contain myself	Let's turn the tap on, bit by bit
I feel empty	Ease a bit of the pressure
I'm about to explode	

Table 7.7 Journey and container metaphors as DIMs and SIMs

Journey and container metaphors – a therapeutic invitation

Goal setting

By positioning the experience in time and place, journey and container metaphors lend themselves well to goal setting. When journey metaphors are used as DIMs it might suggest that the person is without goals. Closed metaphors like *I've had an absolute gutful,* or *I'm at the end of the road* require a deeper discussion about how to *clear the gut* or *find a new road,* or to be aware of a *path* they might not have known. However, the openness of metaphors such as *I'm at a crossroad* facilitates the initiation of mutual goal setting – *let's work out the best path.* A person using SIM journey metaphors suggests that there may be some established goals – your intervention may include eliciting these goals, clarifying them and incorporating them into a treatment plan.

DIM to SIM transformation

Journey and container metaphors provide an opportunity to move from DIMs to SIMs (Table 7.7). One powerful element that is offered by the primary metaphor WELLNESS IS A JOURNEY, is a look into the future – *where can your new flight plans take you?* or *what do you see on the horizon?* Container metaphors that are DIMs should not go uncontested. Consider the patient who tells you *my disc is going to blow.* While this threatening metaphor appears anatomically driven, it may well reflect his beliefs about his mental state and coping abilities. Delving deeper into DIM metaphors may help unveil the root of a problem and offer a SIM-enhancing opportunity to *compose, re-build* or *control.*

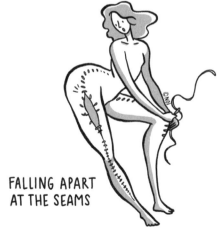

FALLING APART AT THE SEAMS

Figure 7.11 Ontological metaphors provide language for that which is hard to express

Diagnostic metaphors

You may have forgotten that *whiplash* and *heel spur* are metaphorical diagnoses. There are many others that reveal quite evocative sensory imagery. Take *whiplash* for example. Perhaps this diagnostic metaphor evokes imagery that includes a whip, a loud cracking sound, sharp pain if struck by the whip and a power differential – someone might be whipping you. For some, whiplash may even evoke scenes of crash test dummies where a head flies backwards and forward or flies completely off! Consider also the imagery and further metaphors that may arise from a diagnosis of *heel spur – it's digging into me; it's catching; it might snap.*

Many diagnostic metaphors describing pain and disease states are metonyms that are linked to the person who first described them – *De Quervain's Syndrome, Huntington's Disease, LisFranc fracture, Morton's Neuroma, Lorimer's Specific Cortical Stupidity Theory.*[7] Such 'titled' diagnoses may not be a bad thing, but the lack of clarity in the diagnosis could actually be fear-enhancing for some. When the health professional offers a greater explanation of the problem, they may also include a bit on the discoverer to avoid the patient thinking, *did Monsieur De Quervain die from this syndrome?* While some people may be proud to have *golfer's elbow, athlete's foot, tennis elbow* or *jumper's knee,* this doesn't qualify them for an Explain Pain exemption. Others have reflected on how things would be different if Mr and Mrs Awesome, rather than Mr and Mrs Down, had given birth to John. John Down went on to famously name Down Syndrome [20].

Does the existence of diagnostic metaphors suggest clinical and research laziness?

Perhaps these metaphorical diagnoses are embedded because of our laziness. Metaphors inherently mean different things to different people. Being a bit lazy with diagnoses carries the risk of misinterpretation, misunderstanding, literal acceptance (my disc has actually *slipped*) and ultimately danger enhancement. Clinicians using a biopsychosocial framework and reasoned decision making would deconstruct the diagnoses, perhaps under a mechanisms categorisation [21] and provide a more appropriate label or at the very least, a literal understanding of the problem. Labels with the word *syndrome* at the end might suggest a lack of understanding of the pathophysiology – consider *myofascial syndrome* and *complex regional pain syndrome.*

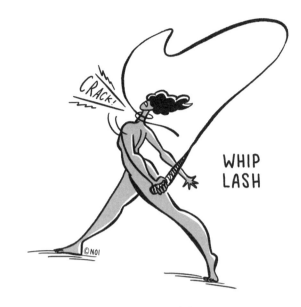

Figure 7.12 Whiplash is a metaphorical diagnosis

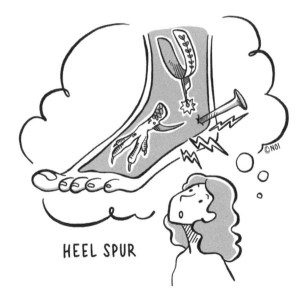

Figure 7.13 Consider the imagery that the metaphorical diagnosis of heel spur may evoke. See Nugget 69 *Heel Spur.*

---

7   Remember this from Chapter 2?

Metaphorical diagnosis	Literal diagnosis – what it actually means
Whiplash	Neck pain associated with an incident of rapid head movement such as a car accident
Frozen shoulder	Reduced movement of shoulder
Heel spur	Radiological evidence of an adaptive strengthening of the bony insertion of the plantar fascia
Hysterectomy	Removal of uterus (nothing to do with being hysterical)
Shin splints.	Pain in the front of the shin
Disc prolapse	Radiological evidence of altered contour of an intervertebral disc
Nerve entrapment.	Less than usual space around the nerve
Compartment syndrome	Swelling of soft tissue surrounded by a fascial layer
Cauliflower ear	Permanent changes to the shape of the external ear as a result of repeated soft tissue damage
Panic attack	Transient episode of increased heart rate, blood pressure, stress hormone release, and associated experience of anxiety

Table 7.8 Common metaphorical diagnoses and their literal meaning

Revise and explain

Many diagnostic metaphors are unhelpful, incorrect, out of date and are rarely, if ever, SIMs. They are often handed out with no further explanation.[8] Each can be revised and explained by simply using the evidence based truth (Table 7.8). We expand on these descriptions in the next Chapter 8 – Nuggets 65 to 71.

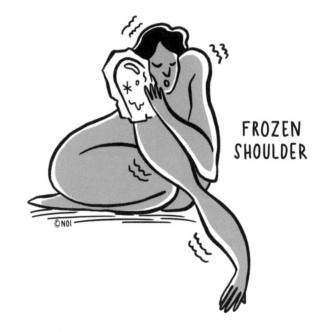

FROZEN SHOULDER

Figure 7.14 Frozen shoulder is an unpleasant diagnosis suggesting permanent shoulder stiffness

---

8   We are well aware that our images could also be DIMs.

Prognostic metaphors

When a person says **my back's completely stuffed**, she has predicted (and possibly limited) her future, and often very confidently! Many prognostic metaphors suggest permanence. However, **I think I am getting a grip on this** and **there is light at the end of the tunnel** provide hope for transformation and goal setting. Prognostic metaphors are often linked to primary metaphors which could be AGE EQUALS TERMINAL DECLINE and INJURY HASTENS AGEING. Critically though, the permanence inferred in these metaphors contradicts the bioplastic nature of our bodies and thus the Target Concept of *We are bioplastic.*

Of course, such statements may be the local vernacular, perhaps an attempt at humour. Old Australians with a few aches and pains often say **cut me off at the neck** and **if I was a horse they would shoot me.** They also say **I'm buggered mate**, or **I'm fucked**. The underlying truth may range from a recent cancer diagnosis to being a little bit tired. Rarely do we think of the literal meaning and if we did, perhaps we would change the metaphor!

Many diagnoses such as osteoporosis, frozen shoulder, fibromyalgia and spondylolisthesis have become metaphors for permanence. The term cancer has become an even more potent metaphor, for example **a cancer on society**.

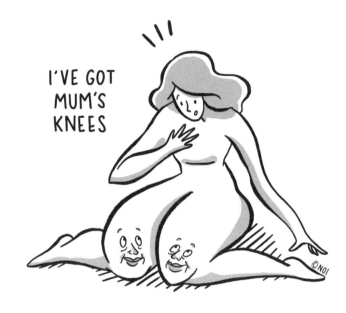

Figure 7.15 'I have my mum's knees' is a prognostic metaphor

More examples of prognostic metaphors
- *The glass is broken*
- *It's bone on bone in there, nothing can be done*
- *I'm riddled with arthritis*
- *I'm ready for the scrapheap*
- *I have the back of an 80 year old, and I'm only 43*
- *I have one foot in the grave*
- *I have nurses' back*
- *I have Mum's knees – I'm fucked*
- *They told me I'd be in a wheelchair soon*
- *Degenerative disc disease*

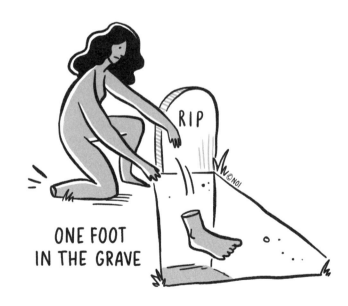

Figure 7.16 You can make your own prognosis via metaphor

Notions of permanence and bioplasticity don't mix

Remember that all of our bodily systems are highly adaptable – a property we call bioplasticity. The permanence of any prognostic metaphor, especially when based on persistent pain, is completely inconsistent with this most fundamental of properties and should nearly always be challenged. Consider the difference between the metaphors *this back pain will follow me forever* and *It hurts today but a new day is just around the corner*. Our language evolved well before we were aware of the remarkable changeability of the brain and the revolutions in pharmacological, surgical, educational and rehabilitation therapies. Might this be one reason that DIMs are so common in health? Perceptions around the notion of permanence are usually DIMs. As a further reminder of this, consider these statements – *the surgeon stuffed up* or *I can't see how it will ever shift* or *it feels as if it will bust open if I bend it*.

Did you or your mates provide the prognostic metaphor?

Health professionals can be sources of prognostic metaphors – *you've got the back of an 80 year old*. We do hear some terrible stories in our travels and collect many more in our email inboxes. A patient with back pain said *they told me I have an obliterated thecal sac,* and sadly, *the physio said that I had a withered arm.* Sometimes these concepts come with powerful visual supports in the form of scans and x-rays. We have all heard – *check out the scans, I'm stuffed.* The internet often doesn't help – *it's repetitive strain injury – I read that it never goes away* or *there is nothing much you can do for fibromyalgia.* In our clinical experience we have noticed that some people believe that the word 'chronic' means forever. Certainly, many people think 'chronic' refers to the future, whereas it really refers to the past.

Chronic pain as a disease?

At the time of writing, we are in the middle of a worldwide debate about whether or not chronic pain should be labelled a disease. There are some powerful socio-political reasons to support this move, but there are equally powerful theoretical and practical reasons to oppose it. Think about how strongly 'chronic pain as a disease' is a metaphor for permanence. This would seem to us to be running the risk of inserting a serious can of worms into the chronic pain space that will, sooner or later, have to be opened. That is one reason we would vote no if it went to a vote.

Transform your prognostic metaphors

A transformative prognostic metaphor is nothing more than the truth. Think about those annoying positive affirmation memes your friends put on Facebook and Twitter – some may be useful. We have shared some of our favourites in the box.

Prognostic metaphors and language with transformative power

- *Your next position is your best position*
- *Don't worry, be happy* – Bobby McFerrin
- *It's a bend in the road, not the end in the road, unless you fail to make the turn* – Helen Keller
- *I skate to where the puck is going to be, not to where it's been* – Wayne Gretzky
- *The man who moves a mountain begins by carrying away small stones* – Confucius
- *When you come to the end of your rope, tie a knot, hang on, and start climbing up* – adapted Franklin Roosevelt
- *Every strike brings me closer to the next home run* – Babe Ruth
- *I'm not afraid of storms, for I'm learning how to sail my ship* – Mary Louise Alcott
- *I didn't fail 10,000 times, I just found 10,000 ways NOT to make a light bulb* – adapted Thomas Edison

More on the artistry of metaphor

We both admit to being seduced by the magic of metaphor on our Explain Pain journeys. We are continually realising their central role in language, links to modulation neurotags and their importance in Explain Pain strategies. We also realise how our favourite treatment metaphors take prime place in our minds, become entrenched and have truly shaped us. Dave is always saying *motion is lotion*. Lorimer is always saying *we are fearfully and wonderfully complex*. We have covered our thoughts on the clinical integration of various metaphor categories but here are our eight top tips for tackling metaphors.

1. Not **another** metaphor – try a literal explanation

As a broad guide we and others suggest that responding to a metaphor with just another metaphor is not advisable [22]. We can do better than *let's thaw it out* in response to *frozen shoulder* and *oil it up* in response to a *stiff old creaking knee* or *let's whack it back in* for *my back is out*. These response metaphors add little and actually support the initial metaphorical DIM. The options here are to negate the metaphor where possible and offer a SIM in response and if possible to power it up.

Take *motion is lotion* – it's a memorable SIM metaphor – it's novelty and rhyme ensure that it's likely to be taken out of the clinic, shared and integrated into life. *Motion is lotion* could be powered up with literal information such as – *our bodies are made to move, movement enhances oxygenation, removes swelling, lubricates your joints, nourishes your brain, makes your blood thinner, reduces your chance of developing diabetes and many other things you don't want – so just get moving and remember that 'motion is lotion'*. Wherever possible, make sure that any response metaphors are positive SIM concepts powered up with literal knowledge.

2. Humour helps

Humour is universal, but the use of it in the health industry varies between countries. We often pass on Norman Cousins' lovely metaphor, **laughter is internal jogging** [23]. Given that laughter will elevate pain thresholds we probably should use it more [24]. Lorimer uses humour in *Painful Yarns* [25] and we added some in the artwork and writing in *Explain Pain* [26] and *The Explain Pain Handbook: Protectometer* [11]. We hope you have detected it scattered through this book. Humour has a diverse range – from metaphorical responses that are quirky, witty and engender smiles, to the more *in your face* statements that we may use at the right time and place and with the right person. We leave the humour bit to you, but we encourage it where appropriate, and remind you that humour naturally links to SIMs. Check out some of our favourite *in your face* statements that we've picked up in our teaching journey below – handle with care!

- *If your back was on your face you would take better care of it*
- *Your head is a drawer – pull it in*
- *You are living your life in your sock drawer – at least go and see what is in the underpants drawer*
- *One foot in the grave – which foot?*
- *At least you're on the right side of the grass and not pushing up daisies*

3. Offer a deeper discussion

Deep learning often requires deep discussion – some learners love this. A more philosophical discussion can often be initiated by sharing a quote from someone well known and mutually familiar to both the learner and deliverer. The more metaphorical the quote, the more likely it can be taken in any direction. Here are some of our favourites:

- *It is not the mountain we conquer but ourselves* – Sir Edmund Hillary
- *It won't happen overnight, but it will happen* – Pantene campaign, circa 1990
- *I can accept failure, everyone fails at something – but I can't accept not trying* – Michael Jordan
- *When the music hits me, I feel no pain* – Bob Marley
- *I skate to where the puck is going to be, not to where it's been* – Wayne Gretsky

- *One can feel many pains when the rain is falling* – John Steinbeck
- *It's surprising what you can build if you do it a little bit at a time* – Henry Ford
- *Pain is ready, pain is waiting, primed to do its educating* – Depeche Mode
- *A man's rootage is more important than his leafage* – Woodrow Wilson

4. Metaphors to keep you on track

Effective chronic pain treatment can be long and sometimes arduous. Catchy and memorable metaphorical statements along the journey can be helpful. Many are linked to pacing activity and compliance.

- *Rome, Adelaide* (insert your town), *wasn't built in a day*
- *You can't eat the whole Toblerone at once (maybe some of you can!)*
- *Good things come to those who wait, as long as you do something while you are waiting*
- *Know pain, know gain*
- *A little bit of pain, lots of gain*
- *Storms make trees take deeper roots* – Dolly Parton
- *Every little helps* – Tesco UK!

Flare ups are inevitable in the chronic pain journey and education will be the foremost treatment. The following may help.

- *Flare-ups happen but don't freak out when they do*
- *You are the one with the keys so you can drive yourself out*
- *It's a bend in the road not the end of the road*
- *Your next position is your best position*
- *Sometimes you need to rest – even God rested (that's when she created football)*
- *Take a break and have a shake*

5. Ditch language that holds back engagement of the bioplastic brain

Much of the language used in day to day descriptions of the brain and its activity is simplistic, mechanical, often derogatory and may hold back effective engagement with neuroimmune pain sciences. Powerful primary metaphors such as MIND IS A MACHINE dominate. They lead to mechanistic secondary metaphors such as the clock-like *my brain has been ticking over* which is somewhat more advanced than *my brain is rusty* or *the cogs are not turning* or *steam coming out my ears,* which clearly dates back to notions from the industrial revolution. These are common – you can *wrack your brain* and *grind out a solution* even if you are *one brick short of a load, one spanner short of a toolbox,* or even *a gherkin short of a cheeseburger* (although this last one is not so much machine-like, clearly!). But you might need to *turn on a light bulb* and even then, *the lights may be on, but no one is home.*

This mechanised view of the brain continues with links to numbers, especially 50%. We hear that *he has half a brain;* we are told about *halfwits,* or *if he had half a brain, it would be lonely* or the oft stated and incorrect *you only use 10% of your brain.* Even the Numeric Pain Rating Scale is powered up by MIND IS A MACHINE – ever thought that we're refining a complex brain process into a number? These mechanistic metaphors can sometimes be derogatory and unhealthy, yet we all tend to use them without a second thought. *Rewire the brain* is a bit trendy these days but you can see the primary metaphor from which it has emerged – that of a hardwired linear system, and we reckon that, ultimately, this will prove to be an unhelpful metaphor.

An IDEAS ARE FOOD [1] primary metaphor impacts on views of the brain – *my brain is fried, mush for brains, spoon-feed the information* or *I'll stew on that* leading to *brain farts* and *shit for brains.* These metaphors not only do little for creating helpful imagery and a contemporary understanding of brain function, they also run real neurotags that have real biological influence. However, *brain food* and *food for thought* could be SIMs.

We might sound here like *wet blankets* – for many people using these metaphors will have no negative impact at all. We all use them in daily language – they're essential for communication, the very tools we use to engage with others. However, remember that there are people for whom their protective buffer makes each and every one of these metaphors potentially important modulators of their experience of life, and of their biological status. Remember too that *EP Supercharged* is about *understanding* our own clinical practice, *understanding* the person in pain, and *understanding* the fearful and wonderful complexity of both.

6. Introduce better brain/mind metaphors

If we search across literature, movies, culture etc. for metaphors for brain function, they all describe an outdated conceptualisation of the brain. Clearly our metaphors (the essence of our communication) haven't caught up! The **brain as a computer** metaphor held up for a few years but has failed principally because computer connections are fixed and the brain's connections certainly aren't. The **brain as the internet** or **brain as a market economy** with notions of supply and demand may be a conceptualisation closer to current understanding. The **mind as an infinite chessboard** [27] works for some. The BODY IS A GARDEN, where the brain is part of an ecosystem may work too. It gives rise to words such as nourish, fertilise, growth, bloom yet on the DIM side, withered, drought, weeds, tangled and overgrown. The brain's parts can be enlivened by metaphor – **dancing dendrites** – and by literal language – mobile microglia.

Before we all throw in the towel[9] however, reflect on the new library of metaphors that are embedded here in *EP Supercharged*. Think of the metaphorical power in **neurotags, competing and collaborating for influence**! Think of the metaphorical power in conceptualising our brain's adaptations as **Darwinian-like**, where the most often **run neurotags gain a bigger influence** over **time**. Which of these metaphors will emerge after their test of time remains to be seen, but their gradual honing as they are passed from one to another, moulded by the experiences and discussions of thousands of clinicians and their patients until they finally 'set' will be exciting to watch!

7. Metaphor and language for the dustbin

We think there are some statements, most of them metaphorical and widely used in society, that should be removed from any health vocabulary (Table 7.9).

8. Don't be ageist

Some metaphors are clearly ageist. They emerge from the primary metaphor AGE EQUALS TERMINAL DECLINE and include **you can't teach an old dog new tricks** and the reverse ageism of **it's easy for you to say that, you're young**. Other examples include **at my age, something has to give** and **I have the spine of a (multiply real age by at least 1.5)**. Our Novella 11 *Oldies are goldies* demolishes the ageist view. Try saying **you can be bolder when you're older**.

---

9 All you smarty pants who are spotting metaphors that we haven't emboldened, that's fantastic – you're getting the hang of it!

Metaphors for the dustbin	Comments
1. *I know what you are going through*	No you don't! We suggest this is replaced with something like I can listen and try to understand what you are going through
2. *You must be a bad/ poor/slow healer*	Just don't say it
3. *Take a cup of concrete and harden up* *Put your big girl panties on*	There's a time and place to suggest toughening up but it must be on a framework of well-developed health literacy, non-sexist, with high level rhetorical skills
4. *Pain is weakness leaving the body*	This statement is bullshit
5. *No one ever dies of pain*	People can die from pain and pain associated problems
6. *Build a bridge and get over it* *Learn to live with it* *Accept your pain and move on*	It's best to honour and acknowledge the current activity of someone's bodily system as that person's best attempt at coping, before offering another approach (Nugget 40 *Honour the output*)
7. *Your glutes are turned off*	This is impossible – it suggests a mechanistic 'turn on, turn off' body
8. *You have no core stability*	See row 4

Table 7.9 Metaphors for the dustbin

Answers to the metaphor questions from page 150

The pain can be a real killer. It goes around and down the inside of the driver muscle to my old knee which I stuffed up years ago. Sometimes it goes into my right ball. That drives me crazy. I get pins and needles in the bloody right foot too. I can't put my finger on why it's happening, but I am ready for the scrapheap! The treatment so far has been bullshit.

Tying up loose ends

Metaphors are powerful language structures that are all around us. You may have forgotten how important they are in life and hopefully you are now aware of their possible meaning and how they involve real life biological substrates. Remember too that metaphors may involve subtle messages that are negative, but you can use them for good too. Helping people strive towards healthy language structure may be as important as guiding them to healthy movement. We will leave you with the following quote:

'Metaphors are as much a product of the lived experience of disease as they are a transforming influence on that experience.' [28]

Notes...

References

1. Lakoff G & Johnson M (1980) Metaphors we live by. University of Chicago Press: Chicago.

2. Lakoff G (2008) The Neural Theory of Metaphor, in The Cambridge Handbook of Metaphor and Thought, Gibbs RW Ed. Cambridge University Press: New York.

3. Burnside JW (1983) Medicine and war - a metaphor. JAMA 249: 2091.

4. Loftus S (2011) Pain and its metaphors: a dialogical approach. J Med Humanit 32: 213-230.

5. Scarry E (1985) The Body in Pain. Oxford University Press: New York.

6. Merskey H (1979) Pain terms: a list with definitions and notes on usage. Recommended by the IASP Subcommittee on Taxonomy. Pain 6: 249.

7. Neilson S (2016) Pain as metaphor: metaphor and medicine. Med Humanit 42: 3-10.

8. Alter A (2012) Drunk Tank Pink. Penguin Press: New York.

9. Grothe M (2009) I Never Metaphor I Didn't Like: A Comprehensive Compilation of History's Greatest Analogies, Metaphors, and Similes. HarperCollins: New York.

10. Donoghue D (2014) Metaphor. Harvard University Press: Cambridge.

11. Moseley GL & Butler DS (2015) The Explain Pain Handbook: Protectometer. Noigroup Publications: Adelaide.

12. Kövecses Z (2010) Metaphor: A practical introduction. 2nd Edn. Oxford University Press: New York.

13. Loggia ML, et al. (2015) Evidence for brain glial activation in chronic pain patients. Brain 138: 604-615.

14. Banati RB, et al. (2001) Long term trans-synaptic glial responses in the human thalamus after peripheral nerve injury. Neuroreport 12: 3439-3442.

15. Watzlawick P, et al. (1974) Change: Principles of Problem Formation and Problem Resolution. Norton: New York.

16. Moseley GL, et al. (2012) The Graded Motor Imagery Handbook. Noigroup Publications: Adelaide.

17. Zamora M & Smith MS (1993) Frida Kahlo: Brush of Anguish. Chronicle Books: California.

18. Sandblom P (1995) Creativity and disease: how illness affects literature, art, and music. Marion Boyars: London.

19. Wittgenstein L (1922) Tractatus Logico-philosophicus. Kegan Paul: London.

20. Leach M (2013) Why is it called "Down syndrome"? (Or, why I wish there had been a Dr. Awesome). Viewed 25th January 2017: http://www.downsyndromeprenataltesting.com/why-is-it-called-down-syndrome-or-why-i-wish-there-had-been-a-dr-awesome/.

21. Butler DS (2000) The Sensitive Nervous System. Noigroup Publications: Adelaide.

22. Lawley J & Tompkins P (2000) Metaphors in Mind: Transformation Through Symbolic Modelling. Developing Company Press: London.

23. Cousins N (2005) Anatomy of an Illness as Perceived by the Patient: Reflections on Healing and Regeneration. Norton: New York.

24. Dunbar RIM, et al. (2012) Social laughter is correlated with an elevated pain threshold. Proc Biol Sci 279: 1161-1167.

25. Moseley GL (2008) Painful Yarns: Metaphors and stories to help understand the biology of pain. Dancing Giraffe Press: Canberra.

26. Butler DS & Moseley GL (2013) Explain Pain. 2nd Edn. Noigroup Publications: Adelaide.

27. Fernyhough C (2006) Metaphors of mind. The Psychologist 19: 356-358.

28. Clow B (2001) Who's Afraid of Susan Sontag? or, the Myths and Metaphors of Cancer Reconsidered. Soc Hist Med 14: 293-312.

8

The Pain Library – Nuggets

Categories of educational interventions

There is no limit to the Explain Pain stories that we can all share with each other. To make them easier to find, use and further develop, we have constructed an Explain Pain library. These stories vary from simple metaphors and quick literal explanations to longer, more complex stories that usually involve some form of multimedia. We suggest two broad categories – *Nuggets* and *Novellas* – based on time, complexity of information and availability of multimedia. We encourage you as the deliverer to build on these stories, inject your own personal flavour and ultimately construct your own.

Category	Description	Misconception target	Delivery
Nuggets	Short stories, usually verbal sometimes with images	Single/multiple grain	More explicit
Novellas	Longer stories using pictures, visual media (eg. YouTube) and props	Multiple grain Sandcastle Lack of emergent frameworks	More implicit

Table 8.1 Nuggets and Novellas

The power in a nugget

Like a piece of gold, a nugget can be thought of as a precious little block of information, a valuable but quick salve, a long-lasting bandage, a dethreatener or a piece of emergency analgesic education. Nuggets are short interventions, say around a minute – they can 'gap fill', challenge inaccurate grains of information and are often metaphorical. Some nuggets could be considered DIM destroyers or SIM enhancers. The information delivered via a nugget is usually explicit – this means the message is face-to-face, clear and direct, there is little room for misunderstanding but it allows room for discussion.

Consider for example, *Take some hug drug* (Nugget 47) where the information is about oxytocin, its effects on the body, how to enhance its production and accentuate self-management. Nuggets don't have to be long and complex, one could be as simple as the direct reassurance that *This will get better* (Nugget 52).

Novellas are longer than nuggets, perhaps requiring 2-10 minutes or more. They often work best when combined with multimedia and are used for individuals or groups. In Chapter 9 we present 15 novellas.

Which story and when?

Selecting the appropriate story and the right time and place for delivery is a clinically reasoned judgement. Once you have established Target Concepts in your curriculum you will be able to pair them up with the best supporting educational stories. Remember you should tailor and adapt your stories to suit you (the deliverer), the learner and the environment (context) – we want to avoid situations where the therapist always thinks *'time to pull out the old phantom limb story again'*. You will have your favourites of course, but they continue to change and are enriched with each person you share them with. Importantly, remember the broad principle – where possible, explain it, dethreaten it and then give the listener something to do about it.

Seventy One Nuggets

How to inspect your nuggets

Each nugget has a jazzy, memorable title. For each nugget, there is a section in italics. This is how we might deliver the nugget, in our language – your language might be different. Under the nugget we've included an account of why you might use each particular nugget and some further resources from NOI. Where appropriate, we have attributed the idea of the nugget as best we can, to the person or groups from whom we first heard it. As far as we know, non-attributed nuggets are our brain children.

Broad pain concepts, neuroscience and neuroanatomy

1. I've got a high pain threshold
2. Pain is a defender not an offender
3. The brain is boss
4. The crown jewels
5. Grandma is distributed in your brain
6. Sensors are like butterflies
7. New neurones until you drop
8. Back pain is like pimples
9. Relax! It's no big deal!
10. Thoughts and beliefs are nerve impulses too
11. The orchestra in the tissues
12. Who farted?
13. Does love come from the genitals?
14. Astrocytes, more popular than the Kardashians

Tissue changes and nociception

15. Well done you old self-healer
16. We stop feeling it way before we stop healing it
17. Cuts heal fast
18. Danger detectors – the great givers of life!
19. Lucky us – no pain endings
20. Security guards on Red Bull
21. Acid tissues
22. Sunburn in the shower

Peripheral neuropathic pain

23. The 62 mini-brains in the spine
24. Pain strips for you
25. Nerves are not like the cord on the toaster
26. Unpinchable nerves
27. Zings and zaps don't mean damage
28. Keep your nerve juice loose Bruce
29. Nervy night pains

Central sensitisation

30. Sensitive sensor lights
31. Turn it up!
32. Your toes are next to your genitals in the brain
33. A fine line between pleasure and pain
34. Mirror pains

Homeostatic systems

35. Stress and swelling
36. The lion sleeps tonight
37. Friends help you avoid the flu
38. Rest and digest
39. Getting sick is a pain in the neck
40. Honour the output
41. You are more powerful than pills
42. Your fingernails grow faster on holidays

Broad treatment nuggets

43. Plasti-cise me
44. Distraction – the most powerful analgesic of all
45. Let the light in

46. Plumbers and poos, electricians and zaps, nurses and needles
47. Take some hug drug
48. It won't happen overnight, but it will happen
49. We are self-lubricating animals
50. It's just a bilby in the bath
51. I ache in the places where I used to play
52. This will get better, this can change
53. A brace/splint/collar is the first step to mobilisation
54. Knowledge is analgesic
55. Stop! In the name of ~~love~~ pain!
56. Make your own anti-inflammatories (not in the garage!)
57. Morphine madness
58. Flush your spinal neurotags
59. When the music hits, you feel no pain
60. Try some Toblerone therapy!
61. You can be sore but safe
62. Don't flare up – but don't freak out if you do!
63. Motion is lotion
64. Be like a chameleon

Scary diagnoses and radiology reports

65. It's not out, it's never out
66. Total knee replacement
67. We grow like trees
68. Spondylolisthesis
69. Heel spur
70. Fibromyalgia
71. Stable platform

Broad pain concepts, neuroscience and neuroanatomy

These nuggets are likely to be used for a lot of different patient situations as they are quite broad. They may relate to any or all of the Target Concepts in your curriculum.

1. I've got a high pain threshold

*So you mentioned that you have a high pain threshold. That's great, you are obviously aware of your personal pain experiences. Let's explore these a bit more. Pain **threshold** is the moment when you realise you are in pain from something that becomes too hot, too stretchy, too cold or too much pressure. But what is really interesting is that a pain threshold changes all the time even in controlled experiments. This really bugs scientists! Pain threshold relies on everything else happening at that time, not just the stimulus. For example males are known to have higher pain thresholds in experiments if run by females. Your pain threshold will change too, depending on your situation at the time, for example how happy or sad you are.*

*Now pain **tolerance** is different. This is the moment when you say 'that's enough', 'stop the test' or 'take the pressure off'. This may occur from a mix of the intensity of the stimulus and how long you've been in pain. Pain tolerance also varies depending on what else is happening at the time. Sometimes people mix pain threshold up with pain tolerance.*

The term pain threshold comes up frequently in clinical situations and people may be proud of their high pain threshold. Most people misconstrue pain threshold for pain tolerance. This offers an entry into discussion about the difference between the two and in particular the power and place of context (Target Concept 6). This discussion may help find DIMs and SIMs that hide in hard to find places and is likely to help clarify the protect by pain line, which is your pain threshold, on the Twin Peaks Model (page 4).

[EP8-21,119]
[EPH11]

2. Pain is a defender not an offender

Attributed to Sicuteri et al., 1992 [1]

Pain looks after you, it keeps you out of trouble. Although it feels unpleasant it causes you to change behaviour when you're in trouble, helps you learn and guides healing. See, pain's a really good thing – we're lucky to have it, but it cops a lot of bad press. It's often thought of as public enemy number one! Did you know that some people are born without the ability to feel pain? They die young because they aren't protected. Imagine what would happen if you didn't know your appendix was infected or you walked on a broken leg. You see, pain is a defender, not an offender – it protects you. When your brain 'weighs the world' and determines that protection is required, pain, the great defender, is called upon. But it's such a good defence that sometimes you can make too much pain.

Understanding the protective role of pain is Target Concept 4 and is appropriate for all Explain Pain interventions. It is the beginning of reconceptualising pain as a measure of perceived threat rather than a reliable indicator of tissue damage. This might be a useful nugget when you hear someone say 'I'd do anything to get rid of pain' or 'I really hate my pain'.

[EP8-25]
[PY39-46]

3. The brain is boss

*The body tells the brain when it is in danger, not when it is in pain. Ultimately the brain is boss – it doesn't **have** to listen to the danger messages that come in from the body and may contribute to pain. Mind you, it is highly likely to listen to the danger messages coming in from a sore tooth when you are at the dentist, compared to the danger messages coming in from yesterday's bruise when you are watching a great movie. There are lots of bosses in the body, but we reckon the brain is the ultimate boss. Remember though, sometimes bosses don't listen, and sometimes they make decisions we find difficult to understand.*

The brain decides when you produce pain 100% of the time. It concludes a danger/safety balance using all the information it has available at that moment. The phrase *'the brain is boss'* emphasises the disconnect between tissue damage and pain. It's a catchy phrase and a short zappy nugget that could help and encourage learners to seek an understanding of the majesty of their own brains.

[EP8-25]
Novella 1 *The majesty of the brain*

4. The crown jewels

Imagine that the royal family has asked you to look after the crown jewels worth a million dollars for a week. Where would you keep them? (Here you are looking for the answer 'in a safe'). Exactly! Just like us – our most precious bit is our brain and we keep it enclosed in the toughest bone we have (tapping our knuckles on our forehead to emphasise the point). *Our spinal cord is extremely precious too because it takes all the messages to and from our body and does a lot of brain work as well. We keep our spinal cord encased within strong, solid bits of bone* (you can draw a cross section to illustrate how well protected it is – like figure 8.1).

Okay – let's say you wanted to protect it even better, what might you install? (Here you are looking for the answer 'an alarm system'). Exactly! And that is exactly what we have – all the tissues near the spinal cord are loaded with alarm bells – little danger detectors that will ring if anything goes even a little bit wrong. They are so close together that we often don't have any way of working out which alarm went off – we just know something did (add lots of little alarm bells to your drawing).

People often believe that their back is weak, fragile and vulnerable. A primary metaphor in society may well be that BACKS ARE FRAGILE leading to secondary metaphors such as *my back is stuffed* or *bad backs are forever*. This nugget reminds people that our backs are 'built for strength' – they protect the spinal cord so well, allowing a little bit of movement at each segment to offer a reasonable amount over the whole length without causing any problems for the spinal cord. This nugget is also helpful to chip away at the influence of scans. People often forget that it is impossible to identify the exact tissue that set off the alarm because the system is so complex. Finally, this nugget reinforces the critical notion that pain is protective.

[EP28-43]

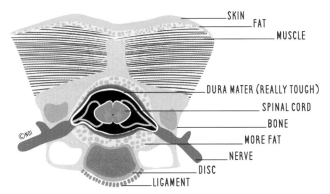

Figure 8.1 The spinal cord is protected by many layers of body tissue

SKIN
FAT
MUSCLE
DURA MATER (REALLY TOUGH)
SPINAL CORD
BONE
MORE FAT
NERVE
DISC
LIGAMENT

5. Grandma is distributed in your brain

If you think about your grandma right now, there will be hundreds of brain parts in action all at once. These brain bits could be related to emotions, memories, sights, other family members, the smell of her famous apple cake, even how grannie moved around her house. Grannie is distributed throughout your brain, there is no specific 'grannie-node'. It's the same with jealousy, happiness, lust, love and pain. If you happened to have your head in one of those fancy new scanners and I pinched your bottom, we would see hundreds of brain parts in action, firing at the same time and connecting with each other. The brain lights up like a Christmas tree when you're in pain or when you think of your grannie or when you think or do anything! There is an individual formula, a neurotag, for each pain experience and because there are so many parts involved, your pain can be changed for better or worse by so many things.

Almost everyone can recall their grandmother or an older family member. An older person can be told how a grandchild is distributed in their brain. The grannie nugget emphasises the power of context in pain (Target Concepts 5 and 6) and reminds us that DIMs and SIMs can hide in hard to find places. Many people may not consider memories, smells and sights amongst other factors, as contributors to their pain state. The nugget also demonstrates collective activity within the brain which may assist the teaching and understanding of emergence.

[EP38-41]

6. Sensors are like butterflies

There are thousands of sensors (detectors) along your nerve cells. Some open up in response to stress chemicals, or to changes in temperature and others open up when you stretch. They sense the world for you, they look out for danger and they report to the brain. But these sensors are like butterflies – they only live for a few days, so your sensitivity is continually adjusting to your environment. So if you are really sensitive now, don't worry – these sensors can change very, very quickly. You can help this process by removing DIMs in your life and seeking SIMs. You can do this all yourself, you don't need any drugs.

This nugget helps to explain the process of sensitivity. It provides hope and reassurance that nerves can quickly change their response properties. It also encourages people to seek out some of the less obvious contributions to their pain states.

[EP28-43]

7. New neurones until you drop

Good news… we now know that we all grow new brain cells right until our last breath! We used to think that the number of brain cells we had at birth was all we ever had. Luckily, we were wrong. We grow brand new ones every day, deep in the brain. However, we know that stress slows down the growth of new cells but exercise, fun, activity, learning and context-rich environments can speed it up. Don't waste this opportunity, dive into life! SIMs enhance the growth of neurones. By the way, did you know song birds grow new brain parts when they learn new songs?

This nugget can be quickly dropped into other nuggets or novellas around the topic of aging or when a person has negative prognostic metaphors such as *I am ready for the scrapheap*. It would be applicable when someone blames their injury on old age, or thinks they can't change.

The story might enhance Novella 1 *The majesty of the brain* and Novella 11 *Oldies are goldies*, and also support Target Concept 8 *We are bioplastic*.

8. Back pain is like pimples

Back pain is like pimples – almost everyone will have an episode sooner or later and with the right approach and plenty of understanding, nearly all of those episodes resolve. In fact, 90% of people will have an episode of back pain in their life that is bad enough to lay them up for a couple of days and have them wondering if they have done some serious damage. But in over 90% of those cases, there is absolutely no identifiable tissue damage! Does this mean they didn't have real pain? Of course not! This reminds us how well our back is protected, which makes complete sense when we remember our back is protecting our spinal cord. The great news is that we now have the right questions and investigations to detect the truly bad things – but they are very rare.

Acute back pain can be super distressing and give an extremely compelling feeling that something is terribly wrong. This nugget can be powerfully reassuring for someone experiencing such an acute episode. Remember to find the right balance between reassuring how common it is and acknowledging how horrible it is; between reminding them that it will get better, that they are not alone, and accepting that right now, it doesn't feel like that.

9. Relax! It's no big deal!

Our Protectometer doesn't just go up when we are in a bit of danger, it goes down when things look safe. Here is a cool experiment:

If someone gives you a little electric zap at the wrist you will probably blink (75% of people do). This is an automatic reflex you can't consciously change. However, if you move your hand close to your face, you really blink hard. But how about this – if you put a wooden board between your hand and your face, your blink reflex decreases again! Your brain is evaluating how much protection your eyes need at that very moment! What's more, it is not about how much protection your eyes ACTUALLY need – if you are tricked into thinking there is a board there when there is not, your blink reflex still decreases.

The mechanism by which these effects are mediated is descending modulation of the brainstem [2]. This example gives powerful evidence that the Protectometer is always being adjusted in response to a range of cues of both danger and safety and we don't know a thing about it. So cool.

Novella 6 *Protecting your turf*
[EP 80-81]

10. Thoughts and beliefs are nerve impulses too

*If you sprain ligaments in your knee, messages will go along nerves to the spinal cord in your back, activate spinal neurotags and eventually, a danger message might arrive at your brain. But these messages are danger messages– you don't know that they are occurring. It's when the brain mixes these danger messages with thoughts, beliefs, memories, future plans and a whole lot of other things that pain **may** emerge. Just like the message from your knee, thoughts and beliefs are real nerve impulses too – they don't just hang around in space or the ether. A thought makes electricity and juice at the end of neurones just like a danger message from a sprained joint does.*

Some learners may need a gentle push to acknowledge that their thoughts and beliefs are as important as the messages coming in from the body. If learners don't accept the physical nature of thought, they may not understand Target Concept 5 *Pain involves distributed brain activity*.

11. The orchestra in the tissues!

There is a huge range of detectors that are scattered throughout the tissues of our body. At any one time the spinal cord and brain will be receiving messages from many of them at once. For the brain to work out that you have your hand on a warm plate not a sharp knife, it looks at the pattern of input, not just the activity of a single receptor. We don't have a 'sharp knife receptor'. The way that the brain uses a wide range of inputs to create an accurate picture is a bit like an orchestra. If you just listen to the tuba, or the viola perhaps, you don't hear the tune, but when you listen to the whole orchestra together, you do. In fact, you only have a full appreciation of the piece of music if all the parts are being played together.

This nugget helps to reinforce how much evaluation is happening in the central nervous system for us to feel anything at all. It is amazing that all of this happens outside of our awareness! Keep in mind, this nugget might be confusing if used at the same time as the *Orchestra in the brain* story [EP78-79].

12. Who farted?

Ever been sitting on the toilet on a particularly smelly day and someone has knocked assertively on the door, making you jump? And how embarrassing it is as the person retreats dramatically at the smell! Scientific experiments show that when we smell something disgusting, our protective reflexes increase. You weren't imagining it – we actually withdraw more quickly when we smell something disgusting!

Here is what the scientists [8] did: using special electrodes placed over muscles on the leg, they recorded the withdrawal reflex that causes you to pull your foot up quickly when you step on something sharp. They then gave people different kinds of smells to sniff – pleasant, neutral and disgusting. When people had a sniff of something disgusting, they had a bigger withdrawal reflex than they had when they sniffed something neutral or pleasant or indeed when they sniffed nothing at all! This amazing experiment shows that when our brain detects anything that might be dangerous to us, it turns up the Protectometer. What's more, we don't know anything about it. DIMs and SIMs can hide in hard to find places.

[EPH22-27]

13. Does love come from the genitals?

Does anger come from your fist? Does lust come from your genitals? Does love come from your heart? Does pain really come from your back? The answer to all the above is 'no'. Pain is a bit like anger, love and lust – it's a conscious experience constructed by your brain, not by your back. Sure it takes into account information provided by the back, but ultimately the brain is boss. So just like you wouldn't look to your genitals for your love problems, or your fist for your anger problems, so too your back can only provide limited answers for your pain problems. You need to consider what's going on in your brain for the best pain treatment.

The love-genitals links makes everybody listen! This nugget encourages understanding of the role of the brain in pain and should help reduce linear and biomedical thinking, and a singular blame for a pain state.

[EP22]

14. Astrocytes, more popular than the Kardashians

One Tweet or Instagram picture from a Kardashian sister may have a million reactions. But a single neurone with all its brother, sister and cousin cells has far more connections than the Kardashian clan. This is because one brain cell is linked to star shaped cells called astrocytes and they form a unit. The pointers on the astrocytes wave around and link with other astrocytes. In this way, activity in one unit can quickly influence two million other units, which quickly influence two million other units, so on, so on…

Let's have a look at the pin-box which represents the neuroimmune units looking after the fingers making a high five. If I touch the index finger, the units looking after the index finger are likely to fire, but the middle finger units shouldn't. But if you believe you've been bitten by a spider on your index finger, the whole hand might hurt, especially if you freak out over spiders. Your brain has turned up the excitement level for its internal model for all the fingers even thought there are no messages coming from the actual fingers themselves. It's these wonderful astrocytes that allow the quick spreading of information with the aim of ultimately protecting you. This is one reason your pain might spread.

This nugget may link into Novella 1 *The majesty of the brain* and neurotag precision and probability discussed in Chapter 2 (pages 24-25). The nugget is easily exposed when linked to the pin-box metaphor.

Tissue changes and nociception

These nuggets relate to changes in tissues that are related to nociception. They particularly address Target Concepts:

- 2 *There are danger sensors, not pain sensors*
- 3 *Pain and tissue damage rarely relate*

15. Well done you old self-healer

Attributed to Tim Cocks, Adelaide 2012

That's a very swollen knee you have there, but in that swelling there's some really good stuff that'll help you heal. The swelling indicates that you've already started the healing process even before you came here, so well done you old self-healer! I'll need to check that there isn't any serious damage, but for now, understand that inflammation is a good thing for you, it's a necessary step towards full recovery and with your great inflammatory response, any injuries you will ever have in the future are likely to heal quickly. It shows the resources your body has when needed. This swelling will go as the tissue heals and if need be, I can help you with that. But for now, take some pride in your body's healing response!

This nugget can shift inflammation from a DIM to a SIM for conditions with acute swelling. *Well done you old self-healer* could also apply to bony changes (like osteophytes) in response to disc changes.

Novella 3 *The kisses of time*

16. We stop feeling it way before we stop healing it

Proof that pain is all about protection rather than about measuring the condition of the tissues comes from minor cuts and scrapes. Think about it - you cut your hand and it really hurts. The next day it hurts a little but you can still clearly see the cut. The next day you hardly notice it but again there is no way it has healed. About a week later someone asks how your cut is. You realise you haven't felt a thing for a few days and you look and it is almost healed. Your brain makes a very calculated guess about whether or not you should protect that tissue by making it hurt. You stop feeling it way before you stop healing it.

Everyone relates to this example and you can go a step further and talk about scars where the tissue is healed but doesn't look perfect and most importantly, doesn't hurt at all.

17. Cuts heal fast

Remember the last time you cut your skin – you watched the redness fade, the wound edges close over and suddenly one day it was all gone – magic! You see, cuts heal fast. Every day you can see the healing happening in front of your eyes. This tells us about the remarkable healing power within our bodies. A cut inside your mouth heals even faster than a cut on your hand. Sprains and strains heal quickly too even though you can't see the healing – and they're not even cut, just stretched tissue! The fact that it's all happening inside and you can't watch the healing progress can sometimes be a little worrying. But rest assured, just like cuts heal fast, so too will your sprain, you old self-healer you!

This nugget helps to dethreaten an injury like a sprain or strain. It helps to emphasise the healing capacity of the body and in some cases, encourages people to consider the question *'Well I've had time for healing, why do I still hurt?'* – could there be any other reasons?

18. Danger detectors – the great givers of life!

We have danger detectors all over our body. They are our first line of defence against anything that threatens the health of our tissues. That is only half their job though – they are also great givers of life and maintainers of health. Imagine an alarm system that also kept the carpets clean and the dusting done! One particularly exciting discovery of this role of danger detectors was made by scientists who study heart attacks and angina – the chest pain that happens when blood flow to the heart muscle is getting a bit low. They found that the nerve endings in heart muscle that fire when oxygen levels are a bit depleted (we can call them danger detectors) also trigger a biological process that results in growth of new arteries! This led doctors to start encouraging people with angina (once clearing them of blockages to major arteries) to not be afraid of some angina because it is a sign that they will be growing new blood vessels.

This aspect of biology has immense power because it reminds us that we adapt immediately in the presence of danger and that the same systems that alert us to danger take the lead in this adaptive change.

---

19. Lucky us – no pain endings

If you stub your toe and it hurts, it makes sense to think that a pain message has been sent from pain endings in your toe and has travelled via pain pathways to your brain. So naturally you rub your toe to stop the pain, which reinforces this idea. But it's not entirely right and it's really important that you understand this next bit. You see, there are no 'pain endings', 'pain pathways' or 'pain messages' despite what you read elsewhere. There are lots of nerve endings in your toe that send danger messages up to your brain and this is what's happening when you stub your toe. These danger messages tell the brain when there is too much stretch, hot, cold or stubbing. But, it's up to the brain to judge everything else going on at the time that you stub your toe and decide whether or not a good dose of pain will be helpful to make you change behaviour. If you stub your toe running across a busy freeway, it's unlikely to hurt – but if you were wandering into the kitchen for a midnight snack and you stub your toe on a chair, it probably will.

This is important stuff to know, supporting Target Concept 2 *There are dangers sensors, not pain sensors.* If you only treat nerve endings for pain states, you're so out of date! Faulty notions of pain endings and pain pathways have created a relentless search for answers to pain states in the tissues – lots of imaging, tests and treatments directed at the wrong place at the expense of a much broader biopsychosocial approach.

[EP32]

20. Security guards on Red Bull

Your danger detectors are like security guards at a club. When you are injured, inflammatory cells are released. The danger detectors become really excited in the presence of inflammation and they respond like a security guard would respond after drinking a few cans of Red Bull. Now no-one wants that kind of security guard on duty unless there is good reason to be really protective of the club. They will go berserk at the tiniest misdemeanour. This is what happens to danger detectors in the presence of inflammation – they become overprotective.

You can use this nugget to explain why things are so much more painful once inflammation has set in, or why rheumatoid arthritis joints can be so painful during a flare-up without evidence of injury.

21. Acid tissues

If you go for a long drive, lie on your side on the couch watching a movie, or do a few hours on the computer without moving, you might feel a bit sore and stiff. What's happened here is that fluid has been forced out of your tissues and your pH has dropped, all making your tissues a bit more acidic and dry. This is enough to excite the sensors in the tissues, sending danger messages to the brain which might contribute to a pain response. Dry acidic tissues might sound a bit scary, but they're easy to fix. Just move, usually in the opposite direction – everyone bends backwards after a long drive. The healthier the tissues the less acidic and dry they'll be. You can flush the stale acidic bits out with movement (works straight away). Remember, your next position is your best position.

This nugget may be relevant for postural pain, for example the kind brought on by sedentary jobs. While 'dry' and 'acid' may be a bit threatening, these evocative words should enhance patient motivation to change. This is a great nugget to dethreaten what is a simple pain state, to give patients a form of self-treatment, a bit of a push to make their body tissues healthier and to understand that there has been no damage to body tissues.

[EP48-49]

22. Sunburn in the shower
Kudos to Winnipeg NOI class of 2001

Remember back when you were a bit younger, at the beach on a hot day, lost your suntan cream and came home sunburnt? Remember too how much a warm shower really stung when you were sunburnt. Much of this is due to nerve endings in your skin becoming sensitive to heat and even the pressure from the water – a great example of what we call peripheral sensitisation. It's very common. Recall your immediate painful reaction to the hot water but also how the pain eased the moment you turned it off. It's the same as when you swallow with a sore throat – it hurts the moment you do it but usually goes when you stop. We call this peripheral sensitisation.

While this nugget will obviously be helpful for someone with peripheral sensitisation, you may also find it a helpful way to introduce central sensitisation. Contrasting is a powerful educational tool. Providing knowledge about peripheral sensitisation can help contrast with the more complex central sensitisation. For example, cold sensitivity is common in central sensitisation and pains don't go away so quickly.

Peripheral neuropathic pain

These nuggets are about your peripheral nerves and nerve roots. They touch mainly on the following Target Concepts:

- 2 *There are dangers sensors, not pain sensors*
- 3 *Pain and tissue damage rarely relate*
- 8 *We are bioplastic*

23. The 62 mini-brains in the spine

There are 31 pairs of nerve roots in your body – multiply that by 2 and you get 62 nerve roots. They emerge from the spinal cord to look after the arms, legs, trunk and head. They each contain a mini-brain which does a lot of local organisation, but is always checking in with the brain. You might know this mini-brain as the 'dorsal root ganglion'. So it's important to keep them healthy with lots of blood and movement.

Just as the brain is well protected by the bony skull, these mini-brains are also well protected. As well as the bony covering, there is tough ligament tissue around them. They only take up about a third of the space in the outlet holes between the vertebrae. So even if you have lost some space in the outlet (very common as you age) there is still plenty of room for the nerve roots. They also move around and love sliding and slithering as you move. The healthier your back is, the more physically healthy the mini brains are.

Nerve root problems can be quite painful, threatening, and even the term 'nerve root' doesn't help. But they are treatable. Information like understanding the space in the intervertebral foramen, and knowing the nerve root's ability to move, glide and adapt will be helpful. Note also that nerve root problems will be reactive to stress such as adrenaline and pro-inflammatory cytokines.

[EP60-67]

24. Pain strips for you

Sometimes pain and sensations such as pins and needles emerge in patterns or strips on the body. Knowing about these strips really helps us understand what's happening. We call these strips dermatomes (here is good opportunity to pull your dusty anatomy atlas off the shelf and show a dermatome map). This is the area of skin looked after by a nerve emerging from the back. Some nerves look after quite large areas of skin. If you feel pain in that area then it may mean the nerve is involved. A touchy nerve reports all it possibly can to the brain about the area it looks after. There is usually nothing wrong with the body parts under the skin even though those body parts might hurt with repeated touching. The nerve may not even be injured either, just sensitive. These pain strips help us understand what's going on. What a fantastic defence system!

Pain felt in a strip along or around the body can be frightening – especially in the more scary zones like L1 and L2, which supply the groin and genitals, or the trunk dermatomes that wrap around the chest. But a quick *Pain strips for you* nugget, after a thorough and appropriate assessment, can help to dethreaten the experience. We've inserted a traditional dermatome map below but don't forget, some patterns link to cutaneous nerve innervation fields.

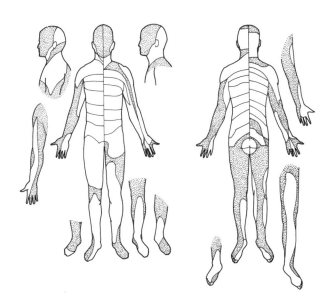

Figure 8.2 Dermatome map [6]

25. Nerves are not like the cord on the toaster

The cord on the toaster is nothing like a nerve. Cut the cord and the toaster is kaput. There won't be any toast – nothing – you might as well put your Vegemite, jam and peanut butter away! But if you injure (cut or compress) a nerve it can react at the site of the injury, along the nerve, or even in the area the nerve looks after. Your nerves are a living and changeable part of you. They can't shut down like the toaster. Even with minimal injury, nerves continue to react when you move too much, too little, are stressed, have the flu or feel hot or cold. If you can understand how nerves behave you and your nerves will be less stressed.

Nerve injuries are paradoxical. You would expect that if a nerve was cut or damaged it would just shut down. But it doesn't. It becomes reactive to many stimuli including local immune activity, temperature changes, movement and psychological stress. The nerve may react in its innervation zone to any or a combination of these stimuli. When someone has had an injury with some nerve involvement but they notice their symptoms worsen when they are sick or stressed, this nugget can be used to explain to them that it's not because the nerve is more injured, it's because it's now highly sensitive. Because it's a living structure – it's changeable.

[EP60-63]

26. Unpinchable nerves

Our nerves are really bendy. Flex your elbow and the nerves in your arm almost do a full 180 – they probably enjoy the workout! But they're almost impossible to pinch because they are so slidey and bendy; pinching a nerve is like catching a lychee with chopsticks – it's almost impossible! The reason we sometimes think we've pinched a nerve is that nerves can become sensitive to movement and sometimes instantly react with a zing or zap. A sensitive nerve usually recovers with some knowledge to desensitise and movement that keeps it wriggling. Feel free to remove the word 'pinched nerve' from your vocab.

The word 'pinch' can make you recoil a little. When you apply it to a nerve as in 'pinched nerve' it's not a healthy metaphor. 'Pinch' means different things to different people. We have known for years that peripheral nerves, nerve roots and sympathetic rami and ganglia can be flattened and a bit ratty, but rarely, if ever, pinched.

[EP60-61]

27. Zings and zaps don't mean damage

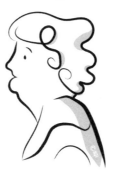

If you have injured or irritated a nerve, when you move around and particularly if you're a bit stressed, sometimes you'll get a 'zing' or 'zap'. A movement might cause a zing one moment, but not the next time – and this is understandably a bit of a worry. Sometimes when a nerve zings and zaps the pain can spread too. But zings and zaps usually go within a short time. Most importantly, a zinging, zapping nerve does not mean that the nerve is injured – it's much more likely that it's sensitive at a particular time and place. And remember, sensitivity is very changeable. Zings and zaps can occur from even minor sensitivity changes – the sort of changes that will never be found on a nerve conduction test but are still very real.

Zings and zaps are usually quite scary and they often lead to secondary postural changes as the person repeatedly tries to avoid the aggravating movement. Forward head posture with secondary muscle and joint changes may result from zings and zaps provoked by neck extension. It's important that the person is encouraged back into gradual neck extension with the knowledge that zings and zaps don't mean damage.

[EP66]

28. Keep your nerve juice loose Bruce

There's juice in all our nerves! Don't try this, but if you cut a nerve it will drip a bit. Nerves are really long and this juice flows up and down the length of your nerve transporting important messenger chemicals. This juice has a special feature – it's much thicker than water and it moves much better when it's kept moving, otherwise it turns to a jelly or thickens like sauce or honey. This is another great reason to keep moving. Total body movements such as yoga, Tai chi, dance or having a good roll around in the grass are great for your nerve juice!

This nugget gives a person yet another reason to exercise and move – nobody wants stagnant axoplasm! It would be appropriate for anyone who is frightened to move, not moving and particularly apt for diabetics – we are aware that their axoplasm is thicker and has a tendency to gel more than that of non-diabetics.

29. Nervy night pains

Night pains are scary. No one likes waking up at night and if you Google 'night pain' you will find that it might suggest a serious problem such as cancer. But night pains are more commonly due to nerve problems. At night your blood pressure drops a little, you don't move as much and sometimes you sleep in an odd position. As a result, some nerve fibres might be starved of blood. Now, nerves adore blood! They love to be moved around and flushed and they'll react when they don't have enough blood. When your blood pressure is high or normal, blood is easily pushed into the nerves thus nourishing them. If your blood pressure is low, for example in pregnancy or at night time, you might notice pains as the nerves are not nourished. This night pain is essentially just a reminder to move, making your body healthier. I'll show you a few stretches, and if you wake up at night, try these stretches then you should be able to go back to sleep.

Of course, night pain is always a red flag, so ensure a thorough examination and referral when appropriate. However, this nugget relates particularly to those whose night pain is peripheral nerve related, such as in carpal tunnel syndrome. This nugget could also be used for a pregnant patient with nerve problems – blood pressure drops in the early stages of pregnancy. The suggested stretches are median nerve mobilising techniques.

Your stories

Got any peripheral nuggets? Pop them below...

Central sensitisation

Most pain states will involve elements of central sensitisation. These nuggets will provide material to address all Target Concepts. You can remind yourself of these on page 128.

30. Sensitive sensor lights

Think of one of those sensor lights that turn on when someone approaches your house. You might notice that your sensor light is coming on all night, keeping you awake, making you worry why people are walking so close to your house at all hours! It starts to freak you out. You eventually decide to keep watch one night and discover it is being triggered by the wind blowing tree branches nearby and by the neighbour's cat. The problem? The sensitivity is set too high. Well, just like the sensitivity on these lights can be set to detect a certain amount of movement, your nervous system's sensitivity can be set too high. It can be triggered any time, night or day, by even minor things. You see, the problem is not intruders in your garden – the problem is the sensitivity of the sensor light.

This nugget is useful when discussing the upregulated nervous system in central sensitisation and the usually overprotective nature of persistent pain.

[EP72-77,82-83]

31. Turn it up!

Attributed to Louis Gifford, c. 1995

One of the most wonderful things about our biology is that it is highly adaptable. We call this 'bioplasticity' (Target Concept 8 We are bioplastic). If the nerves which send danger messages to your brain are active for long enough, they adapt along their pathway and becomes even better at sending danger messages.

This normal adaptation is like turning up a volume knob – the danger volume knob. The obvious result is that your brain receives more messages for the same actual amount of danger. It's a bit like typing a single 'D' on the keyboard, but seeing 'DDDDDD' on the screen. It's like a magnifying glass on the danger message.

This nugget may be helpful for a patient whose pain can be explained by central sensitisation or who is experiencing allodynia or hyperalgesia.

[EP8-25]
[PY39-46]

32. Your toes are next to your genitals in the brain

Have a look at this map showing the brain cells that look after your bodily sensations (show them the homunculus). This is called the homunculus. If you put an Alice band on your head, the homunculus is underneath this area. You'll notice that it's a sort of human shaped. You'll also notice that really important bits for your survival are large, like your fingers and lips. This means more brain cells look after those parts. Notice also how the hands are next to the face and the feet are next to the genitals. That's an interesting mix up! If a leg is amputated, the brain cells looking after the leg are no longer 'exercised', so that area in the brain becomes a little bit fuzzy. Next to it, the area looking after the genitals thinks 'goody, spare brain, we'll take it over' and therefore sensations linked to the genitals are now felt in the phantom foot. Perhaps that's why some people find feet erogenous and love their feet being played with. We even hear about amputees who can feel the sense of weeing in the phantom area and others such as Heather Mills, have reported that their stump is erogenous.

This nugget helps to facilitate a discussion on plasticity and changeability. These stories help us to understand how changeable our nervous systems are and may help explain some odd symptoms that some people may be reluctant to declare.

[EP22-23]

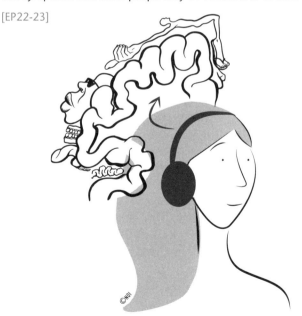

Figure 8.3 The somatosensory humunculus [3]

33. A fine line between pleasure and pain

Recent studies using fancy brain scanners have shown that the brain activity during different sensations and feelings, like pleasure and pain, are similar. We like to say that in the brain it's a fine line between pleasure and pain – the Divinyls sang a song about this. People who are into sadism and masochism are already convinced! This discovery suggests that during pleasurable experiences, you are actually using almost the same bits of brain that you would use when in pain. Therefore, the more pleasure you experience, the more you can coerce these bits of brain away from the pain neurotag, towards a more easily accessible pleasure neurotag. It might even be possible that by experiencing more pleasure (SIMs) you could shift from a pain state to a pleasure state.

This nugget can be used to help people go SIM hunting. The more they understand that SIM hunting can have a strong biological effect on their brain, the more likely they are to keep hunting. The nugget also supports Target Concept 5 *Pain involves distributed brain activity* and 6 *Pain relies on context.*

34. Mirror pains

Mirror pains are pains that are the same on both sides of the body. They are quite common and we now know a bit about them. After an injury (particularly when there are lots of other issues going on) your brain may conclude that you need more protection. It does this by making more sensitising chemicals in your nervous system. There are no fences in the nervous system, so these chemicals can leak and spread around a bit. They can activate and sensitise danger messenger nerves on the other side of your spinal cord, leading to a double-protective pain barrier – mirror pains! It's almost as if your brain wants to keep you doubly safe and has made twice as much of you hurt in order to really protect you! But don't worry, we also know that this sensitivity will settle down – understanding that there is nothing wrong with the tissues under the mirror pain, as well as giving it a bit of time and some healthy movement will all help.

Mirror pains are pains in the same area experienced on the contralateral side of the body. They have been documented after injury to, or inflammation of peripheral nerves and are also experienced in chronic pain states such as CRPS. Sensitivity in the matching contralateral area is actually a normal part of an acute injury. It may cause patients distress and fear if they think their problem/injury is now spreading to the other side and seemingly out of control – so make sure to dethreaten this.

[EP88-89]

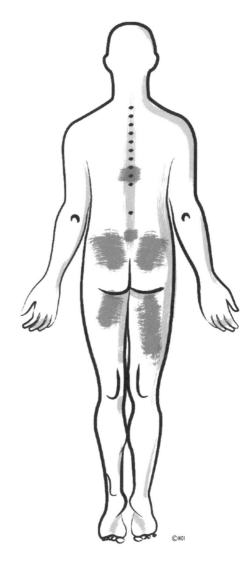

Figure 8.4 Body map showing mirror pains

Homeostatic systems

There are other homeostatic protective outputs such as the motor, endocrine, emotional and respiratory systems that can also become overprotective. Target Concept 7 *Pain is one of many protective outputs* can help explain this process and what you can do about it.

[EP70-90]
[EPH24-27]

35. Stress and swelling

Attributed to Tim Cocks, 2016

Most people think that all swelling comes from the injured body part. Much of it does – but your nervous system also contributes. When you're stressed, freaking out, or just don't know what's going on, your brain can release powerful substances that hype up the inflammation. These substances are all aimed at giving you more protection, but it's often much more then you need to heal. We humans often overdo it! So if you're worrying about work, whether you'll make it back on the football field, if you'll be able to wear your heels at the wedding this weekend, or if you've done serious damage – this will all contribute to the amount of swelling.

A few years ago this information was considered a bit 'out there' but science really backs it up now. Acute swelling after injury is good stuff and important for healing, but too much of it and swelling that persists makes the tissues a bit soggy, boggy and unhealthy – it's best to try to clear it up. You can do this by progressive exercise, stretch, massage, balance and other physical techniques. But you can also engage the power of altering your DIM SIM balance and understanding that you're on the road to recovery! In other words, treat it from both ends – the tissues and the brain.

This nugget emphasises how important it is to understand that pain and all the processes that occur in your body are there to look after you. It also relies on the conceptualisation that inflammation involves an output of the brain, just like pain, feelings, motor and endocrine systems.

36. The lion sleeps tonight

Imagine if you were constantly stalked by a scary animal, say a lion, for a really long time, say six months or longer. The long muscles in your body, like your hamstrings and quads would always be turned on, ready to run or fight. You wouldn't waste any energy on the short stabilising muscles, such as those in the front of your neck or in front of your tummy, so they would probably weaken over time from lack of use. But consider that your 'lion' might be your DIMs stalking you – perhaps work issues, personal stress, creaky knees and fear of health issues you don't understand. So I'll show you how to relax the long muscles, strengthen the short ones and importantly we'll work together to identify the threats (the lions) that have been stalking you and making you adopt this posture. Let's put the lion to sleep.

This nugget helps a learner develop a deeper understanding of how posture relates to stress. It's okay to strengthen and relax muscles, but a biopsychosocial view encourages identification and treatments of concepts that have influenced the postural change in the first place. Clinicians may also notice heightened reflexes as part of the motor system, edgy and quick to react.

37. Friends help you avoid the flu

Many people think that isolating themselves will help them avoid the flu. But we know that spending time with people who make you feel good is healthy for your immune system. We also know that people who make you feel good are potent SIMs that can reduce pain and boost your immune system. So keep in touch, spend some face-time with others, it'll be good for both of you!

There is good evidence that healthy social support networks encourage anti-inflammatory immune states and appropriate immune responses to antigens and pathogens. Encouraging patients to engage in social activity is highly therapeutic and should be a part of a comprehensive pain treatment strategy.

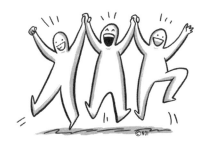

38. Rest and digest

The sympathetic nervous system allows 'fight or flight' in response to acute threat. But we don't hear much about the parasympathetic nervous system which is active when we 'rest and digest' – after a big meal, when you sleep, meditate or relax. It's essential to deal with the natural wear and tear of the day, to nourish and replenish your cells overnight and store energy for the next day.

Since the invention of the light bulb humans sleep about an hour less per day. Since the internet, probably another half hour less again. Maybe we're not having enough 'rest and digest' time and this could explain why you're not healing as well as you could. You can power up your parasympathetic nervous system by scheduling enough rest, sleep and peace. Meditation, yoga, mindfulness practice and fishing will also probably help.

There are multiple active treatment strategies for all and once people know some of the biology behind the parasympathetic nervous system they can appreciate the place of meditative, relaxing and sleep health strategies.

39. Getting sick is a pain in the neck

Have you ever noticed that when you have the flu your old aches and pains come back? Aches and pains may be the first hint that you are getting the flu. Ever noticed that your pain increases when things are really tough at home? One reason this happens is that there are immune cells that modify the efficiency of your danger system. If your danger transmission system is a bit sensitive and then your immune system detects an invader, or you are under threat at home, then wham! The danger system springs into action.

There is another mechanism too – if you sustain an injury at the same time as you are experiencing a psychologically traumatic event, the danger detectors themselves become sensitive to stress hormones. This means that later on, stress hormones themselves can activate the adapted danger detectors. Wow - now you might have pain whenever you are stressed at work but it has nothing to do with danger to your body.

These two mechanisms can explain some pretty intimidating symptoms. They show that we are all single operating systems and that non-tissue threats can activate tissue-bound danger detectors. This information relates to knowledge of the immune set point in Chapter 3 (page 60).

40. Honour the output

Attributed to Daniella Schoeller, Psychotherapist, London c. 2009

Thanks for telling me your story. I can now begin to understand why you have had those thoughts and feelings after what has gone on and what you have had to deal with. I can also see why you have been moving in that way and avoided certain movements and even why you are still swelling up. Your body has done the best it can to try to protect you and to carry you through life. It's almost worth saying 'well done body for now' before we work out some better ways to make your body healthier and to get you going again.

Honouring and accepting the outputs (homeostatic systems) that your patient has used in good faith as their brains have 'weighed the world' and made attempts to cope with life is important. The nugget recognises a person's biological power and healing possibilities before introducing new ways to better manage and treat his or her problem. It also facilitates a broad discussion of homeostatic systems which is likely to initiate a conversation about symptoms (usually DIMs) not considered relevant before.

41. You are more powerful than pills

Most people have short-term relief from opiates like morphine, codeine, oxycodone. However, when it comes to persistent pain opiates pose a problem. There are two reasons for this: one is that for some people they are addictive, the other reason involves two separate effects that opiates have on our nervous system. One effect is to turn down danger messages in the central nervous system – this will normally decrease pain. The other effect is to activate immune cells that make danger pathways more efficient. Your immune system recognises powerful pills as artificial and not 'you'. This kicks off a process making your nervous system more sensitive leading to more DIMs in your body. So when your brain weighs everything in your world and works out that there is more danger than safety it can decide that pain is your best defence and you will start to hurt despite having powerful pain killers on board. You are more powerful than pills! The good news is your body makes its own safe and natural opioids using the drug cabinet in your brain. Why don't you have another chat to your doctor about the pills you're taking for your pain.

This nugget can be used to explain the failure and danger of prolonged opioid use. It can also emphasise the power within us all and is a lead-in to Novella 2 – *The drug cabinet in the brain*. It provides reassurance that there is an endogenous analgesic system in your body if you come off pain medications.

42. Fingernails grow faster on holidays

When you're really stressed, some things in life are just not important and can be put on hold. Let's say you're about to take your first bungee jump. In the hours before, your guts will play up, you probably won't be interested in sex, it's no time to do your algebra homework and any healing can be put on hold. There are more important things for your systems. Instead, your heart will be pumping, blood and energy will be rushing to your muscles, you'll be kept on alert and oxygen will be pouring around your body. All good stuff! The endocrine and sympathetic systems are major players here.

But it's not healthy to wait for a bungee jump for six months – nor is it healthy to be under persistent threat or stress. If these systems stay turned on for a long time, you'll notice things like slow tissue healing, poor digestion, weight loss/gain, loss of libido, affected memory and learning, skin and fingernail changes, increased blood pressure and feelings of anxiety. On the flip side, do you ever notice how your fingernails grow faster on holidays, your hair grows better, your skin looks healthier, your sex drive comes back and you can read some really deep novels? Stress is good, but persistent stress can slow your healing. Now, let's work out what to do about it.

Many symptoms that are common in chronic pain can be linked to the endocrine and sympathetic systems. There is much therapeutic narrative to be gained from understanding the stress response and how it changes from the acute to chronic setting.

Your nuggets

Drop your homeostatic nuggets here...

Broad treatment nuggets

In this section we address Target Concepts:

- 8 *We are bioplastic*
- 9 *Learning about pain can help the individual and society*
- 10 *Active treatment strategies promote recovery*

43. Plasti-cise me

You are now on a journey to change your system – to reduce its hyperprotective setting. Some of this involves training your nervous system. Scientists have discovered four ways to improve the changeability of your nervous system.

1. *Intense exercise – working at a high heart rate even for 30 seconds triggers chemicals in your brain that help you lay down new synapses and prune old ones that are no longer needed. So jump on your bike!*

2. *Learning works best after dinner but before bedtime. During this time you have the best chance of the new connections 'sticking' – sleeping well will top this off. It might be worth learning some sleep tips.*

3. *Having fun will improve plasticity – think of the things you remember most clearly in life – it is the fun times and the horrible times right? Either helps, but you might as well seek out the fun stuff!*

4. *Omega-3s help your brain make new cells. Omega-3s are naturally occurring in a few foods – try flaxseed, walnuts, sardines and salmon for starters.*

This nugget gives the learner some general principles to live by. It also gives them some initial self-treatment strategies. Exercise, sleep, laughter and the right diet will enhance recovery – remember that a balanced diet probably gives us all the Omega-3s we need.

44. Distraction – the most powerful analgesic of all

Have you ever noticed that when you are really engaged in an activity, deep into a good book, helping someone else in a bit of trouble, partying hard or absorbed in a good movie, that your pain is just not there? This is because you were distracted and distraction is one of the most powerful (and cheapest) pain softeners we know of. When your brain is busy doing something else it momentarily stops making pain. Distraction can be used to shake things up and break the constant firing of pain neurotags in your brain – distractions are usually SIMs! You might find that not only does your pain go away when you're distracted, but you move differently, think differently and even breathe differently.

In more technical terms, distraction disassembles pain neurotags, probably by reducing the involvement of the anterior cingulate cortex and the frontal lobe. This nugget also serves to emphasise that there will almost always be a moment when a person with chronic pain has no pain. Finding this moment with a patient will reveal hidden SIMs and can form the beginnings of a treatment plan. It also gives you an opening to discuss the important notion that pain is ultimately in the brain.

45. Let the light in

Nerves and other body tissues love oxygen. Think of oxygen as the light. Many of us get up in the morning, sit down and have our breakfast, sit in the car and drive to work, sit down in front of a computer all day, drive home, sit down and watch TV, then go to bed, still flexed! All the tissues in the front of our body, particularly in our groin and under our arms never really have enough air and light. So remember, bend backwards and let a bit of light into the darkness. Ponder for a moment, when was the last time you had both of your arms high above your head.

This simple nugget targets postural syndromes, which include ischaemic contributions to pain states. It also focuses on areas of the body that are often left out of life.

46. Plumbers and poos, electricians and zaps, nurses and needles

Plumbers are not overly concerned about poos and electricians who get little zaps all the time don't worry too much about them. Nurses don't get too upset over blood and bodily fluids either, though they are very careful with needles these days. Burns don't bug bakers much either. The most common operation on earth is a tooth extraction, probably followed by piercings, but rarely do these procedures lead to a chronic pain state. The common thing in all these examples is that no one is too stressed or freaked out because they understand what's going on and they are familiar with what's happening. Pain is the same – if you understand that it doesn't often mean you have actually damaged yourself, then just like zaps don't bother the electrician, pain won't bother you so much either.

The unfamiliar can be frightening. This nugget highlights the importance of understanding the core concept of Explain Pain – that is, that pain is a measure of the perceived need to protect and not a measure of tissue damage.

47. Take some hug drug

Have you heard about oxytocin? Your brain makes this great juice and it's freely available to you. They call it the 'love drug' or the 'hug drug'. You make it in your brain, it enters your blood, calms you down, de-stresses you, makes you happier, less anxious, less grumpy, settles turbulent guts, makes blisters heal faster and can ease pain too. There are plenty of ways to encourage your body to produce more – having a baby and lactating may help, but if that is not available, cuddle someone you love, sing and dance together or have a photo of someone you love on your desk. Nothing wrong with a lovey dovey movie either. If you can train your dog to gaze into your eyes, oxytocin increases. Gaze back and your dog will get some oxytocin too.

Oxytocin is a neuropeptide produced mainly in the thalamus and released from the pituitary gland. A good dose of oxytocin has analgesic properties. There are scientific studies that suggest that enhanced oxytocin levels may decrease pain via improving mood, decreasing stress, enhancing calmness and lowering cortisol levels.

48. It won't happen overnight, but it will happen

Attributed to Pantene campaign, circa 1990

You've been experiencing pain for a long time now. Unfortunately there is no magic drug, no special massage or manipulation. This is a complex problem and it can only be solved with patience, persistence and courage! Stay positive, understand this may be a long journey, not a quick fix, but we'll make it together!

There's a great saying – 'a ship is safe in harbour, but that's not what ships are for'. When we are in pain we naturally withdraw and seek safety. But it is now known that this can lead to problems in the long term. Part of overcoming pain is venturing back out into the world, extending your boundaries and exploring your whole life – all of it! Start by testing the waters just outside the 'harbour walls'. One way to do this is to start challenging your DIMs and finding your SIMs. It's surprising what you can achieve one little piece at a time.

This nugget, with the saying 'it won't happen overnight but it will happen' provides a base for realistic goal setting and graded exposure. Consider introducing the 'ship is safe in the harbour' metaphor when you notice a patient progressively withdrawing from society and life.

49. We are self-lubricating animals

Without lubrication our bodies will not function – marvel at how your eyelids slide on your eyes, how tendons always glide, how joints are almost friction-free. Discs and the lining of the lungs need it too and sex is really difficult without it as well. Luckily, we are all powerful self-lubricating animals! Much of our lubricating ability comes from a juice called 'lubricin'. The quality and quantity of lubricin improves with movement, but deteriorates with stress. You can build up a lubricin reservoir in your joints with healthy movement.

The lubricin nugget is a powerful story to get patients moving and thinking more fondly about their bodies. It also encourages self-management. Tell them too, that a diet with newly pressed extra-virgin olive oil can also be helpful for lubrication. More recent research points to the relationship between immune imbalances and the quality of lubricin. This nugget links to Target Concept 8 *We are bioplastic* and is a reminder that the body is a part of the 'bio'.

50. It's just a bilby in the bath

Attributed to 'Mr Archimedes' Bath' Pamela Allen, 1998, Harper Collins

Look at this drawing – a bilby (small, furry Australian marsupial) is about to be blamed for the bath overflowing. But it's not really the bilby's fault. Lurking in the bath are some very big animals (DIMs). Sometimes in life, we blame the small, or most recent concerns/ problems/DIMs for pain without recognising the bigger picture – DIMs (even big ones) can hide in hard to find places. Another way of thinking about it might be blaming the last glass of wine for your headache the next day. Your 'bilbies' could be hearing certain words, fearing certain movements or even a worrisome thought. Ponder this – sometimes when you think 'have I got a headache?', just this thought could be enough to tip you into a headache state. Identifying the difference between bilbies and alligators is an important part of recovery. You might not need to worry about every bilby but the DIMs in the bath need your attention.

The story of the bilby in the bath helps explain why minor injuries can become major problems, it powers up the use of the Protectometer, it challenges singular blame, it enhances emergent thinking and it encourages a wider search for contributions to pain states.

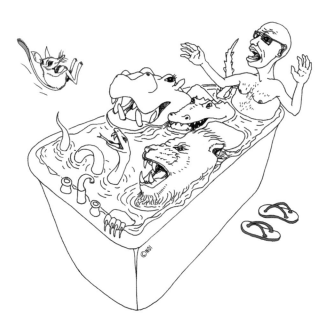

Figure 8.5 The bilby in the bath [4]

51. I ache in the places where I used to play

Attributed to Leonard Cohen, The Tower of Song, 1988

It makes sense that when you have a pain problem it will often be felt in the bits of your body that you use the most. Or parts of your body that are/were really relevant in your life. The bricklayers back, the tennis player's shoulder, the dancer's feet. Consider the area of pain – could it hold a deep connection to your past? You may well put the overall problems of life into the places where you used to play. Let's have a bit more of a chat about the parts that really hurt and what they mean to you.

Leonard Cohen's lyric 'I ache in the places where I used to play' can be a reminder of the powerful aspects of context and meaning to pain and injury. A reminder to see the whole person and his or her rich history. Perhaps we ache for the times when the body part was in all its glorious use. When this happens, it's easy to get angry with it; to reject it, to seek quick, invasive answers to problems with that body part. Maybe we disembody it. If you think about it, graded exposure to activity is really just about playing with the aching parts in different ways and contexts. You learn to re-love the body part that was once vital to so much of your life, and still is.

52. This will get better, this can change

This will get better; this problem can change. We're not into management, we're into treatment.

This is probably the shortest nugget ever. It's appropriate for nearly everyone. It will engender hope, provide motivation and it will matter that they are hearing this from a health professional. It's not said enough!

53. A brace/splint/collar is the first step to mobilisation

Braces, splints and collars are fine for a time. They'll give you support, make you feel safe and protected, allowing you to move all the other parts of your body while your injured area has a rest. There's nothing wrong with a bit of a rest when you've had a shake-up. But nobody needs a brace, a splint or a collar for a long period of time. Think of these supports as the first step to regaining movement again.

This short nugget helps to enhance early activity, limit over-reliance on braces, splints and collars and facilitate goal setting.

54. Knowledge is analgesic

Knowledge can be a 'pain softener', an analgesic – just like an Aspirin (we prefer the term pain softener to pain killer). Can you think about a time when just understanding something took the pain away, or reduced the threat? Not knowing is scary. Imagine sitting at home alone and hearing a noise in the garden. This might mean something different and make you react differently if you have just watched a news report about a burglary on your street – or if you've called for a pizza delivery. You see, knowledge reduces stress and the right knowledge can reduce pain.

This nugget supports Target Concept 9 *Learning about pain can help the individual and society.* Often this is a good nugget to explain early in treatment – when someone understands that knowledge can be analgesic it encourages them to seek more and engage with the conceptual change process.

55. Stop! In the name of ~~love~~ pain!

Okay, let's stand up, face each other a few metres apart. Pretend I am PAIN and everything in front of me is safe, but behind me is tissue damage. You are slowly walking towards me, doing something that is taking you towards damage. As you approach, I say 'slow down, stop. Stop. STOP. STOP!' If you had stopped when I asked you to 'slow down' there would be no trouble, but because it took me to the last 'STOP!' for you to pause in front of me – you now have a flare up. You are in a lot of pain, but can you see you haven't walked past me yet, so I have prevented you from reaching damage? This is how a flare-up works. It tells you that you have come too close, not that you went too far.

Unfortunately, many people think that you only have pain once you are already damaged. This is wrong. In this scenario, I (being PAIN), don't say anything until you have walked past me and arrived at damage. This is NEVER how pain works. Pain stands between you and damage and is always keeping an eye out for you.

By acting out this comparison, we can add visual, auditory and interactive information to the new concept's neurotag, increasing neuronal mass and precision, which both enhance influence (Chapter 2). We might even engage the Diana Ross neurotag in this (ie. the song 'Stop, in the name of love')! This nugget is very useful to dethreaten a flare-up, before or after it occurs and reinforce the protective role of pain.

56. Make your own anti-inflammatories (not in the garage!)

You might have heard of the amazing drug cabinet in your brain. Well, it just got better. Research on mice shows that when a place that is normally safe becomes associated with something dangerous, it can increase inflammation. Let's say a particular mouse cage delivers electric shocks to the mouse so that the cage itself becomes a DIM to that mouse. When the mouse learns that this previously safe cage is now a danger, this knowledge causes an increase in inflammatory molecules. Are there places that you go to that might be doing this? The exciting possibility here is that seeking SIMs could be anti-inflammatory. That is, turning DIMs into SIMs and finding SIMs might be opening up the anti-inflammatory drawer of the drug cabinet. All the more reason to find SIMs and understand their power!

This is a bit speculative but it is certainly possible. We know that learning involves both anti-inflammatory and pro-inflammatory molecules. Of course it seems sensible that identifying the safe elements of life will be coupled with anti-inflammation. The best thing about this speculation is that there is no identifiable risk or side effect of finding SIMs. This nugget might encourage a patient who recognises inflammation as a problem to seek SIMs.

57. Morphine madness

Most people get a few hours of pain relief from morphine. However, when it comes to persistent pain, morphine is a bit of a problem. There are two reasons for this – one is that it is addictive and some people start to crave it. The other reason involves the biological effects that morphine has on our danger pathways. While morphine dampens down danger messages in the central nervous system, thus decreasing pain, it also activates immune cells that make the danger pathways more efficient. This will normally increase pain. Over time, the balance between the anti-danger effect and the pro-danger effect shifts towards an overall danger effect. In this situation, the morphine is actually making the pain worse.

This nugget might be useful for patients using opioids or trying to make sense of why their pain is getting worse even though they are taking more and more opioids. It also provides a stimulus to seek other non-pharmacological options.

58. Flush your spinal neurotags

All our body parts rely on movement for health and your spinal cord with all its spinal neurotags is no different. Healthy spinal movement encourages blood flow to the spinal cord, helps move the cerebrospinal fluid (the fluid around the cord which is so important for nutrition), gives the neurones and other cells in the cord a good workout and makes sure that the tough ligament sheath around the spinal cord has had a good stretch. It probably flushes out some of the stagnant inflammatory compounds in the cord too.

You can be guided here by a clinician who understands something about neurodynamics and sliders/tensioners. You can do stretches such as hamstring stretches (which also gives your nervous system a workout, especially in sitting), chin tucks, knee bends and total body rotations. Aspects of yoga, Tai chi, martial arts and a good roll around in the grass will do it too.

The physical aspect of the nervous system, especially the central nervous system is hardly unrecognised by the health community. But the various components of the nervous system have individual physical properties – for example from neck extension to flexion, the spinal cord is approximately 20% longer and the diameter is 30% less. Neurones fold and unfold during this movement. See [5] and [6] for more on this somewhat forgotten subject.

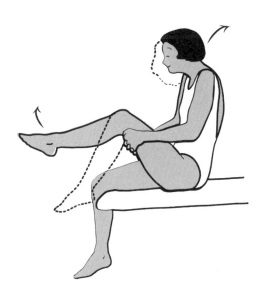

Figure 8.6 Neurodynamic sliders – movement is essential for nerve health

59. When the music hits, you feel no pain

Attributed to Bob Marley, Trench Town Rock, 1975

No one has pain all the time – it's always changing, and it changes the most when your environment changes. Bob Marley said 'One good thing about music, when it hits you, you feel no pain'. Bob might have been smoking a spliff or two, but he clearly understood some neuroscience (including Target Concept 6 *Pain relies on context). You can change your context by going outside, listening to your favourite tune, visiting with friends – it's all about SIMs. So let's find some ways to change your context. Perhaps listen to some of the music you enjoyed before your current troubles began.*

This nugget is particularly relevant when you hear a patient say something like 'my pain is different when I'm out with friends', or 'if I listen to music it doesn't hurt as much'. It makes you want to say, *'yes, Bob Marley once said...'* It encourages a search for SIMs and highly supports the notion that pain is changeable.

60. Try some Toblerone therapy!

Attributed to Helen Slater, Adelaide, 1993

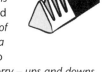

See this Toblerone chocolate bar (seductively unwrap both the yellow cardboard and the silver foil). Your recovery will be a bit like this (tilt the chocolate on an oblique angle and point upwards). You're going to climb out of this, you'll be okay, but there's going to be a few ups and downs along the way (point to the individual chocolate pieces). Don't worry – ups and downs happen to everyone but I'll be here to help. Here, have a piece of choccie.

This nugget might be helpful when your patient asks if they will get better and when they discuss prognosis. It can be used to dethreaten flare-ups and to encourage graded exposure and pacing. This nugget can also help to reduce the fear of the unknown and provide some comforting expectation of recovery.

61. You can be sore but safe

Let's have a look at the Twin Peaks Model image below. Notice on the 'after injury' mountain that the 'tissue tolerance' line is a bit lower than on the 'before injury' mountain. Also notice that the 'protect by pain line' is much lower on the 'after injury' mountain than on 'before injury' mountain. But critically take note that the buffer between protect by pain and 'tissue tolerance' has now greatly increased on the 'after injury' mountain. Activities within the buffer, even though painful, are not harmful – you are so well protected that you are nowhere near tissue damage! See how 'you can be sore, but you are safe' and 'hurt doesn't always equal harm.'

Think about how often you hear someone say *'it hurts, so I must be damaging my body* or *I keep re-injuring myself'*. People often think that experiencing pain, or more pain, is a direct indicator of damaging their tissues. As a result they often stop people undertaking healthy activity. Understanding that you can be sore but safe is a fundamental element of Target Concept 8 *We are bioplastic* and Target Concept 9 *Learning about pain can help the individual and society.*

62. Don't flare up – but don't freak out if you do!

When you flare up, a lot of things happen – the drug cabinet in the brain shuts tight and stops releasing happy hormones, instead it begins to release DIM chemicals that turn up the danger message. Your adrenaline system will go berserk; your motor system jumps into protection mode and this is pretty distressing. This is why it is very helpful to work out how to avoid flare ups. You can learn how to do this. First it is critical that you understand that as long as you are progressing things gradually and haven't done anything stupid (like dosed up on drugs or alcohol so that you can overdo it), a flare-up is simply an uber-protection mechanism. It tells you that you ventured a bit too close to your tissue tolerance, not that you went over it. It tells you your Protectometer ramped up to keep you out of trouble, not tell you you've been in trouble. The best news? Once you really understand what flare-ups are, they lose their power – they are shorter and not as bad. What a system!

Flare-ups are often interpreted as irrefutable evidence that something very bad has just happened in the body. They are nearly always distressing, and are often the thing that sends people back to their doctor, or to a new one, seeking drastic treatment. By changing what a flare-up means, we reduce the likelihood of these behavioural responses. From a biological perspective, flare-ups are probably plasticity-enhancers in a negative way – they switch on all the sensitisation mechanisms – they liberate a whole lot of DIMs. So they are good to avoid. You can integrate this with the Twin Peaks Model (Figure 8.7), principles of graded exposure, and principle of halving the increment after a flare up.

[EP118-119]

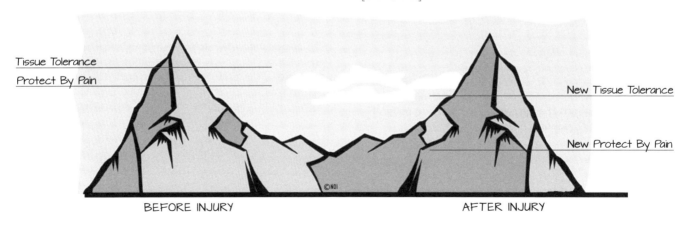

Tissue Tolerance
Protect By Pain

New Tissue Tolerance

New Protect By Pain

BEFORE INJURY

AFTER INJURY

Figure 8.7 The Twin Peaks Model from Explain Pain [7]

63. Motion is lotion

If you can do those few exercises and movements that we've just been through, lots of lovely things are going to happen in your body. You'll put a nice coat of lubricant on your joint surfaces and flush old fluid out of your muscles. Those movements will also make your blood thinner and nourish and awaken the brain cells that look after your body. You'll also push oxygen deep into your lungs. Remember movement is medicine and motion is lotion.

Motion is lotion is a memorable metaphor which may act as a summary of your entire treatment. This is an example of powering up a metaphor with a literal explanation. It should just make you want to get out and move!

64. Be like a chameleon

Attributed to post-graduate student class, La Trobe University, Melbourne, 2009

A chameleon has great power and you can be like one too. Chameleons explore and adapt to their surroundings. They change colour as they move to suit the environment, and they also change colour depending on mood and emotions. If they don't keep changing and adapting they will lose the power to do so. We can all be like chameleons – re-join life, your environment, move and explore your world, try out different environments, practice the power of adaptation. Remember, it's not just about your physical environment, you can move and adapt through your social and emotional environment as well. This is a vital part of rehabilitation and treatment – it's healthy for your body, your brain – healthy for all of you. Go on, be like a chameleon – keep exploring and adapting or, like the chameleon you'll lose the power to do so.

This nugget is specifically for those people who have withdrawn from social engagement and life in general. It might not be for everyone but it does provide imagery to try to entice somebody back into engaging in life. It could be a part of a graded exposure process. Most people think that chameleons change their colours based simply on their environment – a very clever camouflage to hide from predators. And they do. But more than that – chameleons change colour in response to physical, environmental and emotional needs.

Your nuggets

Drop your treatment nuggets here...

Scary diagnoses and radiology reports

There are no rules for the naming of injuries, diseases and pain states. Some of the diagnoses we hear can be scary – Scheuermann's disease with Schmorl's nodes is an example that can be a DIM if unexplained. Others are metaphors, such as whiplash – and metaphors will mean different things to different people. Diagnoses with the word disease attached or which sound very complex, such as spondylolisthesis, or polymyalgia rheumatica can be DIMs without explanation. Phrases with tumour, cancer, sclerosis, heart or ending in 'oma', such as neuroma, can be particularly fear inducing.

Dethreatening a diagnosis is ultimately telling the truth about it, in respect to that particular person (see Chapter 7 pages 160-161). In this way, the DIM can often be turned into a SIM. A suggested process is to explain how the diagnostic term came about, sometimes apologise for it, discuss what it really means for that person and then offer an alternative label.

65. It's not out, it's never out

Despite what anyone says, bits of your body can't go 'out' – not backs, not necks. You can't throw something out – simply there's nowhere for it to go, except in the rare case of dislocation, which is not what you have. 'My back is out' is really a simplification, but it's wrong. We want to offer you a more truthful explanation of what's gone on in your back. It's more likely that your joints are a bit inflamed, stiff, sticky and grumbly – but never out. Perhaps you really mean it's out of sync with the rest of your back? By the way, the models of backs with their plastic discs and bones and even some pictures of spines and discs never show the really powerful supportive ligaments and muscles around them. They can give you a false idea that things can go out.

This nugget is a key part of dethreatening common language. We remind you of the power of metaphor (Chapter 7) including the use of 'out' in orientational metaphors. We also encourage you to remove the term 'out' from metaphorical language. Language such as stable, balanced and on track are likely to be more helpful.

66. Total knee replacement

Total knee replacements are great, especially for older people with significant disabilities and especially if combined with good quality therapy. Everyone should try good quality physiotherapy first, before anything else. But a total knee replacement is a bit of a misnomer. Surgeons don't take the whole knee – all your muscles, nerves, skin, fat, kneecap and most of the knee bones stay. And of course your brain cells looking after your knee also stay although they may be wondering what is going on! Think of a total knee replacement as a joint surface update – it's closer to the truth and doesn't sound nearly as bad. If you know this, the brain cells looking after the knee won't be so stressed.

Reduced stress, knowing the truth about knee surgery and having an understanding of pain must make for a better post-surgical recovery. This is also a reminder that words can be DIMs.

67. We grow like trees

Attributed to Peter Roberts, Adelaide, 2011

The common findings on scans and x-rays are usually related to age changes – the kisses of time. Left and right differences are quite normal. We grow like trees, never the same left and right, adapting to the seasons and the weather. Like trees, we too can be resilient against the irrepressible forces of nature, heal ourselves and can seek appropriate nourishment. Your body and any scans reflect your life story – not necessarily injury or pain. Google an image of Rafael Nadal's (or any professional tennis player's) dominant arm and you will see how different their two arms are.

Patients are naturally concerned about left/right differences in scan findings. 'We grow like trees' can help reconceptualise a persons' body image using positive, ch angeable imagery. This nugget should help change a DIM to a SIM and foster resilience. Find a deeper discussion of scan and x-ray findings in Novella 3 *The kisses of time*.

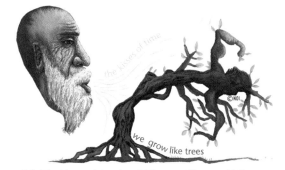

Figure 8.8 'The kisses of time' and 'We grow like trees' [4]

68. Spondylolisthesis

Spondylolisthesis is a really long and complex word! Even health professionals struggle to say and spell it – that's why we often say 'spondy'. But I understand it can be a bit scary to know you have one – and especially if you have looked at those images on Google, which are the cases at the far and rare end of the spectrum. You may have heard or read the words 'break' and 'slip' and these are a bit scary too. I'm going to do a really good and thorough physical exam but I want to share these points first…

- *Spondylolisthesis is really common. Around 500 million people worldwide would be diagnosed with a spondy if they had an x-ray. The great majority of these people would not even know they had something unusual until they had an x-ray.*

- *Research tells us that there is hardly a relationship between having a spondylolisthesis and pain. Even if you don't have pain knowing that you have a spondy could be stressy – unless you know the truth about them.*

- *Many professional athletes have a spondy – many Olympic swimmers and the tennis champion Andre Agassi for example. It didn't stop him winning eight grand slams!*

- *It is important to remind yourself that in nearly all cases, the changes seen on scans didn't happen overnight. They have been there for a long time and well before you knew that an x-ray would report a spondy.*

- *X-rays only show bones – there are really powerful ligaments and muscles around the bones in your back.*

- *Like everyone else on the planet, we can keep our backs healthy – keep the weight off your tummy, keep your back strong and flexible.*

We think that anyone with a diagnosis of spondylolisthesis would welcome this information. And of course this does not negate the importance of skilled examination to identify the rare situations where there is actual neurological injury. All diagnoses should be explained like this – simply the truth.

69. Heel spur

The term 'heel spur' must have been invented by a cowboy, not a biologist! Where a ligament or tendon connects to a bone it usually needs to be very strong. At this point, bone and soft tissue merge into each other. This is how all our soft tissues are connected to our bones. The stronger the connection needs to be, the more the boney bit merges into the soft tissue, for example on your heel bone. When you look at your heel bone x-ray side on, all you see is the bit of the soft tissue that has been strengthened up with extra bone – it can look a bit like a spur. If you were to look at it in real life, it doesn't look anything like a spur – it looks like a tough bit of ligament with a reinforced attachment! It can't catch on anything or poke into anything. It is not sharp and it is not dangerous!

Many people with or without heel pain will have these adaptive changes on x-ray. They are usually normal findings and the same on both sides. The current evidence is that there is no clear link between the presence or size of them and the likelihood of pain. Resolution of pain occurs without changing the x-ray. However, the metaphorical label is highly threatening and almost certainly works as a powerful DIM.

Imagery evoked by the diagnosis could include the sharp spur on a rooster's leg or on a cowboy's boot or even notions of poison, as some spurs such as those on the platypus or the scorpion are poisonous. It is worth spending time to dethreaten the notion of 'spur'. Examine for likely contributors to the pain such as calcaneal nerve involvement [6] or the actual process of adaptation – remember the adaptation process itself, perhaps if hurried by unusual demands, can stimulate some danger receptors – they will settle down once the adaptation process slows. You can even celebrate this remarkable capacity – *'What a fabulous adaptation! Imagine if we could make cars that are stronger when we use them! Imagine if your tyres developed tougher rubber and super grippy tread simply by driving them on rough roads!'*

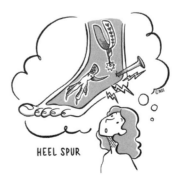

HEEL SPUR

70. Fibromyalgia

Fibromyalgia as a label is influenced by culture – the diagnosis is far more common in some countries than others. While acquiring the label can be fearful for some and a relief for others, we now know what fibromyalgia is. Your central nervous system is super sensitive and output systems such as the immune, sympathetic, endocrine and motor systems are frequently on edge and quickly reactive. All this leads to your body overprotecting itself. Long term over protection leads to changes in the tissues, which send more danger messages into your central nervous system. It's a cycle, but there are many places where you can intervene. It's all about grading movement, understanding pain, removing your DIMs and finding your SIMs.

This nugget forms a broad summary of the biological processes involved in many chronic pain states and the best methods of treatment.

71. Stable platform

Attributed to EP course participant, Atlanta, 2014

So you say you've got a worn out back and the scans show degeneration. Well, I've had a really good look at your back movements and your scans and I think that the findings are more likely related to normal age changes and life events. Even though there is some loss of disc space and bony changes and your back's a bit stiff, it's actually quite a stable platform. I think you'll be able to do most of the things that you want to do on this platform, such as play bowls and work in your workshop. You should not be worried about damaging anything, in fact activity will lessen the chance of any damage happening.

This is an example of a DIM to SIM metaphorical transformation which has followed a sound physical examination and a viewing of any scans. Another example may be somebody who says *'I have a collapsed arch in my foot'*. After an examination, if appropriate you may be able to say *'I don't think you have a collapsed arch. Sure, it's stiff, there are some changes on x-ray, but it's best to consider it as a stable platform. Have a look, it's not much different to the other side!'*

These DIM to SIM transformations are nothing more than the truth. Many patients may have significant fear-avoidance behaviours based on unhelpful perceptions which are repeatedly emphasised by language and thoughts.

Your stories
Pop them below...

References

1. Sicuteri F, et al. (1992) Preface, in Pain Versus Man, Sicuteri F, et al. Eds. Raven Press: New York.

2. Sambo CF, et al. (2012) To blink or not to blink: fine cognitive tuning of the defensive peripersonal space. J Neurosci 32: 12921-12927.

3. Moseley GL, et al. (2012) The Graded Motor Imagery Handbook. Noigroup Publications: Adelaide.

4. Moseley GL & Butler DS (2015) The Explain Pain Handbook: Protectometer. Noigroup Publications: Adelaide.

5. Breig A (1978) Adverse mechanical tension in the central nervous system. Almqvist & Wiksell: Stockholm.

6. Butler DS (2000) The Sensitive Nervous System. Noigroup Publications: Adelaide.

7. Butler DS & Moseley GL (2013) Explain Pain. 2nd Edn. Noigroup Publications: Adelaide.

8. Bartolo M, et al. (2013) Modulation of the human nociceptive flexion reflex by pleasant and unpleasant odors. Pain 154: 2054-2059.

Notes...

9

The Pain Library – Novellas

Novellas!

Novellas are longish short stories.[1] We have hijacked the term to describe Explain Pain stories that are more complex than nuggets, and take perhaps five to ten minutes or even more to tell. Sometimes the Target Concepts are clear and we have listed them with each novella. Other times the Target Concepts may be hidden or implicit. We envisage novellas being used with groups or for individual education sessions, embedded with multimedia support.

If you have read *Explain Pain* (and if not, you need to!) you may have noticed that it's sprinkled with novellas. *Painful Yarns* is a collection of even longer novellas. The narratives within these novellas provide education around many key Target Concepts including the protective role of pain, movement of peripheral nerves, amazing pain stories and the orchestra in the brain amongst others. They are all written in user-friendly language with media to help tell the story.

Fifteen new novellas

Here we introduce some new novellas. These have emerged as our understanding of pain has progressed. Others have come about to answer questions posed by patients and clinicians. We have written these novellas rather loosely – in the conversational manner that we'd use in a clinical situation. We realise they are written from the deliverer's stance in a rather didactic way, so you will need to introduce your own slant, personality and interactional power. Naturally, you will alter the novella to make it relevant to your learner's story. So, here is what you *might* say for fifteen new novellas…

1. The majesty of the brain
2. The drug cabinet in the brain
3. The kisses of time
4. We are gifted copycats
5. Protection has a long memory
6. Protecting your turf
7. Pain on hold
8. Cracks, massage and me!
9. Movement, the SIM-fest!
10. Protectometer for stress, fatigue and anxiety
11. Oldies are goldies
12. Traffic jams, cakes, snowflakes and pain
13. The slidey glidey nervous system
14. Your ever changing brain
15. Smudged maps and what to do about them

---

1   We are very bold here with our use of the term 'novella'. Classics such as George Orwell's *Animal Farm* (1945), John Steinbeck's *Of Mice and Men* (1937) and Hemingway's *The Old Man and the Sea* (1952) are all under 30,000 words and regarded as novellas. Perhaps our stories are novelettes?

1. The majesty of the brain

What an organ!

Our brains have allowed us to fly to the moon, explore the bottom of the ocean, write, paint, make music, harness electricity, love and laugh, sing and invent all sorts of stuff. Our brain works out when we should move or not move, have pain or not have pain, sweat or not sweat, think or not think. It's definitely worth knowing more about – the brain is clearly boss. That's why it's protected by the skull – the toughest bone in our body. Here are a few things to inspire you.

There are over a trillion cells in your brain. Each cell can connect to thousands of others – there are over 1,000 trillion ever-changing connections. It's nice to know that we all have about the same number of brain cells that Albert Einstein had! They combine to make a representation of you. Brain cells wriggle and move, connect and disconnect all the time, all with the goal of making the best possible connections. And it's an energy hog – 20% of all the oxygen we take to make energy is used by the brain.

What an organ! And of course it is only part of your nervous system. Thousands of kilometres of nerve cells and billions of detectors report to the brain all the time. Amazingly, the brain usually has no trouble dealing with all these inputs and working out the best way to respond. Phew!

It's changing all the time

Our brains are changeable and adaptable, more than we ever realised. People who are blind have little use for brain cells organising sight, so touch and sensation use those spare parts. When brain parts are damaged, the original function of the damaged parts can often be looked after by the remaining bits. And the brain will also adapt to look after a bit of damaged body. If you hurt your knee, the brain cells looking after the knee can recruit neighbouring cells to help look after the knee even better. That's one reason why pain sometimes spreads.

The brain's alive! It's electrical, it's chemical and there are messenger fluids constantly moving around in there. We grow fresh new brain cells every day. Every nerve connection is checked out by mobile immune cells on the hour, every hour. You are protected by a full-time internal surveillance system. By the way (and don't be grossed out) living brain is warm, yellow, it moves around a bit when you turn your head and it has the consistency of a nice ripe brie. And it learns and adapts right until your last breath.

But there are bugs in the magnificent organ

Before we are carried away with this glorious organ, look at the incongruent nature of human brain function when it comes to wars and climate change. Why would we do things when we know they are bad for us, or someone else, or the world? Leaving these collective behaviour issues aside, the 'bugs' in brain function can help us understand much on a personal level. People believe and do strange things. We smoke – which sent at least 200 million of us to an early grave last century; we drink incredibly expensive bottled water in parts of the world where the water supply is perfect; we contribute more to hurricane disaster relief funds if the first letter of the hurricane's name is the same as our own.

Illusions trick us all the time, no matter how long you gaze at them. Check out this illusion. It looks like the lines are wonky, but they are perfectly parallel – if you don't believe me, grab a ruler and see for yourself. You would think our brains could work this out. I guess it's no wonder we sometimes make decisions about pain that may not offer the best potential outcomes for us.

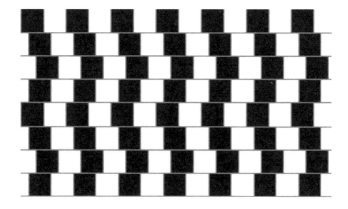

Figure 9.1 The horizontal lines are parallel

What do you know about your brain?

Most people can name a few muscles – quads, hammies, pecs and abs – and even some bones – ribs, sternum, collarbone and shoulder blade. But the poor brain misses out on adequate recognition. Can you name any brain parts? Even worse, we often give it bad press. We talk about it as if it is a machine – *'your cogs are rusty'*, *'steam coming out of your ears'*. Or as if it works like a kitchen – *'stewing on that'*, *'my brain's fried'*. And perhaps you have referred to someone as a *'halfwit'* or *'a brick short of a load'*?

Get to know your brain. It works more like the internet, a market economy, a complex ecosystem or a never-ending game of chess. It has a place for everything you did in the past, for everything you do right now and anything you want to do in the future. The more you know about your brain, the happier, the healthier, the prouder and the stronger you'll be.

Linked Target Concepts

We are bioplastic (8)
Learning about pain can help the individual and society (9)

Additional resources

[EP8-25] *Section 1*
[PY24-38] *Seeing is believing*
The Brain That Changes Itself, Doidge [1]
Brain Bugs, Buonomano [2]

2. The drug cabinet in the brain

Your very own powerful, pain modulating system

Have you ever noticed that you don't seem to hurt when you are in a risky situation, distracted, stressed or really want to keep doing what you are doing? Would you feel pain if you were running away from a furious kangaroo (add your own feared animal here), even if you had an arthritic gammy knee? Over 50 years ago some scientists injected morphine into the midbrain (between your ears) of people with chronic pain. For some of them, the injection eased their chronic pain. Before you are too excited by this, these injections are not used now because they can have massive side effects, so don't ask for a midbrain injection – the response will be a flat *no*! But the discovery was amazing – what these scientists had found was a part of the brain that makes its own morphine-like substance. They went on to show that we all have our very own drug cabinet in our brain – and it's full of powerful analgesics.

Get to know your own drug cabinet

With your very own drug cabinet, you won't be left in the lurch if you're coming off pain medications. You have your own supply. Your drug cabinet is open 24/7, even Christmas day, public holidays and in war zones. It's free, you don't need a prescription, and unlike most synthetic drugs there are no side effects – it's all natural. You may not need as much pain medication if you can make your own. You can keep your drug cabinet healthy and resilient through life and you can help your friends by telling them about it. Sounds good, doesn't it?

Your drug cabinet is made up of millions of brain cells and connections. As well as receiving messages from your body, your drug cabinet links to other brain areas that are involved in things such as planning, memories and thoughts. Close by, it links to a brain part (the amygdala) that is involved in emotional responses and of course, your emotions will change your pain.

Your drug cabinet makes a natural cocktail, which can dampen down danger messages coming in from your body. The cocktail includes serotonin, enkephalin, opioids, dopamine and morphine-like substances and others; it's a powerful combo – call them the helpful happy hormones if you want. They are more powerful than the synthetic pills you buy from the pharmacy. Those drugs don't work so well.

The drug cabinet in action

When your drug cabinet is open, helpful happy hormones flood throughout your nervous system. This dampens down the danger messages as they travel to your brain. Have you ever noticed a bruise on your body after a fun night out and can't remember how it got there? We all know about someone who kicked the winning goal despite a severe injury. The drug cabinet in the brain is surely open in situations like this.

But under some conditions, your drug cabinet can shut up shop. When your cabinet is closed there are fewer happy hormones being produced. Danger messages coming in from your body may be louder. It might be closed when you go somewhere that worries you, perhaps the place where you injured yourself, if you think you have to do something that might hurt you, or if you're generally grumpy. It is as though the drug cabinet is responsive to how safe you feel in general – the safer you feel (ie. more SIMs), the more wide open the drug cabinet. You see, there is a bit of a balancing act going on. The trick is to work out how to open your drug cabinet.

Higher level management

But how can so many different things affect this drug cabinet? Well, just like a pharmacy or drug store is managed by higher authorities, so too is your drug cabinet. A massive network of brain cells dictate whether it opens or closes. Your brain has to work out – *is it worth me having pain now?* To do this it has to 'answer' the question – *how dangerous is this really?*

Most DIMs will close your drug cabinet in your brain. DIMs such as fear, anger and lack of understanding are big closers. Most SIMs will open it, and you want it open! Dethreatening knowledge, having goals, setting your treatment direction, support and understanding are big openers.

The key to the cabinet is ultimately in *your* hands.

Linked Target Concepts

Pain depends on the balance of danger and safety (4)
We are bioplastic (8)
Active treatment strategies promote recovery (10)

Additional resources

[EP8-25] *Section 1*
[EPH44-45] *Use your own drug cabinet*
[PY57-68] *Scratchy & the boring talker*
YouTube clip – *The drug cabinet in the brain*

3. The kisses of time

You've probably had an x-ray, a CT or an MRI. If you've had back pain for a long time, then you might have quite a collection of these scans.[2] Understanding the place of scans and the meaning of their accompanying reports is an important part of your Explain Pain journey. But there is a big dilemma about scans and back pain that we need to discuss.

The scanning dilemma

Overall, we are very grateful that modern scans are as powerful as they are – they can identify problems inside our body that need immediate attention. They save lives. Modern scanning technologies are like really powerful cameras that take finely detailed pictures. Because of the level of detail, these images show up all our unique shapes and 'internal wrinkles' and all the ways in which our bones, joints, muscles and ligaments have adapted to the forces involved in simply living on the planet! We call these adaptations the *kisses of time* and they are usually unrelated to pain.

Unfortunately, these kisses of time are given scary names that sound as though they are abnormal – names like *degenerated* and *osteophytes*. Anyone who has read their own reports would be rightly worried hearing that their back is abnormal. This changes your sensitivity setting – it is a DIM. But in reality we are all bumpy, lumpy and happily worn inside, like a really comfy armchair. Until we share this truth with everybody, our scans will continue to produce DIMs and this is not helpful!

Perhaps you're worried that if you *don't* have a scan your health professional may be missing something really important. Here's the dilemma – some health professionals make a lot of money from ordering and taking scans. Some scan findings can lead to unnecessary and sometimes dangerous invasive treatments. It is highly likely that everything you see on a scan was there before you had pain and will still be there after your pain is gone. There are exceptions to this rule, but health professionals are highly trained to detect situations where scans are really needed.

Addressing the issues

Imaging is so damn good it picks up changes in people who have no symptoms whatsoever. For example, in 20 year olds who have no problems, 37% have 'disc degeneration'

---

2   These scans can actually be recycled for the silver in them!

according to MRI or CT. In 80 year olds this number goes up to 96% – remember these people have no symptoms and no pain – they just agreed to participate in research study! The figures are similar for *disc bulges* too.

Overall, *disc degeneration* and *disc bulges* are related to living on the planet and are often not associated with pain. Some of these changes might actually be useful as they can make the back more stable (Nugget 71 *Stable Platform*). By the way, we have been using the word *degeneration* because of how it was described in the radiology report. Don't let this word automatically link to pain. Degenerative changes are usually normal living changes – skin wrinkles, hair falls out, and the eyes and hearing changes, so does the spine. None of these changes hurt. You would never say that you had 'degenerated' skin, eyes or hair, so why do we say it for spines?

'Okay, well why do I still hurt if you think it's not the disc's fault?'

Remember that pain is always real and it's never just one thing that produces it. Many factors combine to construct pain – including how you *think* about your scans! You see, your ideas and thoughts about your back, like how fragile or vulnerable you *think* it is, are likely to be potent DIMs. So it's what you've inferred from this image of your back that might make you more sensitive, not necessarily the state of the tissues in your actual back.

'But if I don't have a scan, something important could be missed.'

Good point – this is something we all think about. Scans are absolutely necessary sometimes and there are certain patterns of symptoms and impairments that mean a scan should be ordered. I have asked you loads of questions right? All that stuff about night pain, weeing and pooing, numbness, pins and needles, weight loss, funny sensations – remember? Well, those questions let me know if a scan would be beneficial. If there was anything in your answers that even hinted at something more serious, I would suggest a scan. It's also one reason I want to do a good physical examination of muscles, joints, nerves, sensations, movements, strength and endurance. But in your case, there is no need to send for a scan. I will keep a regular eye on things and if any sign at all emerges that you might need further investigation, I will make sure that happens. With this plan, it is very, very unlikely that anything nasty will be missed.

'Well what about an x-ray then? They are cheap and easy.'

X-rays are cheaper for sure, but it's the same story as MRIs and CT scans, except the research was done over 30 years ago. If you take a group of people with pain and a group of people without pain, their x-rays very often look exactly the same. In fact, in some people with knee pain – the report comes back noting changes much worse on one side than the other – but it is the good knee that is worse on x-ray! As your mother might say *'For goodness sake, sonny Jim, spare yourself a little bit of radiation.'*

So we are going to treat *you*, not your scans.

Linked Target Concepts

Pain is normal, personal and always real (1)
Pain and tissue damage rarely relate (3)
Pain depends on the balance of danger and safety (4)
Learning about pain can help the individual and society (9)

Additional resources

[EP13-14,59]
[EPH46-47] *Clean up your language*
Journal article – Brinjikji, et al. 2015 [3]

4. We are gifted copycats

Ever wondered about these things?

Why do you feel exhausted after watching an action movie when all you have done is sit and eat popcorn? Why do we help a young child wee by running a tap? Why are some sporting stars so much better than others? If you see someone yawn, why do you feel the need to yawn?

Clinicians often hear people in pain say *'It hurts to look at that'* or *'thinking about movement hurts me'*. The famous musician Phil Collins has been known to say *'I can't even hold the sticks properly without it being painful'*.

It probably has a lot to do with mirror neurones

About 30 years ago, some Italian scientists found cells in a monkey's brain that were active when the monkey moved *and* when the monkey saw a person doing the same movement. These are called mirror neurones. We now know that most of the brain has this mirroring capacity – we are born copy cats and we can't help ourselves.

Let's think of the example of lifting your arm up. To lift your arm, thousands of brain networks combine together to send the right mix of signals to cause your shoulder muscles to perform the physical movement – and voilà, your arm lifts! Well, if you watch someone else do the same thing, your brain can't stop itself from activating some of the networks that you would be using if you were physically lifting your arm! The same thing even happens if you *imagine* lifting your arm up, or even just plan to. Amazing huh?

There is a dark side too. If lifting your arm is really painful, then *seeing* someone else lift his arm may activate enough of your brain networks that it hurts just watching him. You haven't even done anything! This is a sign of a system that is *so overly protective* that seeing someone else lift his arm is a DIM.

There is good news though – once you understand this, gradually it will stop happening. The brain realises that the DIM is not really a danger at all. A lack of understanding can cause worry and confusion.

Our mirroring ability helps us make sense of another person's movements. We run *their* movement in *our* brain and this helps us to plan our own movements. Let's go back to the action movie – you feel exhausted watching Jackie Chan

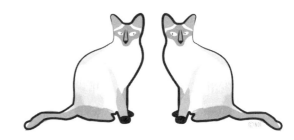

or Harrison Ford because, in some way, you have been running the movie in your own brain. Some people immerse themselves in it – you can tell what is happening in a movie by the constant change of expression on the watcher's face. Thoughts are hard work! Seeing and hearing water flowing mimics urine flowing; sports superstars can read and predict other player's actions really well and keep ahead of the rest. And no wonder you want to yawn when you see someone yawn – it's activating the yawning networks in your own brain.

Emotional mirroring

We also mirror other people's emotions. This mirroring capacity helps us develop empathy, allows us to impersonate other people, to copy their walks, batting style, their mannerisms. When someone smiles, smiling back is almost automatic – it's catchy. Emotions can be contagious. Clinicians sometimes feel sad when we hear patients' chronic pain stories; patients probably do too when they hear someone else's story. Scientists aren't sure that there are special emotional mirror neurones but it seems that making sense of another person's emotions means that you activate your own emotional systems in your brain.

'How can knowing about these mirror systems help me?'

Understanding your own mirroring capacity might help you understand and relieve your pain. If you are in a sensitive state, your pain may be provoked by seeing someone *else* do something that would hurt if you did it. Pain might even be provoked when you think of doing something or when you know you're going to have to do something you don't enjoy.

Tragically, in the past, many clinicians who heard patients say these things presumed that they were a bit odd, or they were lying about it. We now have scientific evidence to understand this phenomenon – you are not odd and we know you are not lying! This mirroring capacity is all about neurotags and once you are aware that mirror neurones can play a part in pain neurotags, it is easy to see how thinking about or watching movements can hurt.

We like to talk about 'sneaking under the pain radar'. Treatments such as Graded Motor Imagery allows you to access your mirror neurones and exercise your brain without turning on your pain. Why not keep the mirror neurones involved in SIMs active too? Watch other people doing fun things, think about doing those things yourself and imagine that you are. Soon you will find that you can start actually doing those things without pain.

One last word on mirror systems

Think about this: if seeing someone in pain or talking about their pain activates our own mirror systems, remember to make sure that when you are with others in pain, you don't spend all your time talking about your pains. Focus together on your SIMs, your effective strategies, your helpful movements, etc. You get the picture...

Linked Target Concepts

Pain is normal, personal and always real (1)
Pain involves distributed pain activity (5)
Learning about pain can help the individual and society (9)

Additional resource

Journal article – Rizzolatti & Sinigaglia 2016 [4]

5. Protection has a long memory

Once bitten, twice shy

Whenever something goes wrong in my house – a jumper is left at school or a prized football is wrecked because it was left outside during a storm – we tend to say *'Okay, what can we learn from this?'* Sounds like parenting 101? Well it is actually a bit daft because nothing can ever happen without us learning *something* from it. There is no way to avoid learning *something* from every stimulus you receive. Once a stimulus has been detected and a signal sent into the mass of cells that make up the central nervous system, it will never be the same again. This is bioplasticity. Rejoice!

Bioplasticity helps protect us against future injuries. The nervous system uses an amazingly diverse set of mechanisms (all of our senses) to detect when we are approaching something potentially dangerous. Sometimes those mechanisms don't stop us from progressing towards danger. That's when pain – the Big Protective Kahuna – can cut in. Pain provides a very effective protective buffer. As pain persists, the buffer grows (check out the Twin Peaks Model on page 4). Sometimes that buffer can be so big, we are protected for a long, long time before our tissues are actually in danger. As the saying goes *'once bitten, twice shy'*.

The immune system remembers too

This emphasis on the nervous system doesn't mean that it is more important than your other equally magnificent systems. Take the immune system for example. Once we are exposed to anything that might put us in danger, such as a virus, bacteria or even a pattern of our own biological responses (eg. fear) to something nasty, our immune system remembers. If it ever comes near us again, we are ready to pounce. This probably sounds familiar, right? It's how immunisation works. Talk about plasticity!

Imagine if we could create a machine or a car that had the plasticity power that we have – if you had a flat tyre from a sharp rock then the tyre would remember what a sharp rock looks like so that next time you encounter a sharp rock, it is pulverised into flat earth without making so much as a dent! Such a car would be incredible! Drive it off road and it would slowly become a four wheel drive. Start pulling a caravan and it would slowly grow bigger pistons. Move to the Middle East and it grows an air-conditioner. If anyone could actually make a car like this, they would surely become very, very rich.

When it comes to pain, really powerful protection happens as a result of the dynamic and intimate relationship between the immune system and the nervous system. It works a bit like this: imagine that you, the organism, come under attack – it might be from the injection of a drug such as morphine,[3] or invasion by a bacteria or virus.[4] It might be a severe physical trauma[5] such as a complicated fracture or being born way too early, or it might be a major emotional trauma[6], such as a massive betrayal of trust by the one person you were relying on for protection, or it might be an episode of profound grief. The cells of the immune system will remember the particular pattern of circulating molecules that occurred at the time of the attack and forever hold them in their memory. They can now be said to be primed so that if that same particular pattern of molecules wanders past again, the immune cells recognise them and turn up your magnificent protective systems, including pain.

Here comes the *boom*. Some of these immune cells that have been primed by previous events in life, or that become responsive to current attacks on your livelihood, also determine the *efficiency* of your danger transmission pathways. This is a big deal because it means that if your danger transmission pathways (nerves) become active, then these immune cells can increase their efficiency. If their efficiency is increased, danger messages are sent more easily. When this occurs, anything that puts you under threat – anything at all – can increase your pain, even when the thing that threatens you has nothing at all to do with your body. Boom – plasticity! Drop the mic!

So how do you work around this protective memory?

The Protectometer is a good place to start.

- This is why the Protectometer asks you to look for threats that hide in hard to find places.

- This is why the Protectometer asks you to look for DIMs in the things you think, say, hear, feel, people you meet, places you go.

- This is why the Protectometer asks you to consider the biological state of your tissues – if you are sick, then chances are your shoulder pain will be worse. If it is hayfever season, you might notice your knees playing up.

The thing is, your immune system has a really, *really* long memory, so it's difficult to escape these protective effects. *However*, if you can identify the DIMs that are involved, we know that they slowly stop causing pain because your nervous system knows that the response is over protective. Again, knowing pain biology generates an endless gaggle of powerful SIMs.

Linked Target Concepts

Pain depends on the balance of danger and safety (4)
Pain is one of many protective outputs (7)
We are bioplastic (8)

---

3   Or in the words of Chapter 3 page 58, a XAMP

4   Or a BAMP

5   Or a DAMP

6   Or a CAMP

6. Protecting your turf

Have you ever found yourself wishing the person you are talking to would just give you a bit more personal space? Ever had to wave your hands around and say *stop crowding me!* Or wanted to leave the party for a bit of fresh air? You are not alone. We all have some sense of our personal space and know when there is someone or something inside it that we don't want to be there!

Our dynamic personal space

Our normal personal space roughly matches the area of space we can touch without taking a step. It is widest around our head and follows our body down to the ground, a bit like a porcini mushroom.

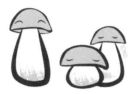

The size of our personal space changes depending on risk and practicality. If you are in a crowded train going to work, your personal space will shrink and you might be oblivious to the fact that the person just 30cm away is picking his nose. Personal space instantly shrinks in elevators. If you are in an empty cinema and the only other person in the whole place comes and sits next to you – 30cm away – you would *definitely* notice him picking his nose and you will probably find his every breath so irritating that you can't stand to stay where you are.

This adaptation for risk and practicality happens all the time. Think about when you are with the one you love, you just can't get enough of each other and this desperation to be together is so strong you feel like any space between you is too much. Next minute you might have an intense argument and all of a sudden you can't stand to sit on the same couch or even be in the same house as one another.

We don't consciously decide when to make our personal space big and when to make it small. We don't decide to be oblivious to the man picking his nose in the train but irritated by the breath of the person who sat next to us in the cinema – it just happens. So how does it happen? Your brain is always mapping the space around you and, if the risk appraisal exceeds a certain level, you want to shift yourself or the intruder. Visual input is really important in constructing these maps, but proprioception (the ability to sense your body position and motion), sounds, touch and even smell can all be involved.

By using tools we can also extend our personal space way beyond what we can reach. An expert painter develops, inside her brain, maps of space that extend to the space around the tip of her brush; an expert tennis player might have a personal space that reaches as far as their tennis racquet does. Some fishermen are thought to develop spatial maps that extend to the tip of their fishing rod! These extensions of personal space clearly have practical advantages.

Your protective space and pain

We tend to be more protective of the space that is closest to our body. If you give a small electrical zap to someone's hand, he has a blink response, which means the muscles around his eyes suddenly contract even if his eyes are already closed. This is a normal protective reflex he can't control. If you zap him on the hand when his hand is near his face, he has a bigger response. He can't help it. But put a wooden board between his hand and his face (a solid, protective barrier), he goes back to a normal blink response. Put a thin piece of paper there (not a solid, protective barrier) and his blink response remains elevated. Have him close his eyes and trick him into thinking the board is there (but it isn't) – his blink response returns. It's all about eye protection. He has no control over any of this – it just happens.

The area of space that we protect aggressively will be bigger if we have more reason to protect it. Take a dog with a wounded paw – if you so much as move your hand near its paw, it might snarl or growl – maybe even if you just look at the paw! We are exactly the same – if you have a painful hand then your brain sets up a protective space. This means that you will be protective of a bigger area of space around your hand. But *protecting your turf* can turn into a vicious cycle. For some people the entire side of their body can become over protected; the brain never has any evidence that things are not that dangerous because nothing ever comes close to the protected area.

Protecting our turf is the same as protecting our body. It is normal, helpful and it happens outside of our awareness and control. Just like pain, it can become a problem if we are *too* overprotected. But as with pain, we can train our systems to be less protective of the space around us. The way we train it is just the same – it's all about understanding this protection, then gradually letting objects and people into the space, gradually going out and mixing with different crowds and by seeking answers to your overprotection in your DIMs and SIMs.

Linked Target Concepts

Pain depends of the balance of danger and safety (4)
Pain relies on context (6)
We are bioplastic (8)

7. Pain on hold

We know that 100% of the time, in every single human ever tested, the amount of pain you have does not relate to the amount of tissue damage. We also know that pain can be related to something you just did, something you did 10 seconds ago, something you did a day or over a week ago. These delays can be very stressful, and they can have you thinking *'what have I done this time'* or *'it must be very fragile – I hardly did anything today'*. There are some reasonably common delays between injury and pain and they are caused by internal processes in your body. Knowing a bit about how these delays work can help to dethreaten them and enable you move on with your life.

Kinds of delay

The 10 second delay: Here you might be performing different activities or a health professional has asked you to perform many movements as they examine you. It might be okay while you are doing the movements but then *whammo!* – it hurts about 10 seconds after, even if you've stopped moving. This is probably due to something called wind-up. If you have a sensitised danger transmission system, repeated movements or activities that are not at first painful can wind-up the system. You might do a few arm movements and then 10 seconds later *boom!* – pain emerges. This is a strong sign that there is a problem in the sensitivity of the nervous system but not necessarily in the tissues.

The next day delay: This often happens after excessive or new muscle activity and is called DOMS, which sounds a bit like a DIM but it means Delayed Onset Muscle Soreness. It happens between 1 to 3 days after activity and goes away on its own. Most explanations link DOMS to microscopic damage in the muscle. We now know that it is also linked to the production of immune molecules and stuff called nerve growth factor, both of which are influenced by stress. So don't let DOMS be a DIM! We also know it is the first sign that you are getting stronger – DOMS comes before the body adapts to become stronger. Remember, the pain will go away quickly and on its own, and you can do a few things such as stretching so that you won't feel it as much.

The two week delay: Injured muscles and ligaments quickly activate danger detectors and often you feel pain soon after injury. Injured peripheral nerves can be a bit different. When a nerve is injured, there are inflammatory mechanisms and normal healing processes that mean the danger detectors can slowly increase their production of danger messages, coming to a peak about a fortnight later. This sort of nerve injury might happen after surgery or maybe after a neck sprain from a car accident. It is the immune system that is driving this delayed sensitivity – all part of the process of nerve healing. It will slowly improve but if you understand that this delayed pattern is a normal part of tissue recovery, it will hurt less and recover more quickly.

The six month or more delay: Any significant tissue injury triggers adaptations within your system. This means you are likely to have 'recurrences' of the pain without reinjuring the tissues. These recurrences simply reflect a heightened level of protection for that body part. They can be triggered by all sorts of things that are completely unrelated to the injury but that are related to the context in which the injury occurred. Or, you might just be under threat – let's say you have the flu or are feeling run down or it's the anniversary of the injury or something unpleasant in life. We know that immune cells can be kept on alert for months and years after an injury to protect us. It makes total sense.

Good news – delays rarely mean re-injury

Here's the good news about delays – they rarely mean re-injury. Pain emerges for other reasons. Many things (DIMs or an absence of SIMs) can keep your protective system sensitive.

Around 60% of people who have had a back injury that was bad enough to make them seek help, will have the same pain re-emerge in the year after. Most people, and some health professionals too, think that this means re-injury. While this is possible and all your systems need a good check out, it is unlikely, unless you have really done something right out of the ordinary like attempting some new bedroom acrobatics, or gardening like you have never gardened before. Remember *protection has a long memory* – it's just the way of the mammal! Perhaps think of this long delay as your brain doing a system checkup, like a fire drill. It will often do this checkup when you're a bit down, flat or have the flu. This might be a convenient time to do it as you will have more sensitising chemicals in your system.

So, if you think about it – delayed pain isn't a sign of re-injury. That's really important for you to know and understand. There's no need to panic – you haven't gone back to the acute injury state when you had really injured your back and there's no need to have all that treatment again.

Linked Target Concepts

Pain and tissue damage rarely relate (3)
Learning about pain can help the individual and society (9)

8. Cracks, massage and me!

So, you've learnt that pain and tissue damage rarely relate. But, I can see what you're thinking – *if my tissues aren't a problem, why does it feel better when my back is cracked, popped or massaged?*

The easy answer is: because these treatments don't just target the tissues. There is much more going on all throughout the body, so let's look into that.

Why does it make me feel better?

First, we need to reflect again on what pain really is – a call for *protective action*. Let's think about when a treatment results in an audible pop or crack. This sound is considered by many therapists as the critical sign that the treatment is working, but many other therapists think it means nothing. Anyway, let's say you hear an audible crack or click during a treatment. There are two likely mechanisms that then lead to pain relief:

1. There is a sudden bombardment of messages from many detectors in your body to your spinal cord. Once these messages arrive at the spinal cord they quieten down the danger messages coming *into* the spinal cord and alter the influences on other nerves that go to muscles. The effects of all this might be enough to give you pain relief for up to a few hours.

2. There are many, many safety cues (SIMs) delivered during this therapeutic encounter, besides the obvious 'treatment'. It is of fundamental importance that you are in the safe hands of a professional. This is a powerful SIM – one of the most powerful SIMs around. It is also important that you *expect* it to work – another powerful SIM. Some health professionals even tell their patients that the audible sound is a sign that the manipulation has 'worked'. The sound itself becomes a SIM. This sound is important for the health professional too – if *they* think the manipulation has worked then they can't help but send some more powerful SIMs your way. There are great experiments that show how powerful a clinician's belief in what they are doing is. Scientific studies have also shown that it doesn't actually matter what makes the sound – whether it comes from the patient on the bed or from a tricky sound maker underneath the bed, it will relieve pain as long as both the health professional and the patient *think* it came from the joint and *think* it is a sign that the treatment did what it was meant to.

All of these processes can have profound effects on networks of cells in the brain. These networks send messages to the spinal cord which dampen down the danger messages going to the brain. All of these things mean that SIMs can greatly outweigh DIMs. This sends the Protectometer down, sometimes taking it right out of the pain zone. These effects can last for a couple of days and in some rare cases, for weeks.

What isn't happening?

The *least* likely mechanism for pain relief from these cracks, pops and massage is a change in the physical properties of the tissues. This is actually fabulous news for both you and your therapist because it means that your pain can be changed, sometimes completely taken away, simply by changing your mix of DIMs and SIMs. Even better, the mechanisms that make this happen are fully available to you 24/7, through the drug cabinet in your brain. Cracks, pops and massage directly access the amazing drug cabinet in your brain, but there are other ways to open the cabinet too. You don't always have to pay someone else to harness the effects of it for you, we can discuss how you can learn to harness it yourself.

So why does my therapist still offer it?

We're not saying that the treatment is bad – but be wary of dodgy explanations. There are still some Jurassic health professionals out there who give people in pain dodgy explanations for why it feels better after cracks, pops and other 'corrections'. These explanations often use words like *out, stuck, jammed, slipped, locked* or *twisted*. Ironically, these dodgy explanations for treatments might actually *increase* their pain-relieving effects *in the short term*, particularly if the therapist truly believes them. But the bad news is, in the long term they will almost certainly lead to a worsening of the problem. That's because these explanations are loaded with DIMs, and when the short-term benefits reside and the pain returns, the explanation leads to an incorrect belief that the problem has also returned.

So be wary if someone offers to *unlock, realign, untwist* or *release* parts of your skeleton. With what we now know about pain biology, there really is no excuse to stay stuck in these DIM-heavy dodgy explanations. If you are given a dodgy explanation like that from your clinician, lend her your copy of EP and change clinicians!

Linked Target Concepts

Pain depends on the balance of danger and safety (4)
Active treatment strategies promote recovery (10)

9. Movement, the SIM-fest!

Movement is the greatest SIM generator. Let's have a look at how.

Start at the joints – motion is lotion

There are specialised tissues in your joints that makes a lubricant-like fluid conveniently called lubricin. This fluid loves movement – and In turn movement makes the joint release this gorgeous juice! Movement keeps the cartilage lining of our joints shiny and smooth, as well as strong and hard. Movement tells our bones how to align themselves to best withstand forces. Just imagine that for a moment! By moving and weight bearing, the internal structure of our bones start to change to best deal with the forces produced by moving! If you took a picture under a microscope of the internal structure of your thumb bone, spent the next fortnight texting all your friends to tell them about it, then took another picture under a microscope, the internal structure of your thumb bone would look different. Your thumb bone adapts to the forces of life.

What about muscles and ligaments?

Even if you are a vegetarian, you might have noticed that all the fibres in a lump of steak run in roughly the same direction. Movement is what makes this happen – it is movement that exerts forces through all our tissues and it is these forces that keep the muscle fibres aligned in the best way, keep them alive, strong and healthy.

Movement keeps blood flowing and flushes out the waste products of life, including the acid that builds up when we don't move. Remember that acid activates danger detectors, so it is helpful to get rid of it. That's not all – movement actually triggers changes in the types of danger detectors we have in and around muscles. This is one reason that when we start an exercise programme it can feel like everything hurts – the danger receptors in the area become more sensitive to the by-products of muscle activity. But don't worry about this – in just a few weeks of regular movement and exercise we very cleverly swap these receptors for a different type that are not activated by the by-products of exercise and so exercise stops hurting! Your muscles, ligaments and danger detection system all adapt to the movement — this is bioplasticity at work.

Movement for an overprotective body

If you have persistent pain, movement may hurt long before you are at risk of injury. This is because of your highly overprotective system and the adaptations that have occurred over the duration of your pain. In this situation movement might hurt but, critically, you are safe. It's guaranteed to slowly hurt less and less if you progress little by little and plan your movement/exercise programme with a good understanding of pain biology and alongside a modern-thinking health professional. Don't forget you are an amazing bioplastic machine.

Movement actually directly affects the danger transmission system in a good way. There are millions of neurones that are activated when we move. In fact, we can activate some of them simply by imagining movement or going out into life and watching people. Thousands of these neurones project directly onto the danger transmission system where they dampen down the danger messages travelling towards your brain.

Movement is a master key to the drug cabinet

Movement is one of the best ways to open the drug cabinet in your brain. It releases a range of analgesics that are pumped all over the body. Movement helps to regulate the basic systems that keep your body functioning, which can be in a bit of a muddle in many persistent pain states. Movement even encourages the production of anti-inflammatory molecules that calm down sensitised danger detectors and danger transmission nerves. It doesn't stop there! Movement allows you to take up more social activities. It triggers new brain cell growth. It makes you think better, improves your memory and reaction time, helps you to work better and, ultimately, play better.

The thing is, movement and exercise are the best things we can do for *all* of our bodily systems – our cardiovascular system, respiratory system, nervous, endocrine and immune systems. As long as you understand your Protectometer, you simply can't go wrong.

Linked Target Concepts

We are bioplastic (8)
Active treatment strategies promote recovery (10)

10. Protectometer for stress, fatigue and anxiety

Pain is not our only protective feeling!

We know that pain is a protective feeling – it makes us do something to protect a part of our body. But we also know that many people with persistent pain are also challenged by other protective feelings, most commonly stress, fatigue, depression and anxiety. While the Protectometer was developed, tested, tweaked and retested, tweaked and retested again, all with people in pain, you might be surprised by how useful it is to address these other protective responses. Some people have had success using the Protectometer to help them understand and overcome problems such as stress, depression, anxiety, phobia, fatigue and even feeling short of breath.

Consider the same pathway

Like pain, these feelings can be considered protective and like pain they are modulated by a range of DIMs and SIMs. As with pain, these DIMs and SIMs will fall under one of the categories on the Protectometer. To see if this works for you, fill in any of the boxes on the Protectometer fold out [EPH].

We suggest the best pathway out is by following the same journey, identifying DIMs and removing and identifying SIMs and using them as best as you can. Once you have packed your bag full of SIMs you can start the slow but steady journey to train your system to be less protective. The Protectometer for pain has a numerical scale. In collaboration with your health professional, you can construct your own scale for any of your feelings. Some broad examples for stress are given in Figure 9.2.

These are all very *reasonable* suggestions and we have learnt from clinicians and punters around the world that this approach has worked for them. However, we haven't done any empirical research on anything other than pain. Until someone does, we can only be sure that the Protectometer works for pain.

Linked Target Concepts

Pain is one of the many protective outputs (7)
Active treatment strategies promote recovery (10)

Additional resources

[EPH24-27] *Other protective systems can load the Protectometer*

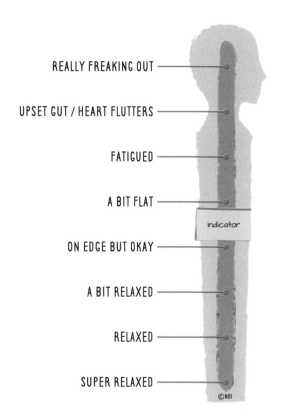

Figure 9.2 The Protectometer for stress

11. Oldies are goldies

We are all living longer – 60 is the new 40, 80 is the new 60...? This is usually a good thing but ageism is in the air. Ageism is a negative perception of getting older and of older people. It's a really big DIM and it needs to be challenged. Young and old people can be ageist, older people can be ageist about themselves. Health professionals and sometimes government departments and companies can be ageist. Let's challenge it, first by obliterating some myths about pain and ageing.

Myths about pain and ageing

Myth 1: Pain is inevitable with ageing.
This is not true but most people including some health professionals think it is. Sure, there may be a few more illnesses and surgical procedures but people over 60 have no more migraines, no more back pain, no more neck pain than younger people have. In fact, the oldies may have less pain.

Myth 2: If you have some pain now, then you will have worse pain later.
This is not true either. Pain comes and goes in older people just like it does in younger people. Even though x-rays and scans may show things such as narrowing of joint spaces, this has *no* relation to increased pain. These are age changes and more age does not equal more pain. Rest easy...

Myth 3: Toughing it out makes it easier to tolerate.
Some of us oldies think *'I can grin and bear it!'* This might be true for a while, but we know that it doesn't make anything easier in the long run and being stoic can lead to depression, which in turn increases pain more in oldies than it does in youngies. You don't have to *'grin and bear it'*, *'suck it up'* or accept it as part of ageing – seek help from an up to date health professional, just as you would if you were younger.

Possible DIMs related to ageing	DIM SIM Category	Possible SIMs related to ageing
I see my wrinkles in the mirror, my scary scans; I hear my uncontrollable farting and hospital smells.	Things I hear, see, smell, touch and taste	My grandkids show me new music; I experience new tastes and smells; I've never had a massage but I might book one.
I do nothing, I just wait, withdraw and get by.	Things I do	I do all kinds of exercise including weight training; I try new movements, laugh lots, watch upbeat movies; I will download the Protectometer App; I'm always curious and rejoice in a good fart!
I am old; it's just old age; of course, it aches when you are old; you can't teach an old dog new tricks.	Things I say	I am ageing gracefully; oldies are goldies; hey, my time's not up yet; I am old and I am staying bold; old dogs love new tricks!
I could fall over anytime and smash my hip; getting older must mean more pain.	Things I think and believe	My body can always heal; I am bioplastic, I can grow new brain cells forever; goals are great; I can wear what I want, I can be who I want to be.
I frequent the same places and retreat.	Places I go	I have my favourite places but like to try new places, different places in comfy shoes.
My health professionals don't know what to do with me; all my friends have the same problems; young people scare me; I avoid computers and social media.	People in my life	I spend my time with positive people, young people, old people and friends – I even share things on Facebook and keep expanding my social network; I'm thinking of adopting a pet.
I stiffen up; I don't seek treatments; I have a poor diet and don't exercise.	Things happening in my body	My fitness is still improving; I enjoy a healthy, varied diet, am optimistic and maintain a good physical appearance. I know which drugs I take, and which ones I don't need.

Table 9.1 Examples of age related DIMs and SIMs

Myth 4: There is nothing you can do for it.
This is rubbish! There are treatments that work for youngies, middlies, oldies and ultra-oldies, such as Explain Pain combined with contextual activity exposure. The Protectometer approach is ideal for oldies alongside appropriate medications.

Age is only a number, it is not an excuse.

The protective power of SIMs

Here is a *really* important study – we know that people who have a positive self-perception of ageing when they are 50 will live on average 7.5 years longer than those who have a negative self-perception of ageing at 50 [5]. Of course, many things will influence self-perception. Positive self-perceptions are SIMs. Table 9.1 shows a list of SIMs and DIMs related to ageing. This list was first put together for an elderly and ageist patient who declared that she was 'ready for the scrapheap'.

A few more good things about growing older

Let's stop for a moment to remember the good things about getting older. You don't sweat as much as those smellier youngsters, if you're bald you can avoid hairdressers (imagine the money you save on shampoo), you can easily see the good and ignore the bad, you problem-solve better than youngies because your brain has more efficient connections, you want less and you have fewer allergies.

Ponder this

Next time you are talking about your sore knee and someone, perhaps it is your health professional, says *'It's just old age'* or you think that yourself, then ask them (or yourself) *'is my right knee older than the rest of me?'*

Linked Target Concepts
Pain and tissue damage rarely relate (3)
Learning about pain can help the individual and society (9)
Active treatment strategies promote recovery (10)

Additional resources
Journal articles – Levy S, Slade MD & Kasl SV 2002 [5]
Thielke S, Sale J & Reid MC 2012 [6]

12. Traffic jams, cakes, snowflakes and pain

Attributed to Tim Cocks, 2016

Have you ever been stuck in a traffic jam, crawling along at a snail's pace and looking ahead for the cause? But eventually when the traffic melts away and you're moving again there didn't seem to be any cause – no hole in the road, no tow truck, no police cars and no ambulances. Traffic jams can seem to have a life of their own – springing into existence then disappearing again.

What about a snow flake? Every snowflake is unique, their beautiful shape and structure is as individual as a fingerprint or DNA. And yet there was no plan for the snowflake to follow, no pattern, no instructions – it just happened, when tiny water droplets blowing in the wind crashed into each other and froze.

A cake just kinda happens too. You take separate ingredients like flour, eggs, milk, butter, chocolate, perhaps a touch of vanilla, mix them together, pour it all in a tin, shove it in the oven and voilà, a delicious cake! The cake that appears from the oven is a completely different kind of thing from the mix that went into the oven. Perhaps this amazing transformation is why kids love baking so much – the excitement and surprise as you see and smell the cake for the first time never diminishes.

These are all examples of things that are emergent – often surprising things, that just seem to happen, like love. There are certain features of emergent things that give them their surprising nature. One way to understand these features is to contrast them with things that are not emergent. Examples of things that are more *linear* include the flow of water through plumbing pipes, a car engine and our digestive system.

Features of emergent things

Emergent things have no boss – there is no one part in control of all the others. Think about the traffic jam – you can't point at one car crawling along with all the others and say that it's that car's fault. But we can look at our plumbing and see that if the master valve is closed, the water flowing through our house will stop.

Another feature of emergence is that the different elements are all doing their own thing without any overall plan. As a snowflake forms, each tiny droplet of water interacts with other droplets nearby and dependent on humidity and wind, a unique pattern appears. In linear things, such as a car engine, each part of the engine works in a very definite way, all with the overall effect of making the car move.

Finally, in emergent things all the parts of the system are interacting at the same time. When you bake a cake the ingredients mix together and interact all at once. Baking the cake may be an emergent process, but digesting the cake is more linear – you chew before you swallow, it slides into your stomach, you break down the food, you absorb the good bits and the waste heads to the storage until eventually it ends up in the loo!

Pain is emergent

Many people incorrectly assume that pain is linear – that pain starts in a muscle or joint after injury and then a pain signal is sent up to the brain where it is registered in a special pain centre. But we now know that pain is more of an emergent phenomenon – there is no pain centre in the brain; no one boss. In fact, there are *hundreds* of brain bits all working at the same time when you experience pain. The different bits are all doing their own thing with no overall plan – some might be increasing danger signals, while others are decreasing danger signals. Your emergent pain experience is the overall best guess from your brain about what is the most appropriate protective output.

One other thing that we know about emergent processes is that you can't understand the whole thing just by looking at one part. You can't understand a traffic jam by looking at one car's steering wheel, you can't understand a cake by looking at butter and dry flour and you can't understand pain by just looking at the muscle or a single brain cell, or even just the brain. Our best bet to understand pain is by thinking emergently – looking at the whole human being, your brain, nervous and other systems, your body, your thoughts and beliefs, the things you do, the places you go and even the people in your life. Sound familiar?

Of course it does, because the Protectometer and the seven categories of DIMs and SIMs is a very emergent way of looking at pain, let's have a look at yours.

Suggested module for teaching emergence

The novella above follows a certain pattern based on the work of Chi [8]. An emergent educational pain module could include (in a somewhat linear fashion!):

1. Contrasting examples of emergent (eg. traffic jam) and linear (eg. plumbing) processes that are non-biological

2. Contrasting examples of emergent (eg. love) and linear (eg. digestion) processes that are more biological

3. Introduce pain as an emergent process

4. Examples of how pain is more emergent than linear using the contrasting features

5. Further examples of the emergent characteristics of pain such as images of distributed processing and use of the Protectometer.

Linked Target Concepts

Pain depends on the balance of danger and safety (4)
Pain involves distributed brain activity (5)
Learning about pain can help the individual and society (9)

Additional resources

[EPS117-119] *Emergent and linear patterns*
Emergence: The Connected Lives of Ants, Brains, Cities and Software, Johnson [7]

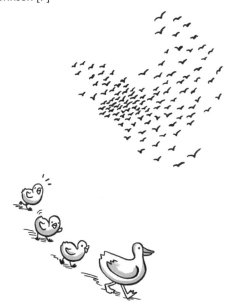

Figure 9.3 Ducklings following the mother duck is a more linear process, a flock of birds is a more emergent process.

13. The slidey, glidey nervous system

We know that nerves are very important in pain because they send messages, but we don't often spend time reflecting on the nerves themselves. You know muscles and joints are not the only movers and shakers we've got! The nervous system compresses, stretches, slides and glides – boy does it move! Knowing about this can help explain a lot of symptoms and maybe make you want to move.

The nervous system is big and tough

Nerves are big and tough – the sciatic nerve in your bum could be as thick as your little finger and it's more than 50% ligament – possibly the strongest ligament in the body. The spinal cord is a thick-walled cylinder of nerves. The outside of the spinal cord is covered by a big thick stretchy ligamentous tube known as the dura mater. This tube continues into the skull and surrounds the entire brain. The nervous system is quite an organ when you think about it – not only does it have to conduct impulses all over your body, it has to be mechanically tough as well. If you put your hand in the air and wave, the nerves in the arm and neck have to move to let you do that. If you bend your spine, the canal around the spinal cord becomes up to 10 centimetres longer. Somehow your spinal cord with all its neurotags, fluids, and spinal neurones has to let this happen. And it usually does.

Your nervous system is a continuous structure – it loves to move

When we move, our nervous system slides, bends and stretches. It could slide as much as 2 centimetres in your arm when you wave it around. But what is important is that it is one single continuous mechanical structure – if you bend your head down, you will move and pressurise your nerves in your low back. Lifting your leg in the air will shift the nerves in your neck. Even a deep breath moves nerves in the arm. Good therapists have worked out ways to check on the physical health of the entire nervous system – check that it can slide and stretch to accommodate all you want to do in life. Another interesting feature is that all the ligamentous structures around the nervous system have danger detectors in them. Like muscles and joints, the nervous system enjoys a good physical workout – it keeps the fluids flushed, gives it a good stretch, disperses any inflammation and gives it a nice oxygenation – yoga, Tai Chi, exercise, dance and a good roll around in the grass all do this too.

People in pain are often sensitive to movement of the nervous system

For people with back pain, lying down and lifting one leg, or even having someone else lift it can be quite painful in the leg or in the back or both. In sitting, tilting your chin towards your chest can bring on back pain! These movements mechanically affect our nervous system. If the health of the nervous system is altered these movements might bring on odd symptoms such as pain or tingling. Strangely, this might occur in a point far away from the body part that is moving. Understanding the connectedness of the nervous system and the parts of the body it supplies can explain this.

There are two main reasons we may be sensitive to movements that tease the nervous system. First, after injury or lack of use, the nerves can be a bit tight or sticky. In this case we need to grade them slowly back into moving again and there are some movements that are especially good for our nerves. Second, your entire nervous system might be sensitised so much that any movement can hurt, even more so if we think the movement is a DIM. Sorting out your Protectometer may help you regain this movement.

Keeping the nervous system mobile

It makes sense to keep your nervous system physically healthy and supple enough to function normally no matter what movements you are doing. The best way to keep the nervous system itself healthy is to keep moving. Sometimes, you might feel extra benefits from specialised exercises that are designed to enhance movement in your nervous system. Ask your clinician about sliders and gliders [10].

Linked Target Concepts

We are bioplastic (8)
Active treatment strategies promote recovery (10)

Additional resources

The Sensitive Nervous System, Butler [9]
The Neurodynamic Techniques DVD & Handbook, Butler [10]

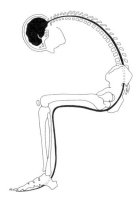

Figure 9.4 The mechanically continuous nervous system [9]

14. Your ever changing brain

Your brain is slightly different now from when you started reading this sentence. Our brains are always changing – we can't stop it – even trying to stop your brain from changing will change it. What's more, the more your brain does anything, the more it changes. We call this learning – learning to ride a bike, learning your times tables, learning to play a musical instrument. The same thing happens with pain. Your brain is really different *now* from how it was before your pain started.

There are some metaphors that capture the effects of a changing brain. Here are three:

1. **The brain as an orchestra**
   Imagine your brain is an orchestra. All of your brain cells are like individual musicians. All the different things your brain does, for example producing pain, are like different pieces of music. The more your brain plays the pain tune, the better it becomes at playing the pain tune. It can become so good at playing the pain tune that the pain tune takes over – the orchestra starts playing the pain tune when it should be playing something else.

2. **Kangaroo tracks in the brain**
   Imagine all the things your brain does are like the tracks made by kangaroos[7] as they hop through the bush. The more kangaroos that follow the same track, the bigger the track becomes, the easier it is to follow and the more the kangaroos and the bilbies and the wombats tend to follow it. You may end up with a major road and then a motorway.

3. **Imagine the brain is a huge cabinet full of maps**
   These could include maps of your body, maps of the places you have been to, maps of where your friends and relatives are and what they look like, maps of different feelings such as pain. The more you go to a certain place, the stronger the map of that place is. It becomes increasingly precise, clear and easy to follow. The longer you have pain, your brain's map for pain becomes more and more precise and clear and easily activated.

These changes are possible because of neuroplasticity. You might have heard of it – it is very trendy at the moment! Another word for it is learning.

We can see the effects of learning when we do brain scans. We have known for over a hundred years that there is one part of your brain that has a map of the surfaces of your entire body – all of your skin and the insides of your orifices – your mouth, nose and other bits too![8] We have drawn it for you. On this map – called 'the homunculus' [or HERmunculus for women!] – the larger the body part, the more brain cells are used to make its map. Or we say 'the more brain real estate is dedicated to that area'. Normally the big areas – the hands and the mouth – are where we have an extra sensitive sense of touch and this extra brain real estate contributes to this extra sensitive sense of touch.

Your actual body parts stay roughly the same size throughout life (unless you work out a lot, are pregnant or have some part of your anatomy artificially enlarged, shrunken or taken off). However, their size in *this* brain map can change every week. People who read Braille have larger maps of their index finger during the week when they are using Braille than they do on the weekend when they are not using Braille. Female dogs that are nursing young have larger maps of their nipples than they do when they are not nursing young. The map of the left hand is bigger in violinists than it is in the rest of us.

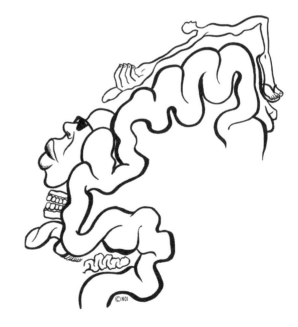

Figure 9.5 The somatosensory humunculus [12]

---

7   Or sheep perhaps. Or kiwis or yaks. It doesn't have to hop.

8   Yep! Your vagina or penis too!

The maps are hard wired and adjusted in real time

All of these maps are the consequence of both a hardwired map and ongoing input from receptors that are in the tissues of our body.

How do we know that the maps are hardwired?

We know that we are born with some basic body maps. About 50% of people who are born without a limb due to a congenital problem still report feeling the phantom limb.

Ever been to the dentist and come out feeling like you have a big fat lip but it looks normal to everyone else? This is common. A similar thing happens when you block blood supply to an arm for 20 minutes, or you have a local anaesthetic that blocks nerve activity in one limb. Scientists now think these feelings occur because the normal ongoing input from receptors in the tissues is suddenly stopped and the brain cells that were 'listening' to that input now start listening to nearby tissues. Scientists don't know why this results in a feeling that the body part is enlarged, but it does.

Having these feelings is not abnormal and does not mean you are going crazy. These 'distorted maps' just remind you that your brain is looking out for you. The great news is that with some clever sensory and movement retraining, you can return these distorted maps to normal.

The best news? Although distorted body maps and the feelings they generate are in themselves actually harmless, they are nearly always DIMs. This means that understanding them, and correcting them, is dumping DIMs and collecting SIMs. Win win!

Linked Target Concepts

Pain involves distributed brain activity (5)
We are bioplastic (8)

Additional resources

Note the educational sequence in this novella:

- understand the idea of maps in the brain – this is the idea of cortical representation

- understand brain changes are normal and occur to 'look after you'

- the brain will change with pain – this can be useful or not

- the brain can change quickly.

[EP22-23] *The Phantom in the body*
[PY47-56] *Twonames and the Magic Button*
Phantoms in the Brain, Ramachandran [11]

15. Smudged maps and what to do about them

Your brain holds millions of maps – maps of your body, the places you go, the things you see, smell, hear, touch, the space around your body, movements, the people you meet and even a snotty nose. The brain uses these maps to give you feelings, orient you to your surroundings, tell you who it is you are speaking to on the phone and allow you to conjure their face in your mind.

The more you use a map, the more precise and efficient it becomes. However, scientists have discovered that there is a limit to this because some brain cells change their properties if they are 'overused'. This is pretty high end biological science, but the principle is easy.

Brain cells and their neighbours

Normally, when you are learning anything, the brain cells that do the learning do two things – they learn how to fire more easily and inhibit (stop) their neighbours from firing. This inhibition of neighbouring brain cells is a key process in learning anything – from how to see as a newborn baby to how to pronounce Worcestershire. Sometimes however, a brain cell 'goes over the edge' and stops inhibiting its neighbours. Actually, it starts exciting them instead. The actual process involves microscopic levels of inflammation, but it is a kind of inflammation that won't change with anti-inflammatory medication or drugs – it needs specific training. More of that in a moment.

This loss of precision results in what we call 'smudging' of your brain maps. Smudging of a map that produces pain might result in your pain spreading. If the smudging involves brain cells that are also in maps for your sense of touch, this smudging will result in your sense of touch worsening. If the smudging involves brain cells used in movement, your movement control will deteriorate. If it involves brain cells used in remembering things, then your memory will deteriorate.

So, if you have experienced these things, then you are not going crazy and your injury is not worsening; you haven't had a stroke and you are unlikely to have some nasty brain disease – you are just smudging a bit. This smudging seems daft, but it might just be serving a very sophisticated biological purpose – to further protect your body. It makes sense but like many things about chronic pain, it really only serves to give you more DIMs.

If you smudge, you can un-smudge

And now for the great news! Smudging is reversible with not all that much training. The smudged bits just have to learn how to be precise again – how to inhibit their neighbours. Helpful training will be individually specific, but an up-to-date clinician will guide you through it. Treatment approaches such as graded motor imagery, mindfulness, tactile discrimination training and of course Explain Pain education capture some of the principles really well.

Replacing DIMs with SIMs in this way shifts your Protectometer level away from pain. And that has to be a good thing!

Linked Target Concepts

We are bioplastic (8)
Active treatment strategies promote recovery (10)

References

1. Doidge N (2008) The brain that changes itself. Penguin: London.

2. Buonomano D (2011) Brain Bugs: How the Brain's Flaws Shape Our Lives. Norton: New York.

3. Brinjikji W, et al. (2015) Systematic literature review of imaging features of spinal degeneration in asymptomatic populations. AJNR Am J Neuroradiol 36: 811-816.

4. Rizzolatti G & Sinigaglia C (2016) The mirror mechanism: a basic principle of brain function. Nat Rev Neurosci 17: 757-765.

5. Levy BR, Slade MD & Kasl SV (2002) Longitudinal benefit of positive self-perceptions of aging on functional health. J Gerontol B Psychol Sci Soc Sci 57: 409-417.

6. Thielke S, Sale J & Reid MC (2012) Aging: Are these 4 pain myths complicating care? J Fam Pract 61: 666-670.

7. Johnson S (2002) Emergence: The Connected Lives of Ants, Brains, Cities, and Software. Scribner: New York.

8. Chi MTH, et al. (2012) Misconceived causal explanations for emergent processes. Cog Science 36: 1-61.

9. Butler DS (2000) The Sensitive Nervous System. Noigroup Publications: Adelaide.

10. Butler DS (2005) The Neurodynamic Techniques. DVD and Handbook. Noigroup Publications: Adelaide.

11. Ramachandran VS (1999) Phantoms in the Brain: Probing the Mysteries of the Human Mind. HarperCollins: New York.

12. Moseley GL, et al. (2012) The Graded Motor Imagery Handbook. Noigroup Publications: Adelaide.

Notes...

10

CURRICULA

Putting it all together

In Chapter 6 we introduced the idea of curricula for Explain Pain and suggested a pathway for constructing your own curriculum. This includes defining aims, objectives and Target Concepts and managing variables related to the learner, the deliverer, the message and the context. We aim to help you create an aligned curriculum to ensure learners do not escape deep learning. You might want to review this section in Chapter 6.

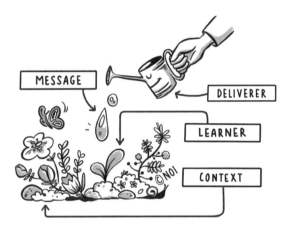

Here are four examples of curricula:

1. A multisession Explain Pain intervention for a group with persistent spinal pain

2. A single session intervention for a group of General Practitioners or allied health providers

3. A multisession intervention for an individual with chronic low back pain

4. A multisession intervention for an individual with complex regional pain syndrome.

How to use the curricula

These four sample curricula are designed to help start you off. We've chosen common educational scenarios and Target Concepts.

Key points

- We have proposed ten Target Concepts in *EP Supercharged* and although we have used all ten Target Concepts in curriculum 1, you will want to adapt, change or use different Target Concepts as you write your curriculum. We suggest that curriculum 1 could be used as an overall guide for other curricula.

- Repetition is inevitable and valuable and all part of an aligned curriculum. Where one element is appropriate in all boxes of a column, it has been emboldened eg. **Formative Assessment** and prefixed by a downward arrow (↓).

- The delivery and resources suggested to support the Target Concepts are produced by NOI. We know and have tested these resources. Some Target Concepts will require additional resources.

- We remind you that these are Explain Pain curricula and in many cases will be delivered alongside other interventions such as CBT, graded activity, GMI and nutritional advice. We invite practitioners delivering these other interventions to consider their own carefully detailed curricula and how they may dovetail with ours.

- Target Concepts are listed in the order in which they are likely to be presented. But remember, a curriculum should be always be adaptable and emergent, so change the order as you see fit.

- We have provided examples of Nuggets (Chapter 8) and Novellas (Chapter 9) in the curricula. You may wish to use others and construct your own.

1. A multisession Explain Pain intervention for a group with persistent spinal pain

The essentials

Learner demographics: The group includes males and females with 'musculoskeletal spinal pain' persisting for longer than two years. The participants are aged between 23 and 52 and are all medically certified unfit for work. Patients diagnosed with severe psychiatric illness have been excluded from the group.

Deliverers: May include physiotherapists, psychologists, occupational therapists, exercise physiologists, nurse practitioners, dieticians and physicians among others.

Number of learners and unique needs: Up to 12. The educational intervention is provided concurrently with graded exposure and a CBT programme.

Number of sessions and time: 8 sessions x 2 hours over 6 weeks.

Delivery Methods: Varied face to face and take home activities including multimedia resources. Participants are supplied with *Explain Pain*, *The Explain Pain Handbook: Protectometer* and have access to *Painful Yarns*.

Place: Ground floor conference/meeting room with accessible parking, access to a garden, coffee and tea making facilities.

Stakeholder considerations:

- Learners will have personal goals and aims. Collective group goals will need to be established.
- Spouses and family – consider involvement during the programme and acknowledge their role and influence.
- Referral sources – regular feedback on progress, learner satisfaction and ideas for further support.
- Employer – will be interested in likely timeframe for recovery and return to work. May need information about the programme.
- Insurer – will be interested in costings, timing, progress, learner satisfaction, and applicability to other groups.

Aims

The deliverer(s) intend to:

- Provide current knowledge about pain and stress biology in relation to persistent spinal pain in a healthy group learning environment
- Engender informed hope
- Provide a framework which integrates Explain Pain with graded exposure and cognitive behavioural therapies
- Use multi-media, storytelling and metaphor to explain and transform the pain and stress experiences of the group
- Make learnt skills applicable to 'whole of life'.

Objectives

At the end of the sessions the learners will:

1. Have knowledge of current pain and stress biology as it relates to them
2. Apply bioplasticity knowledge to set short and long term goals with the expectation of improved outcomes
3. Explore, use and develop personalised functional applications of Explain Pain knowledge
4. Function better with healthy linguistic expression and reduced pain and stress
5. Extrapolate the material and the group skills for future personal pain states of self and others.

Key

*See *EP Supercharged* Chapter 6 page 137 for a description of the columns.

**Ice Experiment: hold block of ice in hand for one minute and think sad, unhappy thoughts – rate pain and record tolerance time. Contrast with holding ice and thinking happy, positive thoughts. Best completed on two separate days.

BIM	– Body in Mind www.bodyinmind.org
CBT	– Cognitive Behavioural Therapy
DIM	– Danger In Me
EP	– Explain Pain
EPH	– Explain Pain Handbook: *Protectometer*
EPS	– Explain Pain Supercharged
fMRI	– functional Magnetic Resonance Image
NNK	– Number Needed to Kill
NPQ	– Neurophysiology of Pain Questionnaire
PY	– Painful Yarns
SIM	– Safety In Me
SLR	– Straight Leg Raise
PNF	– Passive Neck Flexion
ADL	– Activities of Daily Living
ROM	– Range of Movements
OMPQ	– Orebro Musculoskeletal Pain Questionnaire
FBAQ	– Fear Avoidance Belief Questionnaire

3. Explain Pain for an individual with chronic low back pain

The essentials

Demographic: 54 year old male mechanic

Deliverer: Healthcare practitioner

Number of participants and unique needs: One

Number of sessions and time: Currently approved for 8 x 30 min sessions (includes graded activity and functional restoration)

Additional stakeholders and specific needs:

- Partner/family – consider involving partner in future sessions
- Employer – wants to know timeframe for full return to work
- Workers compensation insurer – wants estimate of number of sessions, outcomes and costs

Place: Hospital out-patient clinic, possible hospital café, garden and/ or workplace session

Subjective Ax

- 12 years of numerous episodes of back pain since work incident *'slipping on greasy floor'*
- Most recent flare-up 3/12 ago with gradual increase in pain over several days, then 10/10 back and leg pain, only slightly better now
- *'Sometimes my back feels out'*, *'I just can't get my core stability back'*.
- Pain severely effecting ADLs and no longer enjoys watching mates play footy
- Feeling tired during the day and difficulty sleeping at night
- Noticing skin dryness and rashes in variable locations
- Reports his partner has had to take time off work to transport him to appointments as well as increase home duties
- Cousin died of Multiple Sclerosis which started with *'weird symptoms'* and *'she was always tired'*
- Currently working with restricted duties but is concerned that he will further injure himself if he returns to pre-injury employment
- States his employer is not engaged in return to work process. Reports being angry regarding the injury which *'could have been avoided if my employer had provided the correct equipment'*
- Reports increasing pain during each employment and case manager meeting
- Radiology report states *'multi-level degenerative disc disease with loss of joint space, especially at L4/5 with a left-sided focal disc protrusion at L5/S1, possibly impinging at the exiting nerve root'*

- Has received physiotherapy, massage and chiropractic treatment and reports no benefit. No existing goals
- Has been taking NSAIDs since onset and has been on Oxycodone and Endone since recent flare-up
- Recently referred to psychology, wary about *'seeing a shrink'*
- Surgeon recommended discectomy, patient seriously contemplating surgery
- Seeing a gastroenterologist for alternating constipation and diarrhoea, stomach ache and excessive flatulence
- OMPQ= 130 [1]; NPQ = 6/13 ('strong patho-anatomical understanding of pain biology' [2]); FABQ = 13 (abnormal [3])
- Nil bladder/bowel symptoms; nil History Ca; 6kg weight gain over 6/12

Explain Pain assessment

- Patient reported he is not that interested in learning about pain, just wants his back *'fixed'*; *'don't tell me it's all in my head'*
- Prefers to learn by *'doing'* and enjoys watching YouTube clips about fishing
- Owns a computer with internet access and reports high level use
- Patient reports previous excellent memory, however in last few weeks has forgotten 2 appointments and finds it hard to concentrate at times; *'my wife is getting more upset with me lately'*
- Googled radiology report findings and discussed these with a friend who has had a similar experience; *'I'm obviously in big trouble here'*, *'it looks like I'm stuffed'*
- Pain literacy: est. low-mod based on NPQ, OMPQ and subjective examination
- Level of misconception: est. flawed mental model (sandcastle) level

Objective assessment

- All lumbar movements restricted and guarded (especially flexion) with obvious non-verbal fear of movement
- Sensation✓✓, reflexes (L)=(R) (both hyper-reflexic), weakness (R) L4/5, has trouble walking on heels
- SLR (L) 70°,(R) 35°, LBP / PNF increases LBP
- Recognise back: accuracy (L)=70%, (R)=65% (abnormal [4]); Response time (L)=2.0 sec, (R)=2.2 sec (normal [4])
- Recognise hands: Accuracy (L)=90%, (R)=90% (normal [5]); Response time (L)=1.5 sec, (R)=1.4 sec (normal [5])
- Two-point discrimination over low back region: (R)=85mm (L)=80mm (no significant difference [6])

	MESSAGE			
Target Concept (Linked Objectives)	**Other ways of expressing the Target Concept**	**Content**	**Delivery & Resources**	**Reir**
Awareness of the problem of pain in society (1,5)	• Chronic pain is an epidemic • An individual's pain problems are reflective of problems in society as a whole	• Statistics of pain prevalence, cost and long-term effectiveness of current treatments • Opioid use data including NNK • Awareness of missed groups with chronic pain (eg. stroke and the elderly)	↓Visual media (PowerPoints and handouts)	• Refl part
Pain depends on the balance of danger and safety (1,3)	• Pain is a defender, not an offender • Pain and tissue damage rarely relate • Danger sensors, not pain sensors • The DIM SIM story	• Modern pain definitions [EPH14] • When pain and tissue damage don't relate (eg. phantom limb pain) • Introduce DIMs and SIMs • Protectometer (DIM/SIM balance) • Link to immune balance • Pain is not the only protector	• Definitions [EPH14] • Protectometer [EPH16-18] • Other protective systems [EP43] • Further reading – reassurance [8]	• 'The • Exar tissu • Furt
Pain involves distributed brain activity (1,3)	• No single pain centre • Multiple brain areas collaborate to produce pain	• Introduction to neurotags • Power of contextualisation • DIMs and SIMs are neurotags too • Your virtual body and homunculus • The brain lights up like a Christmas tree • Current brain language is not adequate	• fRMI images • Specific images [EP39,41] • Images depicting interconnected networks (eg. airline flight paths, aboriginal art). • Context [EPH11]	• Link • Refl and • Disc brai
Understanding why and how it hurts is therapy (2, 3, 4)	• 'Knowledge is the greatest pain liberator of all' • Understanding pain changes pain • Education as therapy	• The changeable brain through the life span • Evidence for EP	• Evidence statement [EPS97] • Nugget 5	• Disc • Grou is pe
'Things you hear' and 'Things you say' are categories of DIM SIMs (3, 4)	• Pain metaphors – diagnostic and transformative • Things you hear and say are neurotags • How we talk about pain will influence our experience of pain	• Speech, movement and pain neurotags overlap • Pain related metaphors can be categorised (embedded, invasive, prognostic, disembodied) • The language used to explain diagnosis and conditions can be danger-enhancing and enhance immunological surveillance • Diagnoses needing dethreatening	• Meet the DIM SIMs [EPH16-17] • Examples of pain-related metaphors • Dethreatening exercise [EP83] [EPS161]	• Refl inclu • Disc DIM • Nov • Nu
You can access the endogenous 'drug cabinet in the brain' (2, 3, 4)	• Endogenous/exogenous drugs • The brain produces molecules more powerful than opioids • Alternatives to meds	• Opioids evoke immune defences • The drug cabinet in the brain story including 'keys to the cabinet' and the influence of DIMs and SIMs • Novellas 2, 55, 56	• Drug cabinet [EPH44-45] • YouTube 'Drug cabinet in the brain' • YouTube 'Understanding Pain: Brainman stops his opioids'	• Grou drug
Awareness of multimedia tools for therapeutic pain education (5, 1)	• There are multiple books and Apps to support pain education • Education is multi-disciplinary • Links to stress states	• Introduce EP, EPH, PY and Protectometer App • Awareness of local, national and international pain meetings and groups	• EP, PY, EPH book and App • Provide links (handout)	• Pro GP

...forcement/ Experiential Learning	Assessment Did they get it?	LEARNER	CONTEXT	DELIVERER
		Considerations, practicalities		
...ct on how much pain is a ... of current clinical practice	↓**Formative assessment** • NPQ 11 item scale (answers at end of session and in handout) • Are they interested? ('climate' of the room)	↓**Group will have well developed coherent, pain knowledge (may be inaccurate)** ↓**Preconceived notions of professional scope**	≈ 5 mins ↓**Group will be eating at the same time** ↓**Likely disruptions**	↓**Credibility of allied health professional** ↓**Are they a member of a pain society?** ↓**Time poor professionals – needs to be interesting and to the point**
... Wheel' [EPH15] ...nples of when pain and ...e damage didn't relate ...her reading – EP, PY	• Quality of engagement during 'The Wheel' session • Quality of examples	↓**This information may conflict with pain education received during medical training** • Make a point that this is true for all pain, including pelvic pain	≈ 10 mins	
... Target Concept to context ...ct on the place of context ...pain ...uss 'the orchestra in the ...' metaphor [EP40-41]	↓**Do questions and examples reflect appropriate understanding?** ↓**Is the whole group engaging?**		≈ 10 mins	• Ensure some understanding of fMRI image
...uss opioid evidence ...up discussion of 'knowledge ...wer'	• Reflect on the EP evidence compared with pharmaceutical evidence	• HCPs are known to underestimate patients' ability to understand pain biology [9]	≈ 10 mins	• Be aware of outcome data
...ct on language use, ...ding clinical metaphors ...uss radiology reports as a ...s ...ella 3 ...gets 43 – 64, all SIMs	• This should be the main 'did they get it?' session	• HCPs often use jargon-laden, body-as-machine, danger-enhancing language, but may not be aware of this • Radiology reports containing danger-enhancing language are read by doctor and patient	≈ 15 mins	• Have examples ready
...up quiz activity 'Keys to your ... cabinet' [EPH45]	• Check quiz answers	• GP's are currently receiving instruction to reduce opioid prescription	≈ 5 mins	
...vision of EP, PY and EPH for ...practice library	• 'Where to from here?' discussion	• The available tools are evidence-based. They can be used independently by patients and are time and cost efficient	≈ 5 mins	

Index

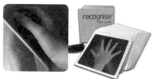

Explain Pain resources

The Explain Pain Handbook: *Protectometer*

This Handbook signifies the next step in the Explain Pain Revolution. Ten years in the making, the Handbook represents the most up to date thinking, and many hours of espresso fuelled debate, from Moseley and Butler. The latest in neuroimmune pain science is distilled into an easily accessible book for patients and introduces the 'Protectometer' – a ground breaking pain treatment tool. This is a patient-targeted handbook combining new material and original artwork.
/available in print format only

Explain Pain Audio Second Edition

Updated and completely re-recorded to reflect the second edition of Explain Pain. David and Lorimer talk you through the science of pain in everyday language, discussing amazing pain stories and how the experience of pain is constructed by the brain, your 'danger alarm system' and the 'orchestra in the brain', the healing processes that occur after injury and why pain sometimes continues long after tissues have healed. Explain Pain Audio Second Edition will give you a deep understanding of pain and help you follow a scientific road to recovery.
/available in print format and audiobook

Painful Yarns

This collection of stories, written by neuroscientist and co-author of *Explain Pain*, Lorimer Moseley, provides an entertaining and informative way to understand modern pain biology. Described by critics as 'a gem' and by clinicians as 'entertaining and educative', Painful Yarns is a unique book. The stories and experiences are great yarns, backed up by metaphors to pain biology. The level of the pain education is appropriate for patients and professionals, the entertainment good for everyone.
/available in print and ebook format

Neurodynamic resources

The Neurodynamics Techniques DVD and Handbook

NOIs international group of faculties presents the definitive manual of neurodynamic techniques for everyday clinical use. This DVD and handbook will help with the assessment and management of physical health and sensitivity issues related to peripheral and central nervous system based pain presentations.
/available in print format only

NTSC English with subtitles in Spanish and Portuguese
PAL English with subtitles in German, Italian, Spanish and Chinese Mandarin.

The Sensitive Nervous System

This text calls for skilled combined physical and educational contributions to the management of acute and chronic pain states. It offers a 'big picture' approach using best evidence from basic sciences and outcomes data, with plenty of space for individual clinical expertise and wisdom.
/available in print and ebook format

Red Wedge

Our wedge is light, strong and allows very localised active and passive mobilisation of joint and neural tissue in the thoracic spine. These techniques are demonstrated in the Neurodynamic Techniques DVD and Handbook and on NOI courses.

Brain training resources

The Graded Motor Imagery Handbook

Written by the principal researchers and educators of the GMI concept, this book will guide you through the science behind and the process of GMI. Essentially a series of brain exercises, GMI involves body part left/right discrimination, motor imagery and mirror therapy. The handbook is suitable for both patients and clinicians.
/available in print and ebook format

Recognise™

Even simple exercises may cause pain if your brain can't recognise whether you are using your left or right side. This can be tested easily and quickly using the Recognise programme. This novel evidence-based programme can provide valuable help in the management many chronic pain states.

App | A measurable, progressive self-management tool for patients. The Recognise App enables you to quickly exercise your synapses on your personal device wherever you are. Test results can be collected and analysed.
/available on iOS and Android

Flash Cards | A great clinical tool and hands-on alternative to the Recognise Apps. Sets of 48 cards available in hand, foot, back, neck, shoulder or knee.

Mirror Box

Mirrors may be used to gain relief and better movement for a variety of pain and disability states, especially those involving the hands and feet. In particular, mirror therapy may be appropriate for problems such as complex regional pain syndrome, phantom limb pain, arthritis, stroke and focal dystonia.

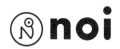 **noi** Noigroup Publications | 19 North Street, Adelaide City West, South Australia 5000
Knowledge driving health | noigroup.com | noijam.com | @noigroup